P9-DHA-482

Contemporary
PRACTICAL/
VOCATIONAL
Nursing

EIGHTH EDITION

Corrine R. Kurzen, MEd, MSN, RN
Former Director
School District of Philadelphia
Practical Nursing Program
Philadelphia, Pennsylvania
Adjunct Professor
Immaculata University
Immaculata, Pennsylvania

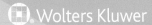
Wolters Kluwer

Philadelphia · Baltimore · New York · London
Buenos Aires · Hong Kong · Sydney · Tokyo

Acquisitions Editor: Kelley Squazzo
Product Development Editor: Shana Murph
Editorial Assistant: Cassie Berube
Production Project Manager: Kim Cox
Design Coordinator: Joan Wendt
Art Director: Jennifer Clements
Manufacturing Coordinator: Karin Duffield
Marketing Manager: Dean Karampelas
Prepress Vendor: SPi Global

Eighth Edition

Copyright © 2017 by Wolters Kluwer

Copyright © 2012 by Wolters Kluwer Health | Lippincott Williams & Wilkins.
Copyright © 2009 by Wolters Kluwer Health | Lippincott Williams & Wilkins. Copyright © 2005, 2001 by Lippincott Williams & Wilkins. Copyright © 2007 by Lippincott-Raven Publishers. Copyright © 1993, 1989 by J. B. Lippincott Company.

All rights reserved. This book is protected by copyright. No part of this book may be reproduced or transmitted in any form or by any means, including as photocopies or scanned-in or other electronic copies, or utilized by any information storage and retrieval system without written permission from the copyright owner, except for brief quotations embodied in critical articles and reviews. Materials appearing in this book prepared by individuals as part of their official duties as U.S. government employees are not covered by the above-mentioned copyright. To request permission, please contact Wolters Kluwer at Two Commerce Square, 2001 Market Street, Philadelphia, PA 19103, via email at permissions@lww.com, or via our website at lww.com (products and services).

9 8 7 6 5 4 3

Printed in China

Library of Congress Cataloging-in-Publication Data
Kurzen, Corrine R., author.
  Contemporary practical/vocational nursing / Corrine R .Kurzen. — Eighth edition.
      p. ; cm.
  Includes bibliographical references and index.
  ISBN 978-1-4963-0764-4
  I. Title.
  [DNLM: 1. Nursing, Practical—methods. 2. Vocational Guidance.   WY 195]
  RT62
  610.7306'93—dc23
                                                                                2015026532

This work is provided "as is," and the publisher disclaims any and all warranties, express or implied, including any warranties as to accuracy, comprehensiveness, or currency of the content of this work.

This work is no substitute for individual patient assessment based upon healthcare professionals' examination of each patient and consideration of, among other things, age, weight, gender, current or prior medical conditions, medication history, laboratory data and other factors unique to the patient. The publisher does not provide medical advice or guidance and this work is merely a reference tool. Healthcare professionals, and not the publisher, are solely responsible for the use of this work including all medical judgments and for any resulting diagnosis and treatments.

Given continuous, rapid advances in medical science and health information, independent professional verification of medical diagnoses, indications, appropriate pharmaceutical selections and dosages, and treatment options should be made and healthcare professionals should consult a variety of sources. When prescribing medication, healthcare professionals are advised to consult the product information sheet (the manufacturer's package insert) accompanying each drug to verify, among other things, conditions of use, warnings and side effects and identify any changes in dosage schedule or contraindications, particularly if the medication to be administered is new, infrequently used or has a narrow therapeutic range. To the maximum extent permitted under applicable law, no responsibility is assumed by the publisher for any injury and/or damage to persons or property, as a matter of products liability, negligence law or otherwise, or from any reference to or use by any person of this work.

LWW.com

CCS0618

Reviewers

Jo Ann Baker, DNP, MSN, RN, FNP-C
Instructional Director, Nursing
Delaware Technical Community College
Dover, Delaware

Mellissa Bess, MSN, RN
Director of Nursing
Chattanooga College for Medical, Dental & Technical Careers, Inc.
Chattanooga, Tennessee

Frances Bivens, BSN, RN
Coordinator School of Practical Nursing
McDowell County Career and Technology Center
Welch, West Virginia

Nakia Blake, BSN, RN
Practical Nursing Program Director
Cambridge Institute of Allied Health and Technology
Delray Beach, Florida

Janyce Collier, MSN, MBA, RN
Nurse Administrator
Franklin County Career and Technology Center Practical Nursing Program
Chambersburg, Pennsylvania

Michele Dickson, DNP, RN, CNE
Associate Professor of Nursing
Prince George's Community College
Largo, Maryland

Diane Duffy, MEd, BSN, RN
Practical Nursing Director
Northwest Technology Center
Alva, Oklahoma

Cassie Flock, MSN, RN
Associate Professor of Nursing
Vincennes University
Vincennes, Indiana

Mary Ann Gaster, RN, MEd, MSN
Instructor of Nursing
Central Carolina Community College
Sanford, North Carolina
Winston Salem State University
Winston Salem, North Carolina

Cheryl Gates, MSN
Director Vocational Nursing and Health Careers
Cerro Coso Community College
Ridgecrest, California

Stacee Gillespie, MS, RN
Practical Nursing Instructor
Northeast Technology Center
Kansas, Oklahoma

Marion Goodman, BSN, MSN, RN
Coordinator Vocational Nursing Program
Lone Star College
Cypress, Texas

Barbie Harbaugh, RN, MSN
Instructor/Faculty
Pennsylvania College of Technology
Williamsport, Pennsylvania

Joanne Heck, RN, MSN
Director LPN Program
Parkland College
Champaign, Illinois

Jenny Holloway, MSN
Nursing Instructor
Vance-Granville Community College
Henderson, North Carolina

Tina Jacques, RN, MSN
Nursing Faculty
Holyoke Community College
Holyoke, Massachusetts

Lea Ann Kathol, MSN, RN, CNE
Nursing Instructor
Northeast Community College
Norfolk, Nebraska

Amy Key, RN, BSN
Practical Nursing Instructor
Tennessee College of Applied Technology
Pulaski, Tennessee

Jeanette Kulifay, BSN, RN
Instructor of Nursing
Hannah E. Mullins School of Practical Nursing
Salem, Ohio

Thirty Lacy, RN, BSN
Vocational Nursing Instructor
Alvin Community College
Alvin, Texas

Stephanie Miller, MSN
Coordinator
Knoedler School of Nursing
Jefferson, Ohio

Marion E. Monahan, MAEd, RN
Director Practical Nursing
Mercyhurst University North East
North East, Pennsylvania

Julie Monsegur, MSN-Ed
Lab/Clinical Simulation Instructor
Pasco-Hernando State College
New Port Richey, Florida

Lauren Mullen, MSN, RN
Nursing Instructor
James Madison University
Harrisonburg, Virginia

Lisa Nolan, RN, MSN Ed, LPN
Instructor
Mercer County Technical
Trenton, New Jersey

Sandra Pangburn, MSN, RN
Practical Nursing Program Coordinator
Hutchinson Community College
McPherson, Kansas

Debra Pitzer, MSN, RN
Faculty
Hutchinson Community College
McPherson, Kansas

Sandra A. Ranck, MSN, RN
Program Administrator
Auburn Career Center
Concord Township, Ohio

Chris Redd, RN, BSN
Practical Nursing Administrator
Washington School of Practical Nursing
Washington, Missouri

Melanie Reeves, RN, MSN
Faculty, Trainer
Hutchinson Community College
McPherson, Kansas

Sarra Reeves, AAS
Associate Professor of Nursing
Coastal Bend College
Kingsville, Texas

Karen Rothschild, RN, MSN
Director, Clinical Development
PruittHealth
Atlanta, Georgia

Mary Russo, MSN
Professor
LincolnLand Community College
Jacksonville, Illinois

Carolyn Santiago, MSN, RN, NP-C
Director of Nursing
Santa Barbara Business College
Bakersfield, California

Darla K. Shar, MSN, RN
Instructor of Nursing
Hannah E. Mullins School of Practical Nursing
Salem, Ohio

Elizabeth Stingo, BSN, RN
Instructor
Fred Eberle School of Practical Nursing
Buckhannon, West Virginia

Karen Taliaferro, BSN
RN-BSN Instructor
Rappahannock Community College
Warsaw, Virginia

Jennifer Waggoner, DNP©, RN
Visiting Assistant Professor of Nursing
Riverside City College
Riverside, California

Preface

Welcome to the eighth edition of *Contemporary Practical/Vocational Nursing*. There have been so many changes in healthcare in just a few years. Advances in science and biology and technology have had a significant impact on the prevention, diagnosis, and treatment of diseases. Legislation has had a significant impact on the healthcare system. The Internet has had a significant impact on teaching and learning and research. Advances and breakthroughs are coming at us very quickly. Much of what students learn now will be obsolete in the not-so-distant future. It is my hope that this book will help practical and vocational nurse faculty impress upon students the importance of lifelong learning and continuing education. While computers and technology will pervade our lives and influence how we live and work, the work of the practical nurse will continue to be one of direct service to others. Personal characteristics and qualities are as important as medical knowledge and nursing skills. The personal characteristics and qualities of nurses that contribute to quality nursing care are covered throughout the book.

Whether to call recipients of health care services *patients* or *clients* or *residents* continues to be discussed. I have generally referred to recipients of nursing care as patients. It would be more appropriate, but extremely cumbersome, to always use the phrase "patient, client, or resident." Regardless of the word used to describe someone who is seeking health care, each person should be viewed as an individual.

Organization

Contemporary Practical/Vocational Nursing is divided into four sections that can be studied as units or as individual chapters. Many of the chapters can be completed independently and several can be completed prior to the beginning formal classroom instruction. The first unit, *Getting Started*, is designed to help the student adjust to his or her role as a student nurse, maintain a healthy personal life, communicate effectively, and recognize that preparation for the NCLEX-PN begins the first day of class.

The second unit, *Understanding Your Profession*, provides an overview of the history of nursing and the roles and responsibilities of nurses in providing nursing care. The last two chapters of this unit explore the complexities of the health care system in the United States including a discussion of the Affordable Care Act, and the contributions and educational preparation of a number of members of the health care team, with particular emphasis on members of the nursing team.

The third unit, *Preparing for Successful Practice*, exposes the student to ethical and legal issues as well as to leadership and management skills.

The last unit, *Moving Forward*, includes a discussion of career planning, a chapter on challenges in the workplace, and it concludes with a look at issues that will confront nurses as they begin a career in nursing.

Appendices provide resources that are valuable long after the basic practical/vocational nursing curriculum is completed.

Text Features

A number of special features are included. They are as follows:

Web boxes that provide suggested resources to enhance the content are interspersed throughout the book.

Critical Thinking Exercise boxes that ask students to use critical-thinking and problem-solving skills to address real-world situations.

Assess Yourself tests that encourage students to begin thinking about how they can capitalize on their strengths and improve in areas that are weak. (These tests are not intended to be used as diagnostic tools.)

Apply Critical Thinking Skills contains discussion questions and activities at the end of each chapter that foster critical thinking and encourage students to take their learning outside the classroom.

Read More About It resource lists present resources from which students can learn more about the issues.

Other pedagogical elements include the following:
- Chapter Content outlines
- Learning Objectives
- Margin boxes that complement and highlight key information in the text
- Ethical and legal case studies

Ancillary Materials

To help instructors prepare class teaching and testing materials, the following ancillary materials are provided on thePoint (http://thepoint.lww.com):
- Learning Objectives
- Pre-Lecture Quizzes
- Guided Lecture Notes
- PowerPoint Presentations
- Discussion Topics
- Journal Articles
- Case Studies
- Student Review Questions
- Assignments
- Test Generator—Multiple-choice questions and the Diploma test generator are available for download on thePoint. With the Diploma test generator, instructors can add their own questions, modify existing questions, and create chapter quizzes, unit quizzes, or comprehensive exams at the push of a button.

The ancillary content available on thePoint is the result of many years of teaching. It is hoped that these materials will enhance and support your teaching experience as well as your students' learning experience.

To the Student

Your decision to become a nurse will undoubtedly change your life. Your experiences will expose you to the sorrows and joys of being human. You will acquire knowledge and learn nursing skills, but beyond that, you will learn how to care effectively.

Although contemporary society does not place a lot of value on providing services or on caring for strangers, you have chosen a career that requires both. Your special ability to care and to provide care for others will be appreciated by the hundreds or even thousands of patients you will serve during your career in practical/vocational nursing.

Your faculty has designed an instructional program that will take you from where you are now to being a nurse—a process that is often challenging. You will spend many hours studying and preparing for clinical assignments. You will experience both success and frustration. You may occasionally wonder whether the effort is worth it. But you will persevere, and you will succeed because you have a special ability to care for others.

It is my hope that you will continue to care as much as you care today. Take pride in what you do and how you do it, and treat all people with dignity and respect. You will feel tremendous self-satisfaction when you know you have done your best.

Corrine R. Kurzen, MEd, MSN, RN

Acknowledgments

Acknowledging those who have helped make the eighth edition of this book possible is an opportunity that I sincerely appreciate. I would like to give a very special thanks to all the teachers and students who reviewed the manuscript in its many forms. I thank students and faculty for making suggestions which are always important to the success of a project such as this. Thanks also to Shana Murph and Kelley Squazzo of Lippincott Williams & Wilkins, for providing the structure and support needed to complete this manuscript.

Contents

List of Self Assessments

GETTING *Started*

Adjusting to Student Life

LEARNING OBJECTIVES

When you complete this chapter, you will be able to:

1. Design a schedule that includes time for study, personal needs, and family, social, and recreational activities.

2. Identify sources of financial aid to assist in paying for your nursing education.

3. Use your understanding of learning styles to increase your rate of learning and retention.

4. Apply critical thinking skills in decision making and problem solving.

LEARNING OBJECTIVES *continued*

5. Incorporate all of the components of classroom instruction when learning new information.
6. Organize your notes and notebooks according to subjects and dates.
7. Use reference sources to locate needed information.
8. Use test-taking skills when taking various types of tests.
9. Explain the relationship between classroom and clinical instruction.

Twenty-three women and men ranging in age from 19 to 53 years became suddenly silent as Mary Henderson entered the classroom. Mrs. Henderson, a registered nurse for "more than 20 and less than 30 years," as she liked to say, walked briskly to the front of the room. She was a handsome woman with a proud bearing that reflected her feelings about herself and her profession.

"I'm your instructor," Mrs. Henderson said with a serious look. "We'll be spending most of the next year together, some of it right here in this classroom. This school has seen hundreds of eager students enter—and I've been around for more graduations than I would like to admit." She smiled brightly. The class responded with a laugh. Mrs. Henderson surveyed the students, face by face. "There are 23 of you in this class today," she continued. "How many of you expect to be here when we assemble on graduation day?"

The room became silent. The students looked around the room at one another. Slowly, 23 hands went into the air. Mrs. Henderson nodded approval. It was exactly the kind of confidence she liked in a new class. She had a good feeling about this group. The students' positive attitude was already beginning to show. She knew it would be invaluable later when they would be deep into their studies and might need a boost through the hard work that lay ahead.

"And how many think the others in this class will be here with you when you graduate?"

Every hand shot up without hesitation.

"Wonderful," Mrs. Henderson exclaimed. "That's exactly what I had hoped. And that's exactly the way it will be if we all work together to stay together. However, it's possible that some won't be here to graduate. I frankly doubt it, with such an enthusiastic group as this, but it could happen. The decision will be yours." She paused. "Every one of you has the potential to succeed in this program. You wouldn't be here if you didn't. And I would not be here if I didn't have faith in you, too. It won't always be easy. But I know the goal is worth it because I've been a nurse for…" She smiled. "I almost said how long, didn't I?" The class laughed.

Once again, Mrs. Henderson looked into the face of each student. "All right, class. We've made our decision. I, your program teachers, and the administration will do everything we can to support that decision. We're all in this together to become nurses. Let's get to work to make it happen." The students broke into spontaneous applause.

Your decision to become a licensed practical/vocational nurse can be one of the most fulfilling choices of your life. In approximately 1 year, you will be ready to enter practice. The knowledge and experience you gain in school will prepare you for an important career that is valuable to society and is also personally rewarding.

The months ahead will be full. You'll work on a busy daily schedule with new ideas, information, and people. You'll be asked to make hard decisions. When asked to do something, you will be expected to do it. Much of what you do will be influenced by rules and regulations. In addition, you will have to balance the demands of your personal life with those of your student life. How well you adjust and learn will become the foundation of your career.

But you've been a student before. Whether that was last year or years ago, being a student again is not a totally new experience for you. A student nurse must work hard and be dedicated to achieving goals, but you've made the first step already.

✔ Going back to school requires making adjustments.

ORIENTATION

Student orientation sessions with faculty and staff are held to familiarize new students with their program's facilities and hospital affiliations. In these sessions, the rules and regulations for class, hospital, and residence conduct are explained. The program's courses and course content are described. If there is a student government, it is explained. Information about important student resources, such as library, health, and counseling services, is given in detail.

The more you know about your program, its requirements, and what is expected of you, the better and more quickly you will adjust as a student. Student orientation sessions are the perfect times to ask questions. If you've already had your student orientation, review the information you were given. If you have more questions, now is the time to ask an instructor for the answers.

PERSONAL ADJUSTMENTS

Adjusting to student life requires more than knowing rules and regulations. It is more than simply studying and learning. Understanding yourself or self-awareness—being conscious of your own feelings and how well you fit in—is equally important. We discuss understanding yourself and self-awareness in depth in the section on Emotional Health in Chapter 2.

✔ Before you can care for others, you must understand yourself.

Caring for others is a big responsibility, and it is often physically, mentally, and emotionally demanding. The better you understand yourself, the better you will be able to care for others.

Understanding oneself improves the quality of the care given because full attention is on what has to be done without interference from personal issues. If you can't take care of yourself, your effectiveness as a nurse will diminish.

Taking care of yourself means being aware of, understanding, and providing for your own physical, emotional, and intellectual needs. These needs may be complex or simple.

Being aware of your needs and what to do about them is your responsibility. But you are not alone. Your instructors and program administrators know that personal, social, and scholastic problems can arise at any time.

Counseling services to help students make adjustments and solve problems may be available to you. Make use of them. If your program does not have special counseling services, discuss your needs with your program adviser, your instructors, or other members of the faculty or administration. Don't hesitate to ask for help or advice—the sooner, the better.

FINANCING YOUR EDUCATION

Many students need financial assistance to achieve their dream of starting a career in nursing. There are many resources that provide financial assistance, but most require something in return for the assistance.

Financial aid offered by health care agencies often requires you to commit to a period of employment in their facility after graduation. Scholarships may or may not require some sort of payback. Federal student loans require students to pay back loans after graduation while financial aid grants generally do not require a payback. Private sponsors, the military, religious organizations, schools, banks, unions, and many other organizations have very specific criteria for awarding financial aid.

Ask your high school counselor, a librarian, or a nursing school counselor for assistance or conduct your own research for financial aid resources. Be cautious when paying someone to do the research for you, and be sure any contract you sign clearly indicates whether you are guaranteed funds or just guaranteed a list of places to apply for financial aid. Remember, the Free Application for Federal Student Aid (FAFSA) is **free** and you should never pay to apply for federal loans or grants.

✔ *You should not pay an application fee for federal financial aid or scholarships.*

If you decide to use financial aid to pay for your education, request only the amount you will need to get through the program. While you may be offered more than you need, you have to pay back some or all of the money you are awarded. Paying back student loans after graduation can be an economic burden for the borrower.

YOUR PROGRAM

Organization and Curriculum

Your school and the subjects (curriculum) you study will prepare you to become a licensed practical nurse (LPN) or a licensed vocational nurse (LVN). LPNs are known as LVNs in Texas and California.

Your program may vary somewhat from other practical/vocational nursing programs, but the foundation of most programs is similar. In general, basic nursing and health care theory and principles are presented in classroom lectures. Clinical instruction is provided in a variety of health care settings, such as hospitals, long-term care facilities, rehabilitation centers, community health agencies, and mental health treatment centers.

✔ *Nursing instruction occurs in the classroom and in clinical settings.*

Programs are approximately 1 year long. Some are sequential with classroom instruction followed by clinical instruction. Others offer a concurrent curriculum, which presents theory at the same time as the clinical rotation in that subject. Community colleges, vocational/technical schools, and hospitals or other types of health care institutions usually sponsor programs.

Basic course curricula for programs include communications, anatomy and physiology, pharmacology, professional issues and concerns, contemporary health issues, fundamentals of nursing, sociology, psychology, mathematics, geriatrics, nutrition and diet therapy, maternal and child health, and medical–surgical nursing. Certification in cardiopulmonary resuscitation and first aid may also be required.

Program Structure

Your success as a student will be improved if you understand and use your program, its organization, and its personnel efficiently. Each part of your program has an objective.

Your school's objective is to provide the overall structure and services needed to be certain that graduates will be safe and competent nurses and that they will pass the licensing examination in practical/vocational nursing.

The administration's objective is to manage the program so that all school policies and procedures are followed and that the course of study meets the local, state, and national requirements.

Your instructor's objective is to guide you in applying the concepts of nursing that you learn in the different courses of study.

Learn why your program is structured the way it is. Find out why each course is included. Ask what you are expected to do. Much of your success will depend on how well you prepare. If you know what to prepare for, doing what is expected will go smoothly.

Get to know your institution and its administration. Learn who the people are who run it. Find out what they do. This information will be invaluable when you need help.

Know your instructors. Find out what they expect of you. Learn their views on class discussion. Knowing who welcomes discussion and who prefers to lecture without interruptions tells you when to ask questions and when to be a good listener. Find out how your instructors feel about their relationships with students. Some may like open, friendly associations. Others might prefer well-defined lines between the teacher and the student. When you know your instructors' preferences, you can avoid the mistake of trying to warm up to someone who views such friendliness as improper.

Familiarize yourself with the importance of grades, quizzes, and tests. Find out how tests are scored and which count more than others. Learn the value of class participation, homework, punctuality, and attendance.

In other words, learn everything you can about your program and the people in it. The more familiar you are with your program, the easier it will be to adjust to it. Your immediate objective is to integrate your student life with your personal life so that you can concentrate on your long-term goal: to become an LPN or LVN.

SCHEDULING YOUR TIME

How you use your time can make the difference between being prepared and falling behind. Almost every day will be full. On occasion, you may wish there were more than 24 hours in a day. Finding the time to get everything done may take some ingenuity. When you do find extra time, you will treasure it. A written schedule is a good way to organize your time so that every hour can be put to its best use.

A good schedule should be realistic. To get the most from your program and still have time for your personal life, make a schedule that fits the time you have, not how much you wish you had. Set your tasks and the amount of time to do them according to what you can reasonably expect to get done.

Use your class schedule as the basis for organizing the rest of your time. A well-organized schedule should let you see a full week, hour by hour, at a glance. For a sample schedule, see Table 1-1.

You can purchase a pocket- or purse-size calendar and use its organization as the basis for your own daily and weekly program. You can create a schedule on notebook paper and put it in your notebook. Or you can download a planner from a Web site that you can save on your computer. Regardless of which you decide to use, it is important that you create and maintain a written daily schedule.

✔ *An objective is like a goal, only more specific.*

✔ *Know what your instructor expects of you.*

✔ *Always stay focused on your goals and objectives.*

✔ *Learn to manage time efficiently.*

✔ *Make a daily schedule and stick to it.*

TABLE I-I Typical Weekly Schedule of a Parent With Two Children

	Monday	Tuesday	Wednesday	Thursday	Friday	Saturday/Sunday
5:30	Get up, dress, prepare breakfast, and organize school bags for self and children.					Sleep.
6:00	Get children up and have breakfast.					
6:30	Drop children off at babysitter.					Get up, shower, and dress.
6:45	Arrive at school's fitness center. Exercise and shower.					Work on school projects.
8:00	Anatomy class	Anatomy class	Anatomy class	Anatomy class	Anatomy class	Get children up and breakfast together.
8:50	Anatomy class	Anatomy class	Anatomy class	Anatomy class	Anatomy class	Household chores, shopping,
9:40	Psychology class	Psychology class	Psychology class	Psychology class	Psychology class	religious services
10:30	Break	Break	Break	Break	Break	
10:40	Nursing class	Nursing class	Nursing class	Nursing class	Nursing class	
11:30	Lunch Review lab procedures.	Lunch Review for Math test.	Lunch Make flash cards.	Lunch Review lab procedures.	Lunch Meet with advisor.	Recreation and time with children and other family members
12:30	Nursing class	Nursing class	Nursing class	Nursing class	Nursing class	
1:20	Math class	Nutrition class	Math class	Nutrition class	Nursing class	
2:10	Vocational relations class	Sociology class	Vocational relations class	Sociology class	Math class	
3:00	Travel from school—memorize medical terminology on flash cards.					Prepare clothes and food for the next few days.
3:30	Pick up children from babysitter/school.					
3:45	Household chores. Prepare dinner.					
5:00	Dinner	Dinner	Dinner	Dinner	Dinner	Dinner
5:30	Help children with homework.					Help children prepare for the next school week.
6:30	Study Nutrition.	Study Math.	Study Nutrition.	Study Math.	Study Vocational Relations.	Help children prepare for the next school week.
7:15	Study Anatomy.	Study Anatomy.	Study Anatomy.	Study Anatomy.	Study Anatomy.	Recreation time with children
8:00	Study Nursing.	Study Nursing.	Study Nursing.	Study Nursing.	Study Nursing.	
8:45	Study Sociology.	Study Psychology.	Study Nutrition.	Study Nursing.	Study Psychology.	
9:30	Relax.	Relax.	Relax.	Relax.	Relax.	Sleep.
10:15	Sleep.	Sleep.	Sleep.	Sleep.	Sleep.	Sleep.

LEARNING THEORY

Since the 1960s, a great deal of research has been done on the brain and how we learn. Researchers generally agree that learning occurs when two neurons (brain cells) communicate with each other and then with thousands of other neurons. These connections between neurons are called neural pathways. As these complex pathways and connections are strengthened through repetition and practice, memory occurs. It seems to be true that the more frequently a neural pathway is used, the stronger the pathway becomes and the longer the memory lasts. Because the human brain has about one quadrillion neural connections, we all have abundant opportunities to store an amazing amount of information in our memory.

✔ *Physical and mental exercises seem to improve memory.*

The results of all of this brain research can be helpful to you as a student. It's important for you to know that you can maximize your learning potential by understanding how you process, learn, and retain information. When you were an infant and a young child who was learning how to learn and remember, you developed preferences about how you like outside information transmitted to your brain. Some of us prefer to get information through our eyes and others prefer getting it through one or a combination of the other senses that includes taste, touch, hearing, or smell.

Major Learning Styles

Of the senses, the tactile/kinesthetic (touch, movement, posture, orientation), visual (seeing), and auditory (hearing) are the primary routes that people use when attempting to learn something. Researchers agree that most of us, whether we realize it or not, learn better and more efficiently when information is presented in our preferred style. Think about the last time you took home one of those "assembles-in-minutes" products. Did you read the directions aloud (auditory)? Did you watch the instructions (visual), or did you just go ahead and try to put the parts together (tactile)?

✔ *Using your preferred learning style helps make learning more efficient.*

The self-assessment test "What's Your Learning Style?" on pages 10 and 11 will help you determine your preferred learning style. Although you have probably come to rely on more than one sense to learn, knowing how you learn most quickly and efficiently will make learning easier and quicker and you will be able to retain information for a longer period of time.

Applying Your Learning Style

If the self-assessment indicates that you're a visual learner, you learn best by "seeing" things. Learning is most efficient for you if you draw a picture, diagram, or cartoon; create a visual image in your mind; watch a videotape or a movie; or create graphic organizers to illustrate main ideas and supporting details.

✔ *Visual learners like pictures, diagrams, videos, and other visuals.*

Graphic organizers are drawings that are helpful to visual learners (and often other types of learners) because they paint pictures of concepts that may be difficult to remember or memorize. Box 1-1 on pages 12 to 15 shows four types of graphic organizers, with an example of how each is used. The complexity and type of the subject will determine which organizer is appropriate. Try using one of these or your own designs to visualize other information you need to learn.

If you learn best through kinesthetic and tactile senses, moving and doing and touching will help you learn. Here are some ideas that might work for you.

✔ *Tactile learners like to touch and handle things.*

✔ *Auditory learners like to hear information.*

As you handle the equipment, say the name of it, spell the word, and say aloud its purpose. Feel textures and relate them to major concepts you need to learn. Make things you can manipulate out of household items (containers, papers, food items, etc.) and office supplies (pens, paper clips, thumbtacks, etc.). Gestures and expressive movements help you learn and remember complex concepts.

If you're an auditory learner, you probably learn best by hearing. You can maximize your learning by listening and reading aloud. When you train yourself to "hear" words in your mind, the quality and efficiency of your learning improve. Discussing and talking with someone will help you learn and retain information. Auditory learners might consider making an audiotape outlining the major points that need to be learned. You prefer verbal instructions but get distracted by surrounding sounds or noises.

Research also shows that memory is enhanced if you use more than one sense. For example, creating flash cards can be a visual, kinesthetic, and auditory activity because you see the word, write it, and then say it aloud. Making a conscious effort to use as many senses as possible to learn new materials will improve your performance as a student.

ASSESS YOURSELF   What's Your Learning Style?

Learning style refers to the ways you prefer to approach new information. Each of us learns and processes information in our own special style, although we share some learning patterns, preferences, and approaches. Knowing your own style also can help you realize that other people may approach the same situation in a different way from your own.

Take a few minutes to complete the following questionnaire to assess your preferred learning style. Begin by reading the words in the left-hand column. Of the three responses to the right, circle the one that best characterizes you, answering as honestly as possible with the description that applies to you right now. Count the number of circled items and write your total at the bottom of each column. The questions you prefer provide insight into how you learn.

1. When I try to concentrate...	I grow distracted by clutter or movement, and I notice things around me other people don't notice.	I get distracted by sounds, and I attempt to control the amount and type of noise around me.	I become distracted by commotion, and I tend to retreat inside myself.
2. When I visualize...	I see vivid, detailed pictures in my thoughts.	I think in voices and sounds.	I see images in my thoughts that involve movement.
3. When I talk with others...	I find it difficult to listen for very long.	I enjoy listening, or I get impatient to talk myself.	I gesture and communicate with my hands.
4. When I contact people...	I prefer face-to-face meetings.	I prefer speaking by telephone for serious conversations.	I prefer to interact while walking or participating in some activity.
5. When I see an acquaintance...	I forget names but remember faces, and I tend to replay where we met for the first time.	I know people's names and I can usually quote what we discussed.	I remember what we did together and I may almost "feel" our time together.

6. When I relax…	I watch TV, see a play, visit an exhibit, or go to a movie.	I listen to the radio, play music, read, or talk with a friend.	I play sports, make crafts, or build something with my hands.
7. When I read…	I like descriptive examples and I may pause to imagine the scene.	I enjoy the narrative most and I can almost "hear" the characters talk.	I prefer action-oriented stories, but I do not often read for pleasure.
8. When I spell…	I envision the word in my mind or imagine what the word looks like when written.	I sound out the word, sometimes aloud, and tend to recall rules about letter order.	I get a feel for the word by writing it out or pretending to type it.
9. When I do something new…	I seek out demon-strations, pictures, or diagrams.	I want verbal and written instructions, and to talk it over with someone else.	I jump right in to try it, keep trying, and try different approaches.
10. When I assemble an object…	I look at the picture first and then, maybe, read the directions.	I read the directions, or I talk aloud as I work.	I usually ignore the directions and figure it out as I go along.
11. When I interpret someone's mood…	I examine facial expressions.	I rely on listening to tone of voice.	I focus on body language.
12. When I teach other people…	I show them.	I tell them, write it out, or I ask them a series of questions.	I demonstrate how it is done and then ask them to try.
Total	Visual:_____	Auditory:_____	Tactile/Kinesthetic:_____

The column with the highest total represents your primary processing style. The column with the second-most choices is your secondary style.

Your primary learning style: _____

Your secondary learning style: _____

Now that you know which learning style you rely on, you can boost your learning potential when working to learn more. For instance, the following suggestions can help you get more from reading a book.

If your primary learning style is **visual**, draw pictures in the margins, look at the graphics, and read the text that explains the graphics. Envision the topic or play a movie in your thoughts of how you'll act out the subject matter.

If your primary learning style is **auditory**, listen to the words you read. Try to develop an internal conversation between you and the text. Don't be embarrassed to read aloud or talk through the information.

If your primary learning style is **tactile/kinesthetic**, use a pencil or highlighter pen to mark passages that are meaningful to you. Take notes, transferring the information you learn to the margins of the book, into your journal, or onto a computer. Doodle whatever comes to mind as you read. Hold the book in your hands instead of placing it on a table. Walk around as you read. Feel the words and ideas. Get busy—both mentally and physically.

More information on each style, along with suggestions on how to maximize your learning potential, is available in the book *Learn More Now* (Hoboken, NJ; John Wiley & sons. 2004).

©*Marcia L. Connor, 1993–2014 All rights reserved.* http//:marciaconner.com

BOX 1-1	Graphic Organizers

VENN DIAGRAM

These figures can be used to show relationships between things. For example, the patient could be at the center (C) and each of the surrounding circles could contain the people or departments who have relationships with him or her. A Venn diagram has two or more circles.

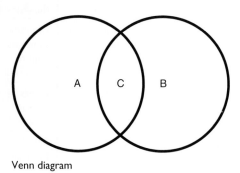

Venn diagram

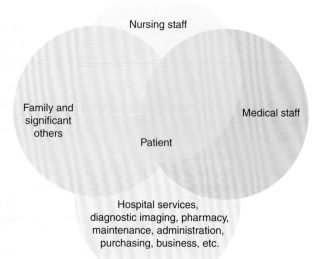

Venn diagram representing some of the people and offices that have a relationship with a hospitalized patient. Note that all of the circles include the patient.

CYCLE

A cycle shows how a series of events proceed in a particular sequence. The suggestion given on how to picture the eight rights of medication administration is an example of a cycle.

BOX
1-1 **Graphic Organizers** *continued*

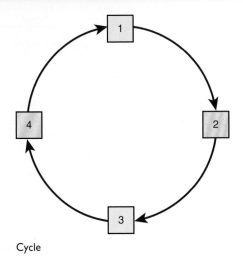

Cycle

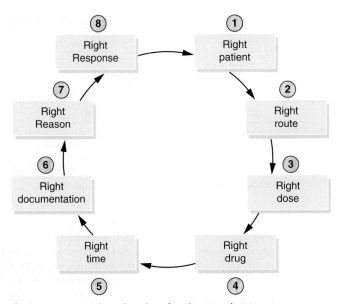

Cycle representing the eight rights of medication administration.

SPIDER MAP

The spider map is used to describe a central idea: a thing, a process, or a concept. For example, the topic, concept, or theme might be personal care. The main ideas could be bathing, oral hygiene, skin care, and documentation. Each of the main ideas would then include details related to the main idea.

continued on page 14

BOX 1-1	Graphic Organizers continued

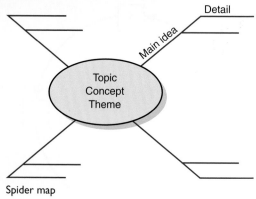

Spider map

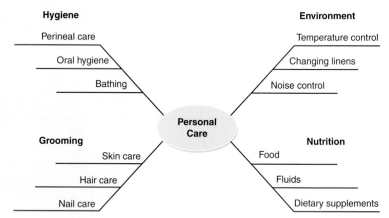

Spider map representing some of the components of personal care.

CLUSTERING

Clustering is an activity that generates ideas, images, and feelings around a particular word. This activity is especially helpful if you need to sort out your feelings or thoughts about a specific subject. For example, the stimulus word might be death. Additional words that immediately come to mind are fear, funeral, terminal illness, and children. Each of these words will cause you to think of related words that can be added to that cluster. This activity helps you more clearly define and separate a broad thought or feeling into its distinct parts.

BOX
1-1 **Graphic Organizers** *continued*

Clustering map

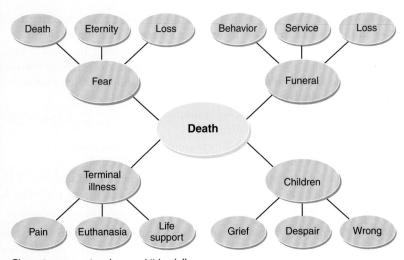

Clustering map using the word "death."

CRITICAL THINKING SKILLS

Critical thinking skills are essential to making good decisions in your personal as well as professional life. There is no room in nursing for poor decisions, so developing good thinking skills is essential for a nurse. You'll also find that applying these concepts to your personal life can help you make better personal decisions.

✔ *Critical thinking skills are the foundation of good decision making.*

Definition of Critical Thinking Skills

It is impossible to be a competent nurse without good critical thinking skills. As you learn in the classroom and as you acquire clinical skills, you will develop a broader knowledge base. As this base broadens, so too does your ability to make connections between what you have learned and what you already know. As these connections grow, you can begin to make projections about what can be expected in very different situations. The more knowledge and experience you gain, the stronger your foundation for critical thinking will become.

Critical thinking is a way of thinking that is clear, accurate, precise, relevant, deep, significant, logical, fair, and broadly based. It evaluates assumptions, inferences, different points of view, information, and concepts, and it considers implications and consequences. It has purpose and is not biased or prejudiced. A critical thinker then is one who is open-minded; does not jump to conclusions; is a good communicator; and consistently monitors, analyzes, and assesses his or her thinking.

✔ *Critical thinkers continually work to improve their thinking skills.*

You'll want to take the facts you have learned and begin by applying those critical thinking skills that include reasoning, inferring, judging, and logic.

Reasoning is the word we use when we mean we are using our mind to make sense of something. Everyone uses reasoning to reach a conclusion; however, only those who are skilled reasoners are good critical thinkers. Characteristics of critical thinkers who have good reasoning skills include those who

- Have a clear goal or purpose for reasoning
- Use reasoning to solve problems
- Are flexible and look at problems from many different points of view
- Base decisions on data, evidence, experience, and research
- Make sure the assumptions they are using are accurate and sound
- Think through the implications of decisions resulting from reasoning to reach a solution to a problem

✔ *Reasoning, inferring, judging, and logic are important critical thinking skills.*

Inferring is the word we use when we are describing the mental act of concluding that something is so because something else is so. If a patient's oral temperature is 101°F, a critical thinker would use his or her inferring skills to come to an accurate and realistic conclusion that there are many reasons why the patient has an elevated temperature. The patient may have an infection, perhaps he just drank hot coffee, she could have just completed a strenuous workout, and so forth. The critical thinker uses good reasoning and inferring skills and decides that more information is required before a decision about the cause of the fever can be made. A person who is not a good critical thinker might infer that an elevated temperature is only and always caused by an infection.

Judging is the word we use to describe the mental act of forming an opinion that can lead to deciding something. Critical thinkers make judgments by using reasoning skills, evaluating inferences, and using good sense. The critical thinker realizes that there are many reasons why patients do not comply with treatment plans. A person who is not a good critical thinker may judge the same patient as uncaring about his or her own health.

Logic is the word we use to describe the mental act of trying to figure things out. Logical thinking is based on using good reasoning, inferring, and judging skills, along with evidence, facts, and truths. Critical thinkers use logic to determine what is relevant and what is irrelevant in a situation. They use logic to decide what supports and what does not support a belief, what they know and do not know, what does or does not contradict an opinion, and what action they should or should not take. Critical thinkers use logic when they are, for example, developing a discharge plan. It would be logical to expect that a first-time mother and her newborn baby would benefit from a follow-up home visit within a few days of discharge. A person who is not a good critical thinker may practice casual and informal thinking and never reach the point of figuring out that the mother and baby should be assessed after discharge.

Using critical thinking skills will help you eliminate those things that don't fit the situation; associate things that go with the situation; put things in order; compare alternatives; contrast findings; evaluate alternatives; and think logically in assessing, planning, implementing, and evaluating nursing care.

Developing Critical Thinking Skills

You can learn to become a critical thinker by working at it. In a given clinical situation, ask questions of yourself, such as "What is the factual basis for my actions? What are the alternatives to my first thoughts? What should I do first and why? Why am I doing this procedure in this way? Did my actions achieve the desired result?"

Welcome questions from your clinical instructor about what you are doing and why. Developing your own questions and questions from your instructor will, with practice, help you take factual knowledge and adapt it appropriately to meet the needs of your individual patients.

✔ *Making good decisions requires coaching from others and lots of practice.*

Box 1-2 describes some of the characteristics of critical thinkers. Constantly working on your critical thinking skills will help you apply the factual knowledge you have attained in a variety of clinical settings and situations.

Applying Critical Thinking Skills

Perhaps the best way to apply critical thinking skills in clinical practice is to "talk through" what you think your options are in a clinical situation. You could talk with a classmate, your instructor, or a staff person whose opinion you value. Ask these people to critique your reasons for choosing a certain action. If what they would do is not the same as what you would do, find out why they would do it differently. In the end, you will have to make your own decisions, but using critical thinking skills will help you make a better decision.

Throughout this book, you will be given opportunities to apply critical thinking skills to situations that will no doubt arise in your nursing career. Practice applying these skills to the "Critical Thinking Exercise" boxes and the "Apply Critical Thinking Skills" section contained in each chapter.

Characteristics of Critical Thinkers and How They Think

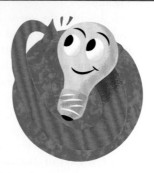

CRITICAL THINKERS ARE

- **Aware of their strengths and capabilities:** They're confident that they can use reason to find answers and make good decisions.
- **Sensitive to their own limitations and predispositions:** They know their weaknesses, values, and beliefs and recognize when these may hamper their ability to assess a situation or solve a problem.
- **Open-minded:** They listen to new ideas and viewpoints and consider the situation from many perspectives.
- **Humble:** They overcome their own tendency to feel that they should have all the answers.
- **Creative:** They are constantly looking for better ways to get things done. They follow recommended procedures; however, they continually examine whether these are the best ways to meet goals and objectives.
- **Proactive:** They accept responsibility and accountability for their actions. They study situations, anticipate problems, and find ways to avoid them *before* they happen.
- **Flexible:** They recognize the importance of changing priorities and interventions when planned approaches don't seem to be getting results.
- **Aware that errors are stepping-stones to new ideas:** They turn mistakes into learning opportunities, reflecting on what went wrong and identifying ways to avoid the same mistake in the future.
- **Willing to persevere:** They know that sometimes there are no easy answers and that there may be time-consuming struggles to find the best answer.
- **Cognizant of the fact that we don't live in a perfect world:** They realize that sometimes the *best* answer may not be the *perfect* answer.
- **Introspective:** They evaluate and correct their own thinking.

CRITICAL THINKERS ALSO:

- **Maintain a questioning attitude:** They ask questions such as "What's going on here?" "What does it mean?" and "What else could it mean, and how else could it be interpreted?"
- **Ask for clarification when they don't understand:** For example, they say, "I'm not clear about this. Can you tell me more?" *or* ask questions such as, "What do you mean by *better*, better in what way?"
- **Apply previous knowledge to new situations:** They see similarities and differences between one experience and another, between one concept and another.
- **See the situation from many perspectives:** They value all viewpoints and watch that their judgments are based on *facts,* not personal feelings, views, or self-interest.

BOX 1-2
Characteristics of Critical Thinkers and How They Think
continued

- **Weigh risks and benefits (advantages and disadvantages) before making a decision:** They avoid risky decisions and find ways to reduce adverse reactions before putting a plan into action.
- **Seek help when needed.**
- **Put first things first:** They ask, "What's the most important thing to do here?"

CRITICAL THINKERS USE LOGIC. THEY:

- **Test first impressions to make sure they are as they appear:** They double-check the logic of their thinking and the workability of their solutions.
- **Distinguish between fact and fallacy:** They take the time to verify important information to be sure that it's true.
- **Distinguish fact from inference (what they *believe* the fact means):** For example, they recognize that because someone is sitting quietly in a corner may not mean that the individual is *withdrawn*; it means that he is sitting quietly in a corner and it would be helpful to find out why.
- **Support views with evidence:** They wouldn't state that the person above is withdrawn without providing additional supporting evidence, such as the individual saying he wants nothing to do with anyone.
- **Determine what's relevant and what's irrelevant:** They recognize what's important for understanding a situation and what's unimportant. For example, the fact that you're a nurse or studying to be a nurse is relevant to how I should write this book; the fact that you are female or male is irrelevant.
- **Apply the concept of "cause and effect":** They look for what's causing a problem to more fully understand the problem itself. They anticipate responses to their actions before performing the action. For example, critical thinkers would attempt to find out the *cause* of pain before deciding how to *treat* it. They would determine how someone might *respond* to a medication before administering it.
- **Withhold judgment until all the necessary facts are in:** They realize the dangers of jumping to conclusions.

Adapted with permission from Alfaro-LeFevre (2014). Evidence-Based Critical Thinking Indicators. Available: http://www.alfaroteachsmart.com/NewCTIReq.htm. No copying without permission.

CLASSROOM INSTRUCTION

You will be spending many hours in the classroom, so preparing for lectures and other methods of classroom instruction is important to your success as a student. The next several pages give you suggestions on how to effectively participate in various types of instruction.

Lectures

Much basic information is presented through the lecture method of instruction. During a lecture, your instructor will present information that will clarify those parts of the reading assignment that may need further explanation, identify important points that you should remember, and assist you in finding relationships in what you are learning.

Lectures will let you know what is expected of you. This setting is where you will have the best opportunity to ask questions. How much you get from lectures will depend on how good a listener you are and how well you have prepared yourself before the lecture.

✔ Prepare for lectures by completing reading assignments in advance.

Listening

Listening and hearing are not the same. Hearing is biophysical, the perception of sounds. Listening is intellectual, a conscious effort to interpret sounds. You may hear sounds being made by someone, but you might not be interpreting those sounds. To understand sounds, you must use listening skills. In lectures and elsewhere, listening takes effort.

Being a good listener is one of a nurse's most useful skills. Throughout your nursing education and career, most of your interactions with instructors, other nurses, physicians, and patients will be verbal. Even the observations you make will depend heavily on what is said to you as well as what you see. Knowing what is said can affect how well you perform.

✔ *Doodling, daydreaming, and talking distract from listening.*

To listen effectively, fix your eyes on the speaker's face. Pay close attention to the words, following them in your mind. Make your written notes while you listen, but concentrate on what is being said rather than on what you are writing.

Taking Notes

Nobody is expected to remember everything, but as a student, and later when you begin to practice, you will be expected to recall a surprising amount of information. The better your memory, the easier this will be. For most people, memory is imperfect. Everyone needs reminding from time to time. The best reminders are well-organized, written notes.

The goal of good note taking is to capture key words, ideas, and concepts in short phrases. Like good study habits, the best note-taking system is the one that works for you. If you already have a note-taking system, use it. If taking notes is not something you normally do, develop a system now. It will be indispensable to you as a student and will continue to work for you after you have graduated.

The advantages of good note-taking skills far outweigh the effort needed to learn them. The main benefit is higher grades. Notes are short, written phrases that capture key points. Well-taken, clearly written notes record important facts and ideas that are buried in books, lectures, films, computer programs, and other instructional materials. Good notes will help you review and remember what you have covered. They are especially helpful when you need them most—for study and review just before quizzes and tests.

Get into the habit of taking notes. Take them in lectures; when you read; when watching films, videos, and demonstrations; during clinical rounds; and in any other situation where you are being given information to learn and remember.

✔ *Be sure you will be able to read your own writing and shorthand.*

If note taking doesn't come naturally to you, or if you have problems keeping good notes, ask your instructor for help immediately. The sooner you begin a set of organized notes, the easier it will be to record, remember, and review the material being taught.

The following are some general rules for taking notes:
- Omit unnecessary words.
- Abbreviate words (but not so you don't know what they mean later).
- Use an outline format.
- Don't repeat what is in a handout or your textbook.
- If you highlight your textbook as you read, highlight information stressed in class in a different color.
- Clarify confusing information with the instructor immediately after class.

An example of outline notes from a pharmacology lecture might be as follows:

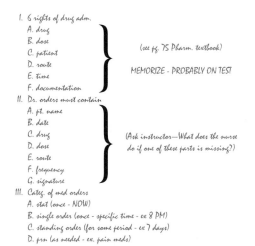

I. 6 rights of drug adm.
    A. drug
    B. dose
    C. patient   *(see pg. 75 Pharm. textbook)*
    D. route
    E. time   *MEMORIZE - PROBABLY ON TEST*
    F. documentation
II. Dr. orders must contain
    A. pt. name
    B. date
    C. drug   *(Ask instructor—What does the nurse*
    D. dose   *do if one of these parts is missing?)*
    E. route
    F. frequency
    G. signature
III. Categ. of med orders
    A. stat (once - NOW)
    B. single order (once - specific time - ex 8 PM)
    C. standing order (for some period - ex 7 days)
    D. prn (as needed - ex. pain meds)

There are many kinds of notebooks. Individual preference will determine which type you use. Some students prefer to use tablets, laptops, a note-taking app, or an audio recording device. Other students prefer keeping all of their written notes in one loose-leaf notebook with subject dividers. A single notebook keeps and organizes all notes for all classes in one place. Making additions or deletions or moving pages or sections from one place to another is simplified. Others prefer a notebook for each subject. An alternative to notebooks is index cards. They allow easy filing and cross-indexing but are less portable and convenient. Students also use tablets, laptops, and notetaking apps that often allow students to record lectures.

For legibility and neatness, use lined paper and write on one side only. The blank facing page can be used for additions or comments to the main notes. Date each set of notes. It's also a good idea to identify each page of notes by date, course, instructor, or subject and to number them if they're in loose-leaf form so that they can be reorganized if they get out of sequence.

When taking notes in class, sit where you can be comfortable and as close to the lecturer as possible. Make sure you have a clear view of the board or screen so that you can read what is written on it. Sit comfortably. Good posture will help you keep alert.

✔ *Getting and staying organized is essential.*

Missed lectures mean missing notes. If you miss a lecture or class, make arrangements to get notes from a classmate to avoid blanks in your notebook and to keep up with the course. Tape-recording a lecture can be helpful if you miss one, but regularly taping lectures wastes time, just as word-for-word notes do.

✔ *Being absent from class for just 1 day can put you far behind.*

Taking notes is easier when reading assignments are kept up-to-date because the information in one reinforces the other. A good general rule is to have your reading assignment done before a lecture. If possible, review assignments briefly, so you will be prepared to take notes on new information that can't be found in your textbooks.

Some guidelines for taking clear notes during lectures are as follows:

1. **Listen.** Pay attention to what is being said; avoid distractions; watch as well as listen.
2. **List.** Write down the main ideas, facts, and supporting data; write down any board notes; write down your questions if something is not clear.
3. **Read.** Read your notes as soon as possible after taking them; fill in with any material you remember but did not write down.
4. **Review.** Review your notes on the day they were made, just before the next class in that subject, and before exams.

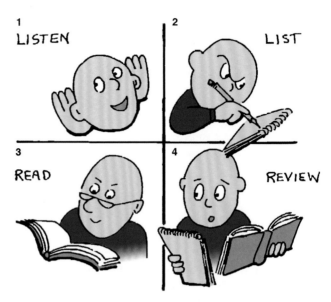

When listening, keep your ears tuned for key words and phrases. Listen and watch for signals that indicate what is considered to be important. Phrases such as "will be on the exam," "studies have shown," "the main reason for," "the important thing to remember," and similar remarks are strong suggestions that what will be said next should be written down.

✔ *Instructors often give clues that certain information is important.*

Other clues that the information is important are pausing, repeating, slowing down, underlining, and emphasizing. If you pay attention, after a few lectures, you will learn the instructor's style and will know when to write and when to listen. During a lecture, be sure to record the notes, diagrams, charts, dates, and other data your instructor writes or projects on the whiteboard or screen.

Your note-taking style should be what is most comfortable for you. But information may come faster than you can keep up with while using normal writing. If you know shorthand or can improvise personal shorthand, you will be able to devote your attention to the information. Use underlining or capital letters for emphasis. Number lists. Eliminate vowels in words to shorten them. Leave out unnecessary words. Shorten sentences.

✔ *Take legible and organized notes that contain information not available from your textbooks.*

The standard abbreviations and terms used in charting that you will be learning can double as shorthand in your note taking. Be cautious when taking abbreviated notes. Although it's easy to abbreviate words, it's sometimes difficult to recall what your abbreviation means. This is especially true when you're building a medical and nursing vocabulary. Completely write or print words that are new to you. If you decide to abbreviate, write the abbreviation in parentheses next to the word. You can use the abbreviation for the new word from that point on because you have a record of what a particular abbreviation means to you.

An example of notes from a nursing lecture might read like this:

Warm Soaks
1. Normal saline solution (NSS)
2. Temp 105 to 110° Fahrenheit (F)
3. Three times a day (t.i.d.)
4. 20 minutes

The next time the lecturer refers to normal saline solution, you need to write only NSS in your notes; when reference is made to three times a day, you need to write only t.i.d., and so forth.

Avoid doodling on your note pages and letting your attention wander. Concentrate on what is being said and condense what you hear into brief, legible notes.

Whereas writing notes is an effective way for most students to learn, others will do better using different strategies or combinations of strategies. Some auditory learners might do best by listening and recording lectures; visual learners might do best by creating graphic organizers. If you know what works for you, continue to use it. If you think you could benefit from a professional evaluation of how you learn, ask your instructor for advice.

Studying

Studying is the process of attentively applying the mind to learn or understand a topic or subject. How much time you have to study will be clear from your schedule. The choice of how to study is up to you.

Study habits are learning tools. Good study habits combined with a desire to learn are essential to success as a student. Both are under your control. If you have study habits that worked in the past with good results, use them. If your study skills are rusty or you don't have a study method, use these guidelines:

- Set regular times for study and mark them in your schedule.
- Establish an area with minimum distractions.
- Set aside a minimum of study time for each hour spent in class.
- Allow enough time to study each subject.
- Schedule your study time by priorities.
- Study the most important subjects first.
- Study hard subjects before easy subjects.
- Set the time you will need for each subject by the difficulty of the material.
- Revise your schedule and priorities according to need.
- Take short rests every 45 to 60 minutes of study time.
- Study just before and right after classes.
- Study when your energy level is up.
- Have all necessary books, papers, notes, and other study material on hand before starting.
- Study dissimilar subjects in each session to help keep you and the material fresh.
- Avoid distractions and interruptions; when they do occur, deal with them quickly.
- Take advantage of instructor review sessions and student study groups.

In general, shorter sessions are less tiring than long ones and allow better concentration and retention of information. Limiting the length of each session makes sessions more productive.

Proper rest and nutrition are important to clear thinking. Be as comfortable as possible, but avoid conditions that make you drowsy.

Where you study can be as important as how you study (Fig. 1-1). Choose places where the lighting is good, the temperature is comfortable, and noise and distractions are at a minimum. Always resist temptations that interfere with scheduled study time.

Once you establish a study pattern, stick to it. There will be times when you will have to make adjustments. Handle them as they come along, and return to your normal pattern when they're done.

Your study schedule should be a part of your life, not all of it. Allow yourself some free time to do the things you enjoy.

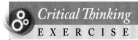

Critical Thinking
E X E R C I S E

You studied hard for a test and just found out that you failed it with a grade of 60%. You feel discouraged and think about quitting school. Choose at least four appropriate Characteristics of Critical Thinkers in Box 1-2 to develop your responses to these questions. Briefly explain why you chose each characteristic and how that characteristic influenced your decision to stay in school or to quit

✔ *Study in a comfortable and quiet place.*

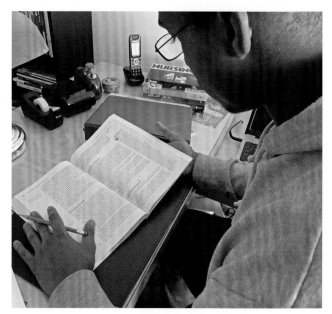

FIGURE 1-1. ● Study in a quiet and comfortable area.

The better organized you are, the easier your life as a student nurse will be. This is especially true if school and study don't come easily for you. If getting organized is difficult, ask your adviser, an instructor, or another student who has these skills for help.

Computer-Assisted Instruction

The use of computer technology is an important component of your nursing education. The sooner you familiarize yourself with computers and what they do, the easier it will be to use them.

Completing computer-learning assignments may be required as a part of your program of study (Fig. 1-2). Instructional computer programs, which aid in

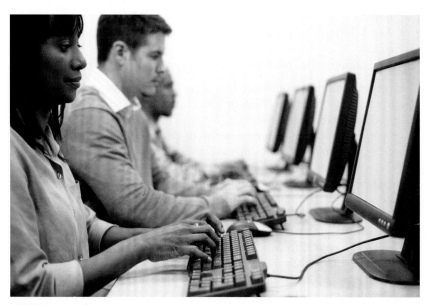

FIGURE 1-2. ● Computer-assisted instruction may be required in your school.

learning, display information on a screen. The user is given step-by-step instructions on how to move from one screen to the next. Ask your instructor, librarian, or computer lab assistant for help if you have problems using computer-assisted instruction.

A computer-assisted learning assignment is usually an independent learning activity, which means that you must do it on your own. Find out what hours you can use the computer lab and whether you need to schedule computer time. Be prepared for the session by having materials such as notepaper, pencils, and textbooks with you.

In addition to required computer-assisted learning assignments, your library or computer lab may have many additional programs on file that will help with your studies. Ask what titles are available and make use of these programs often.

Distance learning, or learning some distance away from the primary classroom, is assisted by computer technology. Lectures, workshops, demonstrations, and even entire courses of instruction offered in one location are broadcast to locations that may be some distance from the primary classroom. Participants can interact with the presenter through telephone, television, and computer technology as though they were in the primary classroom.

Audiovisual Instruction

Audiovisual (A/V) instruction through television, films, DVDs, CDs, streamed media, and other visual media extends your classroom to places and people you might only hear or read about otherwise. Clinical demonstrations, nursing procedures, and your own performance in skills and techniques can be reviewed conveniently and as often as desired when recorded on video media.

Treat A/V presentations with the same approach as you do other sources of information by taking notes and periodically reviewing them.

ASSIGNMENTS

Most days, you will be given assignments to do before your next class session. These assignments are an important part of your preparation and are intended to introduce new material. When you complete assignments before class, you will be able to ask questions to clarify what you did not understand. A few simple guidelines will help you effectively complete reading and writing assignments.

Reading Assignments

Good reading skills are the foundation of successful learning. Whether you are reading a textbook, a journal, or a computer screen, reading is more efficient if you're mentally and physically prepared. Review the study suggestions on pages 23 and 24 because studying and reading go hand in hand. In addition, practice the following:

- Read in a quiet place with a minimum of interruption or distraction.
- Adjust temperature and lighting to a comfortable level.
- Sit upright in a comfortable chair.
- Avoid reading on a full or an empty stomach.
- Place your book or computer screen at a comfortable angle.

To help you to concentrate on what you're reading in books and journals, to increase your reading speed, and to improve your ability to recall what you read, a popular shortcut called the SQ3R (survey–question–read–recite–review)

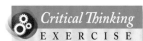
Critical Thinking
E X E R C I S E

Last week, your instructor assigned a project that requires using the Internet. When looking at the project, you think the assignment should take about an hour to complete. You know you have to get this assignment done but haven't gotten to it because your baby has been ill the last couple of days and she has been requiring all of your attention. And now the assignment is due tomorrow morning, and you have to get it done this evening. When the baby finally falls asleep, you go to your computer to work on the project. After several attempts to connect to the Internet, you realize that your modem is not working. Using Characteristics of Critical Thinkers in Box 1-2, write down some of your ideas on how you might be able to complete this assignment before it is due in the morning.

✔ *Remember to take notes during audiovisual and computer instruction.*

✔ *Being able to read well is essential to success in school, in work, and in life.*

method will be useful if you don't have a reading system of your own. Use it as follows:

Survey the chapter or unit by reading the title, objectives, key words, chapter heads, introduction, italicized passages, graphs, illustrations, photos, and end-of-chapter questions before you begin normal reading.

Question what you will be reading. Create questions before you begin.

Read by skimming first to find and look up unknown words. Then read for content. Take notes as you read. Summarize your notes after you have finished reading.

Recite aloud or silently the substance of what you have read. Repeat it as often as needed to get the material firmly fixed in your mind.

Review the material before going on to the next task.

Writing Assignments

Writing assignments, usually in the form of term papers, case studies, and care plans, are a part of your education. You may be given a topic or be asked to choose one. Once you have a topic, the following five steps will help get you through most papers:

1. Collect the material—books, notes, papers, articles, and other reference matter—your paper is to be based on.
2. Organize and then outline the reference material. A sample outline for a short paper follows:
   a. Introduction (states purpose of paper). Say what you are going to say. Open with a topic sentence and follow with a short background or history.
   b. Body (states main ideas and details). Develop the paper's purpose, using research material to substantiate your case. State the main idea and then give details for each main idea you are presenting.
   c. Conclusion (states what was said). Briefly summarize what you have said in the paper.
3. Write your first draft from beginning to end. Avoid rewriting and editing the first time through.
4. Read your first draft, add notes, make changes and revisions, and then write the final draft.
5. Proofread your final draft and make corrections before you hand in the paper.

✔ *When beginning a writing assignment, prepare a clear statement of your topic and then stay focused.*

✔ *Do not wait until the last minute to begin a writing assignment.*

If you write your papers using a word-processing program on the computer, remember to save your work at least every 10 minutes. Also remember to make a backup copy of your work in case you have problems with your computer equipment.

Plan to complete written assignments before they are due. If you have a technical problem with your computer or a personal problem requiring your attention, you will have a margin of time to cope with these unexpected events.

REFERENCE SOURCES

Books

Beyond lectures, other sources of information you will need are found in books. Most of the books you will use will be recommended by your instructors and other authorities. Trust their judgment because they speak from experience.

Choose wisely when buying books other than those your course requires. Nursing books are revised often to keep up with change.

Knowing how to use a book to find what you need is a basic tool for every student. Time spent familiarizing yourself with how to use a book now will save you hours of work throughout your program and career.

Textbooks, reference books, and most other nonfiction books are organized to simplify finding information. A table of contents at the front of a book lists each chapter by title, often with a brief description of the topic covered in that chapter. Page numbers indicate where to find the specific chapter.

An index will be found at the back of most books. The index lists specific items in alphabetical order. Names, subjects, and individual topic-related words are in a good index. If you want to find where in the book to look for psychologists, for example, look under P. The word psychologist will be listed, followed by the page or pages where it is used. Use tables of contents and indexes to quickly obtain the information you need.

✔ *Learn how to use books to find the information you need.*

Appendixes (appendices) are separate sections of related material found at the back of books. A book may have an appendix in which the addresses of nursing organizations are listed, for example. Reference to an appendix is usually made in the body of the book. An item will be followed by a note in this form: See Appendix D, Drug Interactions.

Glossaries are separate sections listing vocabulary words special to the topic of the book, such as a glossary of nursing terms.

Other Materials

Other reference materials include journals, magazines, pamphlets, A/V programs, general reference books such as dictionaries, and information accessed through computer programs or the Internet.

Official journals of nursing and journals published by other health care disciplines provide the latest news and information long before it can be published in books. Your program, library, or instructors may have copies of journals available. You may wish to buy your own online or mail subscriptions, but it's a good idea to become acquainted with various journals first to ensure buying those that fit your needs.

✔ *Be careful to use materials that contain accurate information.*

Some health-oriented books and magazines and popular consumer magazine articles present good, readable, general health information that can be used to supplement your other reading. Follow your instructor's advice regarding nontechnical sources.

When selecting reference material of any kind on your own, see that it's up-to-date, accurate, and reliable. Your instructor is the authority.

Libraries

Modern libraries include many different types of materials that provide learning resources. In fact, the term *Learning Resource Center* is often used to describe what was previously known as the library.

Your program may have its own library or may provide access to one at a nearby hospital or other health care facility. Public libraries, especially central libraries in larger cities, will also have nursing and medical reference material.

✔ *Learn to use the resources in libraries and instructional material centers.*

Using a library is not difficult. It requires familiarity with using a computerized catalog, which lists the titles of materials available in the library. It also requires some knowledge of how materials are catalogued. The process is systematized so that every library is organized in the same basic way. If you have difficulty locating materials in a library, ask the librarian for help. He or she will be more than willing to assist you.

Computers

Whereas many students are quite skilled in using all of the capabilities of computers and the Internet, others will need instructions and assistance. The next few paragraphs and the section on the Internet will introduce inexperienced students to computers and the Internet and some of the ways in which they are used in education. Students who are experienced in using computers and the Internet may choose to skip this section.

If you're thinking about purchasing a computer for your personal use, you should first make a list of what you want to be able to do with the computer. Do you want to be able to write reports and term papers? Do you want to be able to learn math and dosage calculation skills? Do you want to get and send electronic mail (e-mail)? Do you want to be able to work through clinical simulations? Do you want to be able to access a computerized list of drugs and interactions? Do you want to take a simulated licensing examination? Do you want online banking? Do you want to get tutorial programs for your children? Do you need a CD-ROM drive to run the programs you might purchase? Do you want access to the Internet? Is wireless technology an option you should consider? If your school requires that you use a personal computer for instruction, do you have access to a backup computer and do you have someone who can quickly repair your computer should the need arise?

✔ *Know what you want to do with a computer before you buy one.*

After you decide what it is you want to be able to do, you should discuss your needs with one or two people who can provide reliable advice on what you need to purchase. A teacher who uses computers in the classroom, the high school student next door, your child, or a salesperson in a computer store can provide valuable guidance. If you don't have a personal computer, you can often get access to one in public libraries and college libraries or you can rent time in private computer labs, shopping malls, or coffee shops.

Your computer also provides ways for people to communicate with each other. E-mail is an efficient way to send and receive information. Your e-mail address is similar to your postal address. Your faculty may use e-mail to send you messages regarding assignments, schedules, meeting locations, and so forth. If you are assigned an e-mail address, you should make it a habit to check your mail daily. Facebook groups, forums, and message boards can be set up to allow groups with similar interests to "talk" with one another by typing their conversations on a computer. Instructors often create online forums and require students to participate in directed discussions.

The National Council of State Boards of Nursing (NCSBN), the agency that administers nursing licensure examinations, conducts nurse licensing examinations by computer. Because computers are now, and will be in the future, used in so many areas of your nursing practice and in your personal life, it's important that you develop some skill in using this technology. Take advantage of every opportunity to learn to use computers.

The Internet

From one Web site in 1991 to more than 1 billion Web sites in 2014, a world full of information is available to you. To get connected to the Internet, you need either a smartphone or a computer that has a modem to connect to a telephone line, a cable line, Wi-Fi, or a satellite on the roof of your house. Regardless of how you get access to the Internet, here are some general things that you should keep in mind when using the Internet to get information.

✔ *The Internet gives you access to a world of information.*

- ANYONE can put information on a Web site, so information may or may not be accurate.
- Government (.gov) Web sites are some of the best resources.
- Organizational (.org) Web sites provide information about membership, mission, goals, and the activities of that organization.
- Commercial (.com) Web sites usually promote products or services.
- The value of educational (.edu) Web sites depends on the reliability of the people who created them.
- Use Web sites that are organized and easy to use.
- Use Web sites that are frequently updated.
- Be sure that the Web site includes the name and address of a contact person or organization.
- Does the information make sense with what you know?
- Do textbooks and journal articles support the Web site information?
- What are the qualifications of the people who contribute to the Web site?
- Ask your instructor to comment on the quality of a particular Web site.

To access information by using the Internet, type the URL (Uniform Resource Locator) into the blank line on the computer screen. The URL for Web pages is usually http://www followed by the description of the document you are looking for. If you see https:// in the Web site address, know that the "s" means the site is secure making what you are doing on that Web site useless to hackers and eavesdroppers. Those web addresses that begin with http:// are not secure so it is unwise to enter personal information into this type of address.

The following image is from a computer screen with the URL typed in the blank line. Your computer screen might look different from this, but the way you enter the URL is similar for all computers. After you type in the URL, press the enter key to reach the Web site.

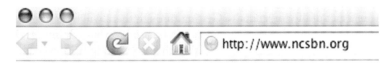

The quickest way to get information from the Internet is to know the Web site URL. For example, to find out more about the NCLEX licensing examination, type in the NCSBN Web site URL (http://www.ncsbn.org) and press the enter key. Within a few seconds, you should be connected to the NCSBN Web page where you can point to a topic and click your mouse button to get information that the NCSBN has made available to Internet users. Appendix A lists a number of Web site addresses that pertain to your nursing education and career. Space is provided to add the address of additional Web sites that you have found useful and accurate.

✔ *Begin keeping a log or bookmarking your favorite Web site addresses.*

When you don't know the Web site address or when you are searching for information rather than a specific site, you can use a tool called a search engine. A search engine is an automated program that is used to find information from many sources on the World Wide Web (www). Type in the URL of the search engine you want to use, press the enter key on your computer, and then type in what you are looking for in the "search" box that appears.

THE *Web*

Here in alphabetical order are five popular search engines and their Web addresses:

AOL	http://www.aol.com
Ask	http://www.ask.com
Bing	http://www.bing.com
Google	http://www.google.com
Yahoo	http://www.yahoo.com

It's important to read and follow the instructions on how to word your search request. The more specific your request, the better the results will match your request.

For example, suppose you want to learn more about the NCLEX-PN but you don't have the Web site address. You could select a search engine and type in your search key words; after a few seconds, you should have a list of choices that might or might not include what you are looking for. Point the mouse on the source you want and click. What comes up may or may not be exactly what you're looking for. You may have to try again. If you're looking for something very specific, you can spend a great deal of time "surfing the Web."

✔ *Disorganized Web surfing can waste valuable time.*

It is easy to get caught up when your search is not very specific. Stopping to read things of interest to you or forgetting what it is that you were looking for will consume time that you might not have. If you have a limited amount of study time and must make the most of it, you probably should not be spending a lot of time looking for information on the Web. Your instructors and classmates can give you direct addresses, so you can use your time wisely and productively. Keep focused on exactly what it is you are looking for and make every effort to avoid getting sidetracked along the way.

TAKING TESTS

Tests are a fact of life for students. Getting through them will be easier if you're prepared. The energy that tests stimulate can be used to your advantage. Direct the energy to preparing for the test, rather than to wasting it in unproductive nervous activity.

Test Anxiety

Test anxiety is a term used to describe the psychological and physical feelings experienced before an examination. Although for most students this feeling actually increases performance, for some, the anxiety is devastating. See Chapter 5 for a self-assessment questionnaire on test anxiety. If the anxiety is overwhelming, following is a list of a few things you can try.

✔ *For most people, a little test anxiety improves performance.*

- Remind yourself that you studied the material.
- Tell yourself that you don't need to get all the answers right.
- Use positive self-talk to improve self-confidence.
- Tell yourself that you will not panic when you don't know an answer.
- Avoid listening to other students talk about what they studied and what they think will be on the test.
- Avoid participating in a last minute review session with other students.
- Avoid taking sedatives or stimulants before the test.

- Get a good night's sleep before the test.
- Practice relaxation techniques.
- Have confidence in your ability.
- Replace negative thoughts about yourself with positive ones.
- Don't panic when other students finish the test long before you do.
- Don't change answers unless you're certain the first one was incorrect.
- Don't put pressure on yourself that doesn't exist. Not doing well on one test will probably not be the end of your enrollment in school.
- Use your reasoning ability and life experience to answer questions that you think you don't know the answer to.

If using these tips doesn't help you overcome excessive anxiety, consider professional help. A professional can offer many strategies that will be individualized to meet your specific needs.

✔ *Professional counseling may help if you experience extreme test anxiety.*

Preparation for tests includes planned study and review sessions. Be sure of the exact location and time the test will be given. Know the kind of test it will be (e.g., true/false, essay, multiple choice) and the subjects it will cover.

Strategies for Taking Tests

A general strategy for taking a paper-and-pencil test includes the following:

1. Before the exam begins, make sure you understand the directions and what you're supposed to do. If you're uncertain, ask questions before you begin.
2. Look over the whole exam before you begin to answer questions to estimate how much time each section will take. Make a note of your estimate so that you can gauge your progress once you're under way.
3. Be certain you understand the relative grading weights of different sections. Some parts of a test may count more than others. Use this information to determine where to spend more or less time.
4. Differentiate between hard and easy sections or questions.
5. Once you have done steps 2, 3, and 4, make a test-taking plan based on your evaluation and stick to it. For example, you can go straight through the test or do either the hard or easy material first.
6. When you have a plan, proceed with the test. Pay just enough attention to the time to keep to your plan.

✔ *Find the test-taking strategies that work best for you.*

Some test-taking hints are as follows:

On Mixed Easy-to-Hard Questions

- *Do easy questions first to build confidence.*
- *Mark hard questions with an x and harder ones with xx, and answer them in order as time allows.*
- *Hard and easy are determined by what you know.*

On Multiple-Choice Tests

- *Find out before the test if you will be penalized for guessing.*
- *When guessing, trust your first response as correct.*
- *Eliminate two or more answers before guessing.*
- *Use what you learn from one question to help answer others.*
- *Answers with "all," "never," and "always" are generally incorrect.*

On Essay Questions

- *Think through each answer before writing.*
- *Make a brief outline.*
- *Allot an appropriate amount of time for each answer.*

- *Answer the easy questions first.*
- *If time is short, get important information down first.*
- *After completing an exam, use any remaining time to review your answers.*

A general strategy for taking a computer-administered test includes the following:
- *Know how to use the mouse, cursor, space bar, enter, delete, and escape keys and any other special keys that will be used during the test.*
- *If available, complete a tutorial prior to the actual test to familiarize yourself with the test format.*
- *Read, understand, and follow the directions for every question on the test.*
- *Answer every question in each section.*
- *Pace yourself so that you have enough time to answer every question. Pay attention to the number of questions and the amount of time remaining during your testing session. Do not spend too much time on a single question.*
- *In some computer-administered tests, you cannot omit questions or go back and change answers. Be sure you know the rules for the test you are taking.*
- *If you do not know the answer to a question, eliminate any answer choices that are obviously incorrect and choose the best of those that remain.*

✔ Taking computer-administered exams will help you prepare for the NCLEX-PN exam.

Standardized Examinations

Classroom exams are designed to test your knowledge of specific subjects learned over a limited time. Standardized tests show how much of a range of subjects you have learned through all or a portion of your education. They compare your knowledge with students around the country. The comparisons are usually given in percentile rankings. An evaluation of your progress can be based on the comparison.

✔ If you cram for quizzes and exams, you probably won't do well on standardized tests or the licensing examination.

Although there is no real method of preparation for standardized exams, you will do better if you complete assignments when scheduled and if you also apply what you learn in the clinical setting. You will do better if you don't cram for the exams given by your teachers. Most students know that cramming does not result in long-term retention of information. Standardized tests draw on a broad range of material learned over a long time. Before taking a standardized test, you may find it helpful to review a similar test to familiarize yourself with the format and types of questions asked. Also, a general review of material that is to be covered in a standardized test will help you recall what you have already learned.

When taking a standardized test, be sure you understand the directions and follow them. Don't make any extra marks on the answer sheet and be certain to mark the boxes or bubbles that go with the questions. If you get out of sequence, every answer will be wrong.

✔ Always read all of the directions before beginning a test.

Standardized tests may penalize you for guessing. The test directions or the person administering the test will tell you. If you're uncertain, ask. Read all the answers before making a mark on your answer sheet. If the test doesn't penalize for guessing, eliminate the answers you know are wrong and guess from those remaining. Avoid skipping questions even if you're not sure of the answer. If you finish the test before the time is up, go back and review the test.

The two most common standardized tests for practical nursing students are the National League for Nursing (NLN) achievement tests and the NCSBN NCLEX-PN licensing examination. NLN achievement tests are given at various points in the nursing program; the NCLEX-PN is the examination that in part determines whether a person receives a nursing license. Chapter 5 provides a detailed discussion of the NCLEX-PN. Depending on your school policies, the NLN standardized examinations are administered either on paper or on the computer. The NCLEX-PN exam is only administered on the computer.

CLINICAL INSTRUCTION

Clinical instruction is arranged by the faculty to give you practical experience in the care of people in various health care settings. Your first clinical assignment might be in a long-term care facility or in a hospital. Regardless of where you're assigned, you will be expected to integrate and apply what you learned in the classroom to the care of the patient (Fig. 1-3).

Before you begin to care for your patient, you should review your textbooks and notes to be sure you correctly understand the patient's condition, the treatment being given, and the procedures you will be performing. In the beginning, your instructor will help you define what you're permitted to do. As you gain experience and clinical skills, you will be expected to identify those skills you can perform independently and those that require instructor observation.

Most often, your day will start with a short preconference. During this time, your instructor will review the instructional plan for the day. You and your classmates will be given an opportunity to ask questions about your assignments. Your instructor may give specific instructions about new treatments or procedures that you may be expected to complete during your clinical time. It's important that you write these notes on a pocket notepad. It's easy in the rush of the clinical environment to forget the directions your instructor gave you. It's also easy to forget what you're expected to do for your patients.

✔ *Be prepared to take notes and complete assignments during clinical instruction just as you would in the classroom.*

The majority of your clinical time will be spent learning to care for patients. Your instructor is usually responsible for your activities in the patient unit, and you must keep him or her informed of any changes in your patient's condition. Your instructor will frequently ask you questions about your patient's disease, treatments, procedures, family situation, and so forth. This is really an oral quiz. You should be prepared to answer these questions at any time.

Meal and break times are assigned by your instructor or the nurse in charge of the unit. Assignments are made to ensure that adequate nursing personnel are

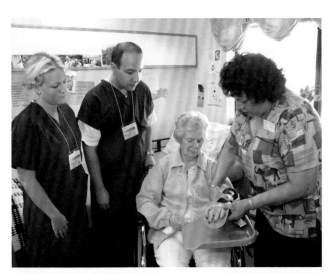

FIGURE 1-3. ● Clinical experience gives you a chance to practice what you learned in the classroom and in the nursing lab.

Critical Thinking
E X E R C I S E

You have a dilemma. You are assigned to go to lunch at 11:45 am. Your patient is scheduled to go to the operating room at 12:15 pm. The patient and his family are very apprehensive about the outcome of the surgery. Not knowing the time you are assigned to go to lunch, they ask if you can stay with them until it is time to go. Using Characteristics of Critical Thinkers in Box 1-2, write down some of your ideas on how you might be able to go to lunch and also stay with the patient until he goes to the operating room.

always present on the patient unit. It's easy to understand why it's important to plan your activities so that you can leave the unit on time and return on time.

Your clinical day may conclude with a postconference. A variety of activities usually occur during postconference. Students may present preassigned reports to the class, the instructor may discuss the care of a particular patient, a guest speaker may present a topic of special interest, or new equipment or procedures may be demonstrated. Note taking is important. You are responsible for learning the material presented during your clinical day, just as you are for learning the material presented during a classroom lecture.

Attendance during your clinical assignments is crucial to developing nursing skills. Your classmates and the nursing staff depend on you. Being late is disruptive to the care of the patient, to your own organization, to the nursing staff, to your classmates, and to your instructor. Your absence requires that your assignment be given to someone else, often at the last minute. Being on time is an essential personal trait of a nurse.

There are occasions when something unavoidable happens and you must be late or absent. Your instructor will tell you how to handle these situations. You'll be expected to comply with your program regulations.

SUMMARY

You are beginning a journey that will sometimes be fun, often be difficult, and always be challenging. You will probably study more, take more exams, and write more care plans than you ever thought possible. But in the end, your willingness to learn the required knowledge and skills along with new ways of thinking and doing will lead to your goal of becoming a licensed practical or vocational nurse and a career that is personally rewarding.

APPLY
Critical Thinking Skills

1. In the opening story at the beginning of this chapter, Mrs. Henderson said, "We're all in this together to become nurses." What do you think she meant by saying this?

2. What do you think will be the most difficult adjustment you will have to make to attend school? What do you think you will do to make the adjustment?

3. Construct a schedule similar to the one in Table 1-1 and follow it closely for 1 week. What changes do you think you should make in your schedule and why?

4. Compare your note-taking system with those of some of your classmates. Look for ideas that will help you with your notes.

5. Discuss study techniques with other students in your class. Which techniques might you be able to use that you had not thought of before?

6. What adjustments could you make in your study schedule to compensate for a short-term personal or family emergency?

7. What are the policies and procedures for using your library facilities, and how can you get assistance in finding information in your library?

8. Share techniques that you and your classmates use to handle anxiety associated with taking exams.

9. Use a search engine and the key words "nursing humor" to add some humor to your tired student life.

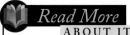
Read More
ABOUT IT

Alfaro-LeFevre R: Critical Thinking, Clinical Reasoning, and Clinical Judgment, 5th ed. Philadelphia, PA: Elsevier, 2013.

Connor Marcia L: Learn More Now: 10 Simple Steps to Learning Better, Smarter, and Faster. Hoboken, NJ: John Wiley & Sons, 2004.

Dunham KS: How to Survive and Maybe Even Love Nursing School: A Guide for Students by Students, 3rd ed. Philadelphia, PA: FA Davis, 2008.

Kesselman-Turkel J, Peterson F: Note Taking Made Easy. Madison, WI: University of Wisconsin Press, 2003.

Kesselman-Turkel J, Peterson F: Secrets to Writing Great Papers. Madison, WI: University of Wisconsin Press, 2003.

Kesselman-Turkel J, Peterson F: Study Smarts: How to Learn More in Less Time. Madison, WI: University of Wisconsin Press, 2004.

Kesselman-Turkel J, Peterson F: Test Taking Strategies. Madison, WI: University of Wisconsin Press, 2004.

Nugent PM, Vitale BA: Test Success: Test-Taking Techniques for Beginning Nursing Students, 6th ed. Philadelphia, PA: FA Davis, 2012.

Paul K: Study Smarter, Not Harder, 3rd ed. Bellingham, WA: Self Counsel Press, 2009.

Pax-PN Secret Study Guide: Nursing Test Review for the NLN Pre-Admission Examination (PAX), 1st ed. Beaumont, TX: Mometrix Media LLC, 2013.

Schuster PM: Concept Mapping: A Critical Thinking Approach to Care Planning, 3rd ed. Philadelphia, PA: FA Davis, 2012.

The Student Nurse as a Person

CHAPTER CONTENTS

LEARNING OBJECTIVES

When you complete this chapter, you will be able to:

1. Name the five levels of human needs described by Maslow.

2. Identify at least six factors that should enhance your personal health.

3. Describe several personal characteristics that contribute to maintaining good mental and emotional health.

4. Explain the role of socializing and recreation in developing positive physical and mental health.

5. Describe your personal values and beliefs related to health.

6. Listen respectfully to the views and opinions of others.

7. Recognize your own physical and mental limits and live within those boundaries.

LEARNING OBJECTIVES *continued*

8. Use a systematic plan to solve problems.

9. Use your understanding of workplace competencies and foundational skills in planning your career.

10. Develop and maintain a career portfolio.

Linda, a licensed vocational nurse working nights in a long-term care facility, was summoned to her patient's room by the blinking light over the room door. The corridors were silent. She stepped into the room, which was lighted by the glow of a small lamp. Her patient, Mrs. Mulrooney, was awake. "Can I help you?" Linda asked.

Mrs. Mulrooney nodded. "I'd like a glass of water," she said.

Linda poured a fresh glass and put it to Mrs. Mulrooney's lips. She noticed that the woman was trembling. "Is something wrong?" Linda asked.

Mrs. Mulrooney looked to the side of her bed. "The bed rails are broken," she whispered.

Linda smiled. "No, Mrs. Mulrooney. They were repaired just today. Remember?"

The woman looked puzzled. "Was that today?"

Linda put the glass on the nightstand. "Yes," she said. "You don't have to worry." She tucked the blanket under her patient's chin.

The woman smiled and said she felt safer with the bed rails up. She then touched the nurse's hand. "You make me feel so good," she said.

Linda returned the gesture with a gentle touch. "I'm glad," she said. "You're very important to me."

Mrs. Mulrooney beamed. "I am?" she asked. Linda stroked her patient's forehead. "Of course you are. You're important to all of us."

For a moment Mrs. Mulrooney said nothing. She was thinking. Then, she smiled. "I guess I am," she said proudly. "I should be. I lived a good life. I have two wonderful children and five grandchildren…."

Linda stepped to the door as the woman's eyes began to close in sleep.

"I think I did with my life what I was supposed to," Mrs. Mulrooney said.

"I think so, too," Linda whispered into the room. Mrs. Mulrooney was asleep. Her face was calm. She was smiling.

HUMAN NEEDS

All people have needs. Because these needs are necessary for survival and health, they are called basic human needs. The story presented above illustrates five categories of human needs identified by Dr. Abraham Maslow, an authority in the field of psychology. They are as follows:

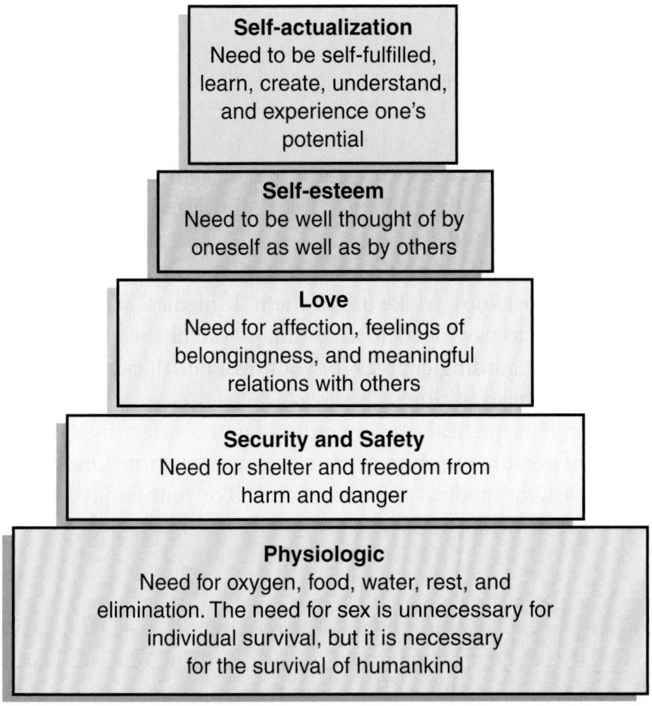

Self-actualization
Need to be self-fulfilled,
learn, create, understand,
and experience one's
potential

Self-esteem
Need to be well thought of by
oneself as well as by others

Love
Need for affection, feelings of
belongingness, and meaningful
relations with others

Security and Safety
Need for shelter and freedom from
harm and danger

Physiologic
Need for oxygen, food, water, rest, and
elimination. The need for sex is unnecessary for
individual survival, but it is necessary
for the survival of humankind

FIGURE 2-1. ● Maslow's five levels of human needs.

1. Physiologic ("I'd like a glass of water.")
2. Safety and security ("I feel safer with the bed rails up.")
3. Love and belonging ("You make me feel so good.")
4. Self-esteem and recognition ("You're very important…")
5. Fulfillment ("I think I did with my life what I was supposed to.")

According to Maslow, these five categories of needs can be ordered from simple to complex. Figure 2-1 illustrates Maslow's five levels of human needs. Physical survival and safety come before love and belonging, followed by the need for self-esteem and for self-actualization or self-fulfillment.

✔ *Meeting basic human needs is necessary for survival.*

Working with others requires understanding their needs. It also requires understanding your own needs. Unless your needs are recognized and satisfied, it's difficult to give full attention to the needs of others. Ask yourself what your needs are in each of Maslow's five levels. Are enough of your personal needs being met to allow you to be concerned about the needs of others?

✔ *Self-actualization (knowing yourself) is critical to being able to care for others.*

The more you work with people, the more opportunity you will have to learn about yourself. The opportunity begins now. Your self-actualization will grow if you know what your needs are and what you must do to satisfy them.

YOUR PHYSICAL HEALTH AND WELL-BEING

Physical health is the absence of disease, pain, or abnormal conditions. It is in a constant state of change as the body adapts to conditions and events affecting it. Good physical health is important for anyone working in health care. Good health makes it easier for you to perform your duties. Being healthy is an example you should try to set for your patients. To be healthy, you have to pay attention to your body as though you were your own patient.

✔ *You are a role model for your patients.*

When you begin caring for patients, a question you often will ask them will be, "How are you feeling today?" The answers your patients supply will help you develop a plan of care for them.

It is not necessary to ask yourself this question. You already know the answer. But you do have to respond to what your body tells you. Waiting for a problem to develop is not the best way to ensure good health—preventing problems, whenever possible, is. Health problems can be minimized through regular physical examinations and dental checkups.

Your program may offer health-related services to its students that include examinations and checkups. Make use of them. If medical services are provided, you will be expected to pay for them according to established policies. Whenever you have questions regarding charges for your own health care, don't be reluctant to ask about them ahead of time.

If charges for your medical care are reduced as a courtesy by a treating physician, it's a sign of good manners to express your appreciation. On the other hand, it's improper to ask for medical advice for yourself or your family from the physicians you work with while on duty.

Diet

"You are what you eat" is more than a clever saying; it's true. Your daily performance is directly affected by what you eat or don't eat. You will learn the fundamentals of diet and nutrition. The consequences of poor eating habits versus balanced nutrition are a matter of scientific record. Your own experience tells you that heavy meals produce drowsiness, hunger disrupts concentration, too much caffeine causes jitters, alcohol impairs judgment, and too many calories lead to excess weight.

Nurses and others whose work is demanding, often intense, and sometimes awkwardly scheduled may be open to breaking the rules of good nutrition. Students may also adjust their eating habits to meet the daily requirements of classes, study time, and their personal life, even though both their mental and physical activities demand peak performance. As a student, you will benefit from good eating habits.

✔ *Maintain good eating habits regardless of your school or work schedule.*

Start each day with a balanced breakfast. Eat small, balanced, nourishing meals to maintain energy and stamina through the rest of the day. Avoid snacks with high sugar content. They produce unstable blood sugar levels while adding calories. Whatever your weight, calories that don't help you to study, keep you alert, or ward off exhaustion have no place in your diet. Learn your ideal weight and maintain it. A nurse who is overweight will have difficulty advising patients to diet. If you have to diet, avoid crash diets and diets that exclude variety.

✔ *Physical activity and a healthy diet promote good health and reduce the risk of chronic diseases.*

Every 5 years since 1980, the U.S. Department of Agriculture (USDA) and the U.S. Department of Health and Human Services (HHS) have jointly published *Dietary Guidelines for Americans*. The 2015 Dietary Guidelines for Americans will be released in the fall of 2015. The 2010 Dietary Guidelines for Americans recommend that for good health and optimal functionality, people should consume a diet that is energy balanced and nutrient dense. Specific recommendations include reducing obesity and increasing physical activity; increasing to a more plant-, dairy-, and seafood-based diet with moderate amounts of lean meat, poultry, and eggs; and reducing the intake of sugars, solid fats, and refined grains. Use the Dietary Guidelines to learn more about recommended nutritional practices for yourself, your family, and your patients.

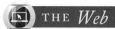

THE *Web*

The 2015 Dietary Guidelines for Americans is available at http://www.health.gov/dietaryguidelines

The 2008 Physical Activity Guidelines for Americans, published by the U.S. Department of HHS, provides science-based guidance to help Americans aged 6 and older improve their health through appropriate physical activity. This same agency issued a midcourse report in 2012 that includes strategies to increase physical activity among youth ages 3 to 17. There is strong evidence that physical exercise lowers the risk of early death, high blood pressure, type 2 diabetes, depression, falls, and a host of other chronic illnesses.

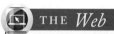

THE *Web*

The *Physical Activity Guidelines* for Americans can be accessed at the U.S. Department of Health and Human Services Web site http://www.health.gov/paguidelines

Figure 2-2 includes a sample moderate aerobic activity schedule for an adult between the ages of 18 and 64 years. Other moderate aerobic activities include water aerobics and riding a bike. Moderate muscle strengthening activities include lifting weights, yoga, and doing exercises that use your body weight for resistance. The important thing is to find either a moderate or vigorous physical exercise program that you enjoy and stick to it.

Following the USDA and the HHS recommendations for diet and exercise and using good common sense will help provide the energy you need to study and concentrate, work and play, and maintain good physical health.

Rest and Exercise

Studying and clinical experience may create a double drain on your energy because of the demand for both mental and physical activity. Having to

	Monday	Tuesday	Wednesday	Thursday	Friday	Saturday	Sunday	Physical Activity TOTAL
Example 1	30 minutes of brisk walking	30 minutes of brisk walking	Resistance band exercises	30 minutes of brisk walking	30 minutes of brisk walking	Resistance band exercises	30 minutes of brisk walking	150 minutes moderate-intensity aerobic activity **AND** **2 days muscle strengthening**
Example 2	30 minutes of brisk walking	60 minutes of playing softball	30 minutes of brisk walking	30 minutes of mowing the lawn		Heavy gardening	Heavy gardening	150 minutes moderate-intensity aerobic activity **AND** **2 days muscle strengthening**

FIGURE 2-2. ● Sample moderate aerobic activity routines. Adults need at least 2 hours and 30 minutes of moderate-intensity aerobic activity and 2 days of muscle strengthening activity each week. (U.S. Department of HHS.)

concentrate while keeping up with a busy schedule may make you more tired than usual. You may require more rest. Watch for signs of fatigue, indifference, sluggishness, personality changes, or a drab physical appearance, such as sallow complexion, breaking nails and hair, and a loss of skin turgor and color. If you notice these symptoms, take immediate measures to prevent the situation from growing worse (Fig. 2-3).

✔ *You cannot catch up on missed sleep.*

Mental alertness and physical endurance are qualities you must have as a student and throughout your career. They depend in large measure on how well you rest. You can't "save up" on sleep. The amount of sleep needed varies with the individual, so only you will know if you're getting enough. About 7 to 8 hours a night is average, although some people manage on less and others need more. Experiment to learn your own limits, and then stay within them to maintain a consistent level of energy.

Restful deep sleep is better than tense light sleep. How well you slept is indicated by how rested you feel after you've been up for a short time in the morning. How one prepares for sleep is a personal practice, but, in general, to ensure quality sleep, relax before going to bed, avoid eating or drinking before retiring, sleep in a comfortable bed, and adjust the room temperature and ventilation.

✔ *Relax in a quiet place a few minutes during the day.*

To increase your endurance during the day, take scheduled rest breaks. It's not necessary to nap, but if you can, let your body and mind enjoy a few moments of peace by reducing or eliminating physical and mental activity.

A scheduled program of specific exercise also helps to keep the body working efficiently. Even though your work may be physically demanding, if parts of your body are neglected, the effect on them is the same as having no exercise at all. Walking, swimming, aerobic workouts, jogging, and bicycling are exercises that use a full range of body activity. To help keep your energy levels high, your body tone good, and your weight under control, engage in a sport or exercise that matches or slightly exceeds your ability. You may find it helpful to join a group of other students or friends in scheduled exercise sessions two or three times a week.

✔ *Physical exercise will energize your tired brain and body.*

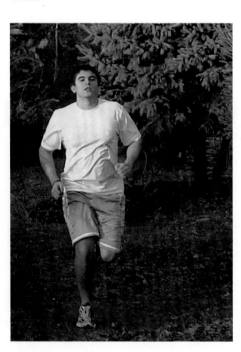

FIGURE 2-3. ● Regular exercise promotes physical and mental well-being.

Oral Hygiene and Dental Health

You will be working closely with patients, staff members, and others who will appreciate the attention you give to keeping your teeth clean and your breath fresh. A pleasant smile can be an asset.

Regular dental checkups will uncover problems such as cavities, decay, and gum disease; daily brushing and periodic freshening will help to ensure a clean, healthy mouth. Consider seeing a dentist or orthodontist if cosmetic treatment is indicated for dentition problems (poor bite), particularly if they affect your self-confidence or the image you'd like to project.

Personal Hygiene

Cleanliness in health services begins with personal hygiene. It affects your image and may affect your susceptibility to infection and disease. Your personal care must reflect the higher overall standards expected from people who work in health care.

Basic personal care includes clean skin, clean, neatly combed or brushed hair, and the absence of body odor. Hands and nails must be clean. If your program (and later your employer) has policies about the use of makeup and body fragrances, length of nails, use of nail polish, and types of hairstyles, follow them. Body fragrances, scented deodorants, and hair sprays may create discomfort in patients and can aggravate allergies. If the decision on grooming aids is up to you, a moderate approach is best. If you're unsure, ask for advice from someone whose opinion you respect.

Clothing and Uniforms

Your uniform is a symbol of your vocation. It is often the first thing people notice, especially patients, who identify it with their stay in a hospital or health care facility. It makes a statement about you, what you stand for, and your authority. It should be worn only at work.

✔ *First impressions are often lasting impressions.*

Maintain a positive impression by wearing uniforms and other clothing that are clean, pressed, and fresh. Shoes are also a part of your uniform and should be clean and in good repair. They should be comfortable and of a style that is consistent with your work and image.

Pins, name tags, and other devices that identify you, your institution, or your affiliations should be worn in accordance with policies set forth by your employer, your state, or the associations they represent.

Posture

How you stand, sit, walk, and carry your body is a matter of habit by now. If your habits are good, there's no need to change them. On the other hand, if your posture is not good, changing it usually improves your appearance, performance, and energy level.

The key to basic good posture is to hold your body straight. When standing, keep your back straight and your head up. Walk with your shoulders back and your head erect. When sitting, keep your back straight and both feet on the floor. Be relaxed in your posture, not rigid. Keeping muscles tense will tire you quickly.

✔ *Your posture says a lot about how you feel about yourself.*

Body language, which is how you hold and carry yourself, can reflect how you feel physically, some of what you feel about yourself, and some of what you feel about others.

For example, standing straight expresses self-confidence. Slouching reduces your authority. Talking to someone with your arms folded tightly across your chest puts people off. Facing them directly in a straightforward, relaxed manner encourages a positive response.

Smoking

People who smoke give many excuses for their habit, but nobody can claim that it's good for health. The public is keenly aware of the negative effects of smoking. Studies clearly show that some heart disease, lung cancer, chronic obstructive pulmonary disease, and other ailments can be directly linked to smoking. You will learn more about the health dangers associated with smoking as your knowledge about health increases. You will see patients whose only reason for being ill is related to smoking; some of them, tragically, are terminally ill. Others will have illnesses that smoking complicates by making manageable conditions worse and marginal sickness serious. In the air or on one's clothes, smoke is an irritant. For a patient whose well-being depends on optimum conditions, the smell of smoke, whether firsthand or secondhand, is contraindicated.

There is another side to the smoking question for you as a student nurse. As a highly visible member of the health professions, your example to others can affect how they view their own smoking. A health practitioner who smokes gives unspoken approval to the habit.

If you smoke, you have an obligation not to do so when or where it will affect others in any way. For your good health and the health and comfort of those around you, look closely at your excuses for smoking and its consequences. You will find plenty of reasons to quit. Tobacco Free Nurses is an organization funded by the Robert Wood Johnson Foundation and is the first national program focused on helping nurses to stop smoking. Its Web site provides free resources and support that have helped tens of thousands of people quit smoking.

Chemical Dependence

The use and abuse of substances such as alcohol, narcotics, barbiturates, sedatives, tranquilizers, depressants, inhalants, hallucinogens, and cannabis can lead to serious problems that affect people from every walk of life. For some, addiction (uncontrollable, compulsive dependence) and habituation (psychological and emotional dependence without addiction) occur quickly, and trying something "just this once" may lead to untold misery and unhappiness.

Nearly every day, we read or hear about the devastating effects of substance abuse. The drunk driver killing an innocent person, the teenager dying from an overdose, the apparently successful husband (wife, mother, father, sister, brother) committing suicide because of an addiction, and the person being murdered for a few dollars to buy drugs are all tragedies indicative of the seriousness of substance abuse.

The use and abuse of these substances can lead to the loss of family, job, and self-respect. Drug-related convictions can prevent a person from receiving federal student financial aid, from joining the armed services, from holding public office, and from holding a number of good jobs.

✔ *The abuse of alcohol and drugs can result in loss of your nursing license.*

The illegal use or possession of controlled substances can also be cause for denying, suspending, or revoking a nursing license. Your school and the clinical facilities with which you affiliate have policies on drug use.

The firsthand knowledge of the effects of drug and alcohol abuse that you gain through your program should be a constant reminder to you to protect your health and career. Others who are not so fortunate may approach you because of your access to drugs in a hospital or institution. Make it very clear to them that you don't use, approve of, or supply or administer any drugs for any reason unless prescribed by a physician for your patients.

There is a high rate of drug and alcohol abuse among nurses. This dependence is doubly tragic because it affects not only their own lives, families, and careers but also the lives of their patients.

Whatever your personal beliefs and feelings about the use of alcohol and drugs, there is never justification for using these substances at work or for abusing them at any other time. Your education and the experiences you will have will reveal the disastrous effects of drug and alcohol abuse on people's lives and health. The likelihood of serious disciplinary action in your program or by an employer in the future (many use random drug screenings) is ample reason for you to avoid their use and abuse.

As a nurse, you have a twofold relationship with drug and alcohol use. You must be very cautious of substance use in your own life, and you must also empathize with your patients who have a problem with substance abuse.

Almost all State Boards of Nursing have a rehabilitative program for nurses whose practice is impaired because of drug or alcohol addiction. These programs are designed to prevent the revocation of the nursing license by designing and monitoring treatment programs. Nurses who don't comply with the voluntary program are subject to more severe disciplinary action, including the loss of their nursing license. Your local telephone directories and your State Board of Nursing can provide the names and telephone numbers of agencies that work with people who suffer from various addictions.

The National Institute on Drug Abuse (NIDA) is a government agency that provides information on abuse and addiction for medical and health professionals, students and young people, and parents and teachers in both English and Spanish. Its Web site includes a description of many abused drugs, their street names, and the effects of these drugs on the body. The NIDA is a reliable source for information and teaching materials related to addiction.

Personal Illness

The same standards of care and protection you use when working with patients with transmissible illness apply to you when you're ill. The difference is that, although you may be informed about your patients' health, they know nothing of yours.

✔ *Attending classes or going to your clinical assignments when you are sick is unfair to classmates and patients.*

It is your obligation to avoid contaminating the clinical environment when you have any illness that could harm or affect a patient's health or well-being. This rule applies to transmissible diseases, from common colds to serious infections, to conditions that have a negative psychological effect, such as coughs, rashes, and other symptoms of disease.

Your program or clinical facility policies may be explicit on matters of personal illness. If not, your good judgment will tell you when to avoid exposing coworkers and patients to your illness. Your awareness of the state of your health is your best guide to protecting yourself and others.

Sexually Transmitted Infections

More than 110 million Americans have sexually transmitted infections (STIs). These infections were previously known as sexually transmitted diseases or venereal diseases. Syphilis, gonorrhea, chlamydia, acquired immunodeficiency

✔ *The first case of AIDS in the United States was identified in 1981.*

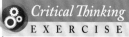

Critical Thinking
E X E R C I S E

One of your very close friends who knows you are in nursing school calls and says he thinks he might have AIDS. He says he doesn't know what to do or whom to trust. He wants to meet you after school tomorrow because he needs to talk to someone. You know you will be there for your friend, but you realize how little you really know about AIDS. Use appropriate Characteristics of Critical Thinkers in Box 1-2 on pages 18–19 to develop your responses to these questions.

✔ *The best way to control STIs is through education.*

syndrome (AIDS), herpes, human papillomavirus, trichomoniasis, and hepatitis B are just a few of the more common STIs. Complications can be serious and may lead to death. Those that aren't directly life-threatening can lead to infections and illnesses that are. Many STIs cause sterility, chronic pelvic pain, and poor pregnancy outcomes.

The U.S. Centers for Disease Control and Prevention estimates that an additional 20 million Americans become newly infected with one or more STIs each year. In addition to the human cost of these diseases, the financial cost of treating these new cases plus those that have become chronic (lasting over a long period of time) is estimated to be more than $16 billion annually.

The emergence of AIDS in the United States in 1981 greatly increased public awareness of STIs. However, there is still a lot of misinformation and fear about STIs. Providing health information to others is a service performed by nurses. As a student nurse, you may be asked questions about STIs. When providing information, be sure you give accurate answers and suggest reliable sources for counseling and treatment.

The extent of STIs in the United States is enormous, as shown by the following approximate figures from the U.S. Centers for Disease Control:

- Nearly 20 million new cases of STIs occur each year.
- Approximately 50,000 new cases of human immunodeficiency virus infections are reported each year.
- Nearly 3 million additional people acquire chlamydia each year.
- 1 in 4 sexually active Americans teenagers is infected with herpes simplex virus type 2.
- 14 million new cases of human papillomavirus are reported each year.

Although some STIs can be transmitted by blood transfusions and other means, transmission is generally associated with human sexuality, a subject that many find difficult to discuss. Your willingness to be open, frank, and honest about STIs is important to patients and others who seek information because education is the best method to control these diseases. As a student nurse, what you have to say is valuable.

You should not make judgments that will keep information about STIs from those who need it. STIs can be acquired by anyone who is sexually active, and there are no social, economic, racial, or other barriers. Because STIs always involve two or more people, the sex partners of anyone with an STI should be informed so they can seek medical attention. Because reinfection of a partner is likely if only one is treated, all partners must get treatment to contain the chain of infection.

Learn accurate, scientific information about what causes STIs, what their incubation periods are, how they are transmitted, how to identify them, and what to do to prevent and treat them. Armed with this information, you can do much to promote good health for yourself and others. For further information on STIs, refer to the Centers for Disease Control and Prevention's Web site (http://www.cdc.gov/std/) and your nursing textbooks.

YOUR EMOTIONAL HEALTH

Mentally and emotionally healthy people are able to effectively cope with the pressures and stresses that are a part of everyday life. It is essential that those who are aspiring to become nurses be mentally and emotionally healthy so they can provide the compassionate nursing care that patients expect to receive.

As a nurse, you will be confronted almost daily not only with personal pressures and stresses but also with those of your patients. Nurses who are focused entirely on their own problems and concerns will not be able to recognize the needs of the patient. Everyone experiences upsets in life. It's not the degree of upset but how it is handled that determines the state of one's mental health.

✔ *Good mental and emotional health is an essential trait of a nurse.*

Many people have personality quirks that are managed appropriately and aren't considered mental disorders. However, as many as 1 in 10 Americans needs professional help for mental disorders, whether they seek it or not. The degree of your own mental health will be evident in how you interact with others. It will influence your success in life and work.

Mentally healthy students see a need to act and then act responsibly. They will act independently if the duty is clearly theirs or willingly under the direction of others when asked. If uncertain, they are willing to ask questions and request help when needed. They deal with problems as the problems are, not as they wish the problems were. When confronted by an unfamiliar task, they know not to attempt it without consulting their instructor or a supervisor.

✔ *Work to develop the traits of a mentally and emotionally healthy person.*

Mentally healthy students also have the ability to accept constructive criticism. Students who use correction and comment to improve themselves and their work don't personalize the criticism but recognize it as a part of the education they have paid for and expect.

Mentally healthy students keep an open, analytical mind. They see the positive side in situations and people that others may not see and work to promote it. They are open, caring, and friendly, and they respect their peers, supervisors, and other members of their health and administrative team.

Because nurses have the responsibility to care for people whose attention is fully on themselves and the effects of their illness, they must continually work to maintain their own mental health. Some techniques for maintaining good mental health are to understand yourself; to assess your personality; to examine your personal values, beliefs, and prejudices; and to learn to cope effectively with stress.

✔ *If you feel you cannot cope, seek professional help.*

Understanding Yourself

One gains or develops maturity and good mental health through self-understanding. A willingness to look at yourself and your life objectively (self-evaluation) and to squarely face what you find will influence how well you succeed.

All of life's experiences, whether good or bad, affect how you see yourself and provide an opportunity for self-understanding and self-improvement. For example, adapting to divorce can lead to better self-understanding, just as adjusting to being married can. Raising a child alone can provide valuable lessons for living, just as sharing the responsibility with a spouse can. When you evaluate yourself, look at every side and use what you see to build yourself up, rather than tear yourself down.

✔ *You will need to learn to leave your personal problems in the parking lot when you go to work.*

Without self-understanding, you can't reasonably expect to understand others and therefore to help them. You aren't expected to be free of faults—nobody is. But your obligation as a nurse is to care for others. To do that, you have to make the effort to limit your self-concerns during your workday so that they don't prevent you from attending to the needs of your patients.

Developing self-awareness is a lifelong process that produces rewards from the beginning. How deeply you probe is a matter for you to decide. To start, ask yourself how well you really know yourself. Does what you know agree with how others see you? Are you willing to make changes?

Personality

Personality is the collection of behaviors and attitudes that sets one person apart from everyone else. You were not born with the personality you have today. You developed it gradually, consciously, and unconsciously, as a way of adapting to the circumstances of your life and environment. Personality is not character. Character relates to the conscious, consistent way one reacts to ethical and moral customs and the standards of society.

It is easier to change personality traits than character traits, but neither is altogether easy. It's your personality that interacts with others. Your personality is where to look for traits that need to be refined, changed, or eliminated.

As a nurse, how well you interact with others is important. The personal nature of your work requires you to do more than just get along. You also must inspire positive relationships. Supervisors will expect you to work with minimum supervision. Peers and associates will expect you to do your share of what needs to be done. Your patients will expect you to see to their physical and emotional needs without being asked. To relate positively takes conscious effort, especially in a health care setting, where there is a broad mix of age, culture, and background. Your personality will not work on "automatic pilot" with such diverse populations. You have to be willing to adapt as new situations occur.

✔ *Identify one or two personality traits that you would like to work on changing.*

It takes time to change personality traits, especially deep-seated ones, but they can be changed if you know what they are. Study yourself as though you were someone else. Make notes of traits you think are positive and those you think detract from a healthy personality. Look among the people you respect for traits that make them stand out and use them as models. You don't have to adopt them entirely; just use the parts that suit you.

Get input about how others see you from people whose opinions you respect. Make it clear how important their insight is and that you're not looking for flattery. Be willing to accept what they tell you whether you agree with it or not. Use what you learn to change the parts of your personality that would hinder you from becoming a better person and a better nurse.

Personal Values and Beliefs

As individuals we behave independently, but much of our behavior is a result of learned social customs. These learned social customs taken as a whole provide a simple definition of culture. Culture is the sum of values, ideas, customs, attitudes, roles, behaviors, and arts of given groups of people during specified periods. It is the pattern of overall behavior that is passed from generation to generation.

✔ *Nurses must recognize that people have customs and values that are different from their own.*

Within a culture, various groups share a religion, race, common ancestry, or other specific similarities. These groups are subcultures and are termed ethnic groups. An example of a cultural custom is the institution of marriage. The way a given group of people within a culture celebrates weddings is an ethnic difference. For example, a traditional Western European wedding dress is white, and a traditional Chinese wedding dress is red. Many people spend much of their lives in the comfort of their own ethnic or cultural heritage, with people who share their similarities. However, as a nurse, you will come into contact with people from widely differing backgrounds.

✔ *Nurses must accept and even encourage people who are seeking health care to practice their cultural and religious beliefs.*

Because of the nature of nursing, nurses care for a full range of people from cultures and ethnic groups different from their own. How you handle patient differences will be a measure of your compassion, understanding, and maturity. It will also depend on your willingness to accept individual differences regardless of your personal opinion.

The foundation of your service to your patients is the acknowledgment that their basic needs are the same as everyone else's, including your own. Your patients experience hunger, but their choices in food may differ from yours. They need clothing, but the styles they wear may not be found in your wardrobe. They need shelter, although they may not be your neighbors. They need human kindness, but they may be strangers to you. Everything about your patients may be a "world" away from your own, but when all their cultural and ethnic differences are removed, you are their nurse, they are your patients, and you live in the same world.

To be an effective nurse, it's necessary to examine yourself to see if you have any prejudices that might compromise how much and what kind of care you provide to those in need.

Prejudice

The term *prejudice* describes the attitude of people who reject another person or ethnic group's differences in favor of their own group's values. Prejudice is not confined to race or culture, for it can also be directed at people of a certain gender or social class or with a certain sexual preference. Prejudiced people believe that their beliefs and values are right and that those who don't hold the same values or beliefs are inferior or wrong.

✔ *A nurse cannot provide or withhold care based on any prejudice.*

Prejudice is not something one is born with but a behavior learned from others usually early in life. It comes easily because it takes no work or effort. It only needs one's willingness to go along with someone else's negative beliefs about individuals or groups of people. The result is widely accepted misinformation and misunderstanding about an ethnic group's values, customs, and behaviors.

To provide effective nursing care, a nurse must work to consciously value the differences inherent in different cultures and ethnic groups. Learning about other groups and incorporating cultural sensitivity in your nursing practice will enhance communication with your patients. When your patient trusts you to respect their beliefs and values, the resulting plan of treatment will be culturally acceptable to the patient, as well as medically sound. Learning to work with and care for people from many different backgrounds and beliefs requires special skills and is the topic of Chapter 9.

✔ *Learning about others provides us with an opportunity to know more about our world.*

Stress

Stress is a condition of tension between two opposite forces. The forces can be physical, psychological, economic, or social, alone or in combination. A simple yet descriptive example of physical stress is a hot-air balloon tied to the ground by a rope. The balloon wants to rise. The rope wants to hold it down. Tension created by the opposition between the force to rise and the force holding the balloon down makes the rope stretch. If a rope is stretched too far, it will break.

Because so many situations in life are so similar to this analogy, stress has become a word in everyone's vocabulary. A child experiences stress when he or she wants to go outside but is stopped by a parent because the weather is wet and cold. A student facing an important exam experiences stress. A stomach that is overfilled with a holiday meal produces stress. A couple having an argument undergoes stress.

Not all stress is harmful. Limited stress before an exam can raise energy levels, for example. But too much stress may result in anxiety, physical illness, psychological distress, fatigue, and other emotional and physical responses. Stress requires a response. The nature of the response—how one copes—determines whether the stress is relieved or worsened.

✔ *Stress and tension can have serious physical effects.*

Complete the self-assessment test "What Is Your Stress Index?" on pages 50–51. Note that the results of this test will vary depending on your frame of mind at the time you take the test. If you take the test several times over a period of weeks and your score indicates that you're vulnerable to stress, you might consider professional counseling. Counselors can often help you learn to make changes in your life that will reduce your level of stress.

✔ *Share relaxation tips with a friend.*

The connection between the mind and body is underscored by stress. A stressful situation always produces a reaction in the body. If the reaction is too great, the odds increase that something will hurt or break. Tension headaches and some ulcers are related to stress. Nervousness and anxiety result from stress. It's to anyone's advantage to learn to control stress.

✔ *Find a favorite stress relaxation technique and use it as often as necessary.*

Stress that gets out of hand can be harmful. When anxiety or other stress-related conditions begin to dominate your life and your efforts to manage stress by yourself aren't working, look to others for help. Talking to a friend may be enough. A chat with your instructor may help. Professional counseling is always a good idea when the stress in one's life exceeds the ability to cope.

ASSESS YOURSELF   What Is Your Stress Index?

Stress can be difficult to understand. The emotional chaos it causes can make our daily lives miserable. It can also decrease our physical health, sometimes drastically. Strangely, we are not always aware that we are under stress. The habits, attitudes, and signs that can alert us to problems may be hard to recognize because they have become so familiar.

How high is your stress index? Find out by scoring your answers to the questions below.

Do you frequently.

	Yes	No
Neglect your diet?		
Try to do everything yourself?		
Blow up easily?		
Seek unrealistic goals?		
Fail to see the humor in situations others find funny?		
Act rude?		
Make a "big deal" of everything?		
Look to other people to make things happen?		
Complain that you are disorganized?		
Avoid people whose ideas are different from your own?		
Keep everything inside?		
Neglect exercise?		
Have few supportive relationships?		
Use sleeping pills and tranquilizers without a doctor's approval?		
Get too little rest?		
Get angry when you are kept waiting?		

	Yes	No
Ignore stress symptoms?		
Put things off until later?		
Think there is only one right way to do something?		
Fail to build relaxation time into your day?		
Gossip?		
Race through the day?		
Spend a lot of time complaining about the past?		
Fail to get a break from noise and crowds?		
Total your score (Score 1 for each "YES," 0 for each "NO.")		

SCORING

1–6 points: There are few hassles in your life. Make sure, though, that you are not trying so hard to avoid problems that you shy away from challenges.

7–13 points: You've got your life in fairly good control. Work on the choices and habits that could still be causing you some unnecessary stress in your life.

14–20 points: You're approaching the danger zone. You may well be suffering stress-related symptoms, and your relationships could be strained. Think carefully about choices you have made and take relaxation breaks every day.

More than 20 points: Emergency! You must stop now, rethink how you are living, change your attitudes, and pay careful attention to diet, exercise, and relaxation.

Adapted with permission from Canadian Mental Health Association, National.

Relaxation

The most effective way to control stress is to release the tension before it gets out of hand. Managing stress, whether your own or your patient's, can be accomplished by a number of techniques combining physical and mental relaxation (Fig. 2-4). In principle, these techniques cause the mind and body to slow down for a brief period or quietly force a change of attention. A progressive relaxation technique, for example, uses a 15- to 30-minute process in which one's attention is focused on every part of the body, one part at a time, while one is consciously thinking and feeling relaxation. In another technique, called guided imagery, the person who wishes to relax uses his or her imagination to think himself/herself into a pleasant situation, such as lying in the warm sun on a sandy beach.

Aromatherapy, massage, humor or music therapy, breathing exercises, qigong, Reiki, Tai Chi, yoga, meditation, jogging, and strenuous physical exercise are just a few techniques that can be used to control and reduce the effects of stress. You can practice stress management and relaxation techniques on your own or in a group. Group sessions are helpful because they let you share an experience with others, which itself reduces tension. Many relaxation techniques are done alone, can be completed in just a few minutes, and should be made a part of your daily routine. A number of good suggestions on relaxation techniques are provided on the American Holistic Nurses Association Web site.

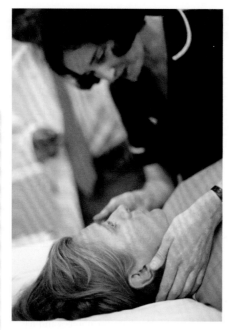

FIGURE 2-4. ● Massage is one way to promote relaxation and manage stress.

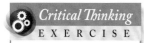

List three situations or events that occurred over the past 6 days that made you feel "stressed out." If you had the opportunity to be in the same situation again, how might using some of the character-istics of critical thinkers change your physical and emotional reaction to the situation? Use appropriate Characteristics of Critical Thinkers in Box 1-2 on pages 18–19 to develop your responses to this situation.

Because the work of a nurse is often mentally, emotionally, and physically demanding, it is important to develop a plan of self-care early in your career. The better you care for yourself and your own needs, the better able you will be to care for others.

Problem Solving

Your physical and mental health can be improved by learning to apply skills that help solve problems. Poor problem-solving skills can contribute to a sense of frustration, low self-esteem, and feelings of inadequacy.

Not knowing exactly what to do in a specific situation is a problem. Problems can be complex, with many parts and many consequences, or simple, with just one answer. As a nurse, you will have your share of each kind of problem. Knowing how to solve them will make you a better adjusted person and will also make you more effective as a nurse.

It is not a good idea to respond to a problem without thinking about it first. Applying the Characteristics of Critical Thinkers that were discussed in Chapter 1 (Box 1-2) will help you as you think about and begin to define a problem.

✔ *Use a system to solve problems.*

Although it may sometimes be faster to act without thinking, you will do better if you use a system to solve all problems to avoid making errors. The first step in solving problems is to make sure you understand the problem. State the problem in your own words as accurately as you can. Once you know what the problem is, determine its cause. There may be more than one reason for the problem. Find as many reasons as you can before attempting a solution. Make sure your information is accurate to avoid acting on hearsay, rumor, or someone else's misinterpretation of facts. If the problem is related to a single individual, it is best to attempt to solve the problem with that person and not involve those who are not part of the problem.

✔ *Keep an open mind when looking for solutions.*

After pinpointing the causes, see whether the problem has more than one solution. If so, study each to find which one will solve the problem with the least negative effect on those involved. Avoid letting your motives or emotions influence the solution.

Once you have a solution that seems to best fit the problem, decide who is best suited to put the solution into action. Be careful not to use automatic solutions that are based on presumption. You may not have all the facts, or you may be seeing the problem or its solution from an inaccurate point of view. You can use your own past experiences to evaluate new problems, but avoid the trap of assuming that the solution that worked in the past will work every time. It may, but if you don't look closely at the problem, you could miss a key difference.

When you must question someone's authority to solve a problem, do so carefully. Give a clear, intelligent statement of the problem and its solution in a way that will keep the issue neutral. Problems can be worsened if the people involved are forced to defend their position or attack yours.

Following is a general guide to problem solving. Use it, but treat every problem as unique and solve each on its own merits.

1. Define the problem in your own terms.
2. State your own objectives realistically.
3. Get as many facts as possible.
4. Get advice from your instructor and others, if necessary.
5. Examine alternative solutions carefully.
6. Give yourself room to change solutions if necessary.
7. Choose the best solution in your judgment.
8. Take responsible action.
9. Evaluate the consequences of your action.
10. Choose another solution if your action did not solve the problem.

To become a good problem solver, you must work at it. Remember these steps and make every effort to use them when faced with a problem you must solve. After a while, when confronted with a problem, you will automatically apply these steps. You will find that you're feeling more confident that the solutions have been the best, given the circumstances and the problem.

✔ To become a good problem solver, you will need to practice.

YOUR CAREER

Just as attention to your physical and emotional well-being will help you attain a healthier and happier life, carefully planning your career will help you have more rewarding work experiences.

Skills for Career Development

You might say that it's too soon to be thinking about the future and career planning. Your goal right now may be to just get through nursing school and pass the licensing examination. However, career developers say that career planning must begin well before graduation. Those who have the most rewarding careers and those who get the jobs they really want are those who have planned ahead—sometimes years in advance.

✔ Now is the time to begin planning your career in nursing.

The opportunities for employment as a new licensed practical or vocational nurse are abundant for those who have the skills that are crucial in the workplace. Although clinical skills are essential, other workplace skills are equally important to potential employers.

Box 2-1 outlines the findings of a U.S. Department of Labor report titled "What Work Requires of Schools." This document identifies characteristics of workers that are considered essential for solid job performance.

Basic skills, thinking skills, and personal qualities are the foundation skills needed by workers in high-performance workplaces such as health care. Being able to learn; to solve problems; to get along with people; and to read, speak, listen, and perform mathematical functions are a few of the essential foundation skills.

✔ Employers are looking for employees who have clinical skills, foundation skills, and workplace competencies.

| BOX 2-1 | Workplace Know-How |

The know-how identified by Secretary's Commission on Achieving Necessary Skills (SCANS) is made up of a three-part foundation and five workplace competencies needed for solid job performance. These are as follows:

FOUNDATION SKILLS

Competent workers in the high-performance workplace need the following:
- **Basic skills**—reading, writing, arithmetic and mathematics, speaking, and listening
- **Thinking skills**—the ability to learn, to reason, to think creatively, to make decisions, and to solve problems
- **Personal qualities**—individual responsibility, self-esteem and self-management, sociability, and integrity

WORKPLACE COMPETENCIES

Effective workers can productively use the following:
- **Resources**—They know how to allocate time, money, materials, space, and staff.
- **Interpersonal skills**—They can work on teams, teach others, serve customers, lead, negotiate, and work well with people from culturally diverse backgrounds.
- **Information**—They can acquire and evaluate data, organize and maintain files, interpret and communicate, and use computers to process information.
- **Systems**—They understand social, organizational, and technologic systems; they can monitor and correct performance; and they can design or improve systems.
- **Technology**—They can select equipment and tools, apply technology to specific tasks, and maintain and troubleshoot equipment.

The full document is available at http://wdr.doleta.gov/SCANS/whatwork/whatwork.pdf

Workplace competencies are equally essential. The workplace competencies listed in Box 2-1 include skills in five distinct areas. If you look closely at the examples included with each of the five competencies, it becomes quite clear that workers need to know and be able to do more than just perform tasks associated with a job.

Workers need to be able to work with people from diverse backgrounds, they need to know how to use resources that are often very expensive, they need to use computers to process information, and they need to use and maintain equipment.

Those who hire practical/vocational nurses say they look for all of these qualities when interviewing potential employees. It's important that now, early in your career, you work every day to improve these skills. Doing so may make the difference between getting, keeping, and losing a job in the future.

Continuing Education

To make sure your skills and knowledge don't become obsolete, it's important to include continuing education as a part of your career development and planning.

Continuing education is the term used to describe planned learning that occurs after a formal certificate or degree program. It includes workshops, seminars, conferences, staff development, journal reading, and some on-the-job training programs. It can also include enrollment in advanced courses at colleges and universities. Detailed information on continuing education is provided in Chapter 16.

Many states have laws that determine the number of hours of continuing education you need each year to renew your nursing license. You may want to focus your attention on a specific area or a specific clinical specialty or you might want to divide your time between several different interests. You should know that a person who has broad skills is usually more valuable to an employer than is one who has very narrow skills. It's not too soon to begin focusing some attention on the area of nursing in which you think you might want to work.

You might also consider enrolling in a full- or part-time degree program at some time in the future. If you decide to do this, you will need to choose a major area of study. Be sure to do some research to be sure that what you want to study will lead to employment opportunities after graduation.

Career Plans

A career plan is a well-thought-out plan that describes where you expect to be and by when. It is certainly subject to change as the employment picture changes, and as you grow and develop as a nurse, but without a plan, your career may never have a clear focus. A career plan will help you manage your own career and will help you develop characteristics identified with employability. If, or more likely when, your employer makes changes that affect you, you will be prepared to make the transition and to move on to the next level in your career.

A career plan should be written and it should describe what you expect or would like to be doing 5 and 10 years from now. Outline what you need to do to achieve those long-term goals and be specific in identifying the time frames in which each step should be completed. List the activities you must complete to reach your goals. Box 2-2 provides an example of a career plan for a student who has been enrolled in a practical nursing program for 2 months.

You should take some time now to outline your own plan. Then, look at your plan every few months. Make changes if you need to, but remember to keep a clear focus on your future as a nurse.

Portfolios

A career portfolio is a collection of documents that showcase your performance and accomplishments over time. It's something that you can hand to a person who is interviewing you for a job or to accreditation agencies to document continuing education. The portfolio can also be submitted as a part of your performance appraisal.

You should begin your nursing career portfolio now because if you wait, you will forget to include information that might make the difference in getting the job you really want. Keeping a portfolio is an ongoing activity and one that should be kept up-to-date.

Portfolios can be loose-leaf binders with plastic sleeves in which you place important information. Portfolios can also be in electronic format using Microsoft Office or a commercial career portfolio development Web site. If your portfolio is on paper, keep a complete copy in a safe place. If your portfolio is electronic, be sure to properly back up your data using a cloud-based storage service or an external hard drive so that if your computer breaks down, you will still be able to retrieve your information. Whatever format you choose, the portfolio should be divided into at least four sections. The first section should include your résumé, letters of reference, certifications, licenses, and any letters of commendation you received from your instructors or from patients. It may be too soon to get letters of reference, but it's certainly not too soon to insert your cardiopulmonary resuscitation certification card or other certifications that were required before you started school.

The second section should contain a list, by date, of all of your continuing education activities. Include the dates you attended, the names of the presenters,

✔ *Participating in continuing education is important to your future as a nurse.*

Critical Thinking EXERCISE

Imagine for a few minutes that you have been working in the same job for 2 years. You love the people you work with, and everyone pitches in and helps everyone else. The unit supervisor just called a team meeting to tell everyone that the facility was sold yesterday and it would be closed within a month. What do you think your first reaction to this news would be? What can you do to be prepared for something like this? Use appropriate Characteristics of Critical Thinkers in Box 1-2 on pages 18–19 to develop your response this situation.

✔ *The portfolio will show prospective employers that you are committed to a career in nursing.*

BOX 2-2   Career Plan for a Student Who Has Been Enrolled in a Practical Nursing Program for 2 Months

LONG-TERM GOALS

- Within 1 year, I expect to graduate from practical nursing school.
- In 2 years, I expect to be working full time as a staff nurse in Greenwoods Retirement and Long-Term Care Center.
- In 4 years, I expect to have my long-term care (LTC) certification and be working full time as a nurse manager at Greenwoods.
- In 7 years, I expect to finish community college and have my RN license.

STEPS TO ACHIEVING MY CAREER GOALS

September 2014

Enroll in PN school.

Join Health Occupations Students of America (HOSA).

Subscribe to *Journal of Practical Nursing*.

Participate in at least one "extra" activity each month (preferably something related to older people and preferably at Greenwoods Retirement and Long-Term Care Center).

August 2015

Graduate.

Take licensing exam (AND PASS!!).

September 2015

Get a job in an LTC facility (preferably at Greenwoods Retirement and Long-Term Care Center).

September 2015 to September 2017

Work as a staff nurse, progress to giving medications and complex treatments, and then become unit manager.

Attend at least one staff development/month.

Attend four conferences related to management in LTC.

Study for the LTC certification test.

Volunteer in the local senior citizen center one evening a week.

July 2017

Apply to Gateway Community College Registered Nurse (RN) program.

September 2017

Start part-time classes at Gateway.

Maybe work part-time at Greenwoods?

Apply to be an NCLEX-PN test question writer.

September 2018

Take the LTC certification test.

Become a nurse manager hopefully at Greenwoods.

June 2021

Finish requirements for RN license.

Assess future at Greenwoods.

Revise career plan.

and a paragraph describing the topic of the activity starting with the most recent first. There will be many opportunities while you're in school to participate in such activities. Keep a record of these in this section of your portfolio.

The third section should contain a list of all of the school- or nursing-related activities in which you're involved. Include the dates, names of the organizations, and a brief paragraph describing your activities. Examples of activities that would be placed in this section include Health Occupations Students of America (HOSA) activities, school committee activities, health-related community events in which you participated, and so forth.

The fourth section of your portfolio should include any miscellaneous information that would be relevant to your career in nursing. Highlighting your ability to speak more than one language could be important to potential employers. Other information that could be included in this section is a record of immunizations and blood test results. You might also include in this section a copy of your long-term career plan. Presenting a neat and comprehensive notebook or computer link to a prospective employer indicates that you're serious about your career. It may be the edge you need to get that great job.

SUMMARY

Being a nurse is a rewarding but demanding career. You must attend to your physical health and well-being every day by paying attention to what you eat and when and to getting sufficient sleep, rest, and relaxation. You must attend to the emotional part of yourself so that the burdens of those you care for do not overwhelm you and cause stress that can devastate your own health and destroy your relationships with others. And you must actively plan your future so that where you end up in your career is where you chose to be. Having a rewarding career requires planning ahead and now is the best time to get started.

APPLY

Critical Thinking Skills

1. In the opening story at the beginning of this chapter, Linda told Mrs. Mulrooney that the bed rails were "repaired just today. Remember?" Suppose Linda didn't know the bed rails were repaired. List other responses to Mrs. Mulrooney that would be comforting and appropriate.

2. List 10 to 15 of your needs and then place them in one of the five appropriate categories of human needs described by Maslow.

3. Think about how you might handle a situation when you know for certain that a classmate is using illegal drugs or is addicted to drugs or alcohol.

4. Describe the personal traits or characteristics that contribute to becoming an effective nurse.

5. What can you do to identify and adjust personal prejudices?

6. What are some effective methods you might be able to use to reduce stress and anxiety?

7. Select a problem related to either school or your personal life, and use the problem-solving techniques presented in this chapter to find one or more solutions. Did this process clarify your thinking?

8. After having read about career development and planning, start putting documents in your portfolio.

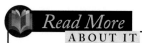

Blonna R: Coping with Stress in a Changing World, 5th ed. Columbus, OH: McGraw-Hill Higher Education, 2011.

Cano X: Resumes That Stand Out!: Tips for College Students and Recent Grads for Writing a Superior Resume and Securing and Interview. Author, 2014.

Garnesby S: Career Planning & Development: The Path Towards Your Dream Job. Author, 2013.

Handsfield H: Color Atlas & Synopsis of Sexually Transmitted Diseases, 3rd ed. New York, NY: McGraw-Hill Professional, 2011.

Milliken ME, Honeycutt A: Understanding Human Behavior: A Guide for Health Care Providers, 8th ed. Independence, KY: Cengage Learning, 2011.

Morgan H: The Infographic Resume: How to Create a Visual Portfolio That Showcases Your Skills and Lands the Job. New York, NY: McGraw-Hill, 2014.

Payne WA, Hahn DB, Lucas EB: Understanding Your Health, 12th ed. New York, NY: McGraw-Hill, 2012.

Womble, DM: Introductory Mental Health Nursing, 3rd ed. Philadelphia, PA: Lippincott Williams & Wilkins, 2015.

Communication Skills

CHAPTER CONTENTS

LEARNING OBJECTIVES

When you complete this chapter, you will be able to:

1. Apply your knowledge of communication skills to enhance relationships with others.

2. Conduct periodic self-assessments in communication skills.

3. Use techniques that enhance communication with patients.

4. Communicate empathy in the health care environment.

5. Avoid blocks to effective communication.

6. Use knowledge and resources to effectively communicate with people with special needs.

> **Natasha and John were talking about the clinical units to which they were assigned while they waited for their teacher to start class.**

John started the conversation by complaining, "I can't wait to get off of 6 West. It has to be the worst place in the world. I really hate going there. I can't wait for my next assignment."

"What exactly do you mean, you hate going there?" asked Natasha. "Is it the patients, or is it the staff, or is it your classmates? Can you be more specific, John? Maybe if you figure out exactly why you don't like it there, you'll be able to do something about what's bothering you."

"Well," said John, "leave it to you to make me explain myself. I think it's a lack of organization or something. The charge nurse is supposed to put our time for lunch on the assignment sheet, but she forgets to do it almost every day. Then, when we remind her, she writes down one time and tells us another time. She creates chaos."

"That doesn't seem like such a huge problem to me," said Natasha. "Just have your clinical instructor talk to her. That should solve the problem."

"It's not as simple as you make it sound, Natasha," said John. "There are lots of other things. In the team conference, she jumps from one patient to another and never seems to finish a sentence. We all feel as though we know less about our patients after the conference than we did before. I guess now that I'm talking out loud to you, I'm getting a clearer picture of what the root of the problem might be."

"I'm glad talking has helped you," said Natasha. "What do you think might be the cause of the problem?"

"I think," said John, "that the charge nurse has very poor communication skills and it affects everyone who works on the unit."

✔ *Good communication skills are absolutely necessary in nursing.*

Good communication skills are absolutely necessary in nursing because how you communicate affects what you communicate. Both will influence your relationships with peers, supervisors, patients, coworkers, and physicians.

DEFINITION OF COMMUNICATION

Communication can be defined as the exchange of information. In 1928, I. A. Richards, an English literary critic, offered the following definition of communication:

> *Communication takes place when one mind so acts upon its environment that another mind is influenced, and in that other mind, an experience occurs, which is like the experience in the first mind, and is caused in part by that experience.*

✔ *Communication involves an exchange of information.*

Although Richards' definition sounds simple, you know that getting what is in your mind into the mind of another person is not so easy. The more complex the information or concept, the more difficult the task.

You have probably often had conversations with people to give instructions about what or when to do something. The person you were instructing said something back to you that led you to believe he or she understood you. In the end, you found that what the person did was not at all what you thought you had asked. Why does this happen and what can you do to improve your communication skills?

COMMUNICATION SKILLS ASSESSMENT

Assessing the way you are now communicating is important in understanding what you may need to do to be a better communicator. Complete the following self-assessment test "How Effective Is Your Communication Style?" to determine the effectiveness of your present communication style.

ASSESS YOURSELF	How Effective Is Your Communication Style?

Indicate how often each statement applies to you by choosing a number from 1 (rarely) to 5 (always).

	Rarely				Always
1. I make direct requests for cooperation.	1☐	2☐	3☐	4☐	5☐
2. I describe my actions by using the facts rather than using vague statements.	1☐	2☐	3☐	4☐	5☐
3. I ask for change by describing the desired result or behavior.	1☐	2☐	3☐	4☐	5☐
4. I express my wants, feelings, and expectations clearly and directly.	1☐	2☐	3☐	4☐	5☐
5. I am able to handle conflict with confidence.	1☐	2☐	3☐	4☐	5☐
6. I generate trust and understanding when I give and receive feedback.	1☐	2☐	3☐	4☐	5☐
7. I trust those with whom I communicate.	1☐	2☐	3☐	4☐	5☐
8. I keep to the point in conversations.	1☐	2☐	3☐	4☐	5☐
9. I ask for information in a way that promotes confidence and cooperation.	1☐	2☐	3☐	4☐	5☐
10. I suggest solutions to problems.	1☐	2☐	3☐	4☐	5☐
11. I am responsible for my communications.	1☐	2☐	3☐	4☐	5☐
12. I respond nondefensively to comments and criticism.	1☐	2☐	3☐	4☐	5☐
13. I listen to clarify information and understand the other person's point of view.	1☐	2☐	3☐	4☐	5☐
14. I resolve conflicts by communicating instead of ignoring problems.	1☐	2☐	3☐	4☐	5☐
15. I get more information by asking questions.	1☐	2☐	3☐	4☐	5☐
16. I talk about my feelings confidently in difficult situations.	1☐	2☐	3☐	4☐	5☐
17. I communicate my goals to my family, friends, and coworkers on a regular basis.	1☐	2☐	3☐	4☐	5☐
18. I treat everyone with respect in all of my interactions.	1☐	2☐	3☐	4☐	5☐
19. I resolve conflicts without taking control.	1☐	2☐	3☐	4☐	5☐
20. I make direct requests for cooperation.	1☐	2☐	3☐	4☐	5☐
21. I give and receive feedback without taking it personally.	1☐	2☐	3☐	4☐	5☐
22. I ask for information and listen until they are finished.	1☐	2☐	3☐	4☐	5☐

96–110 points: Most of the time you communicate your ideas, opinions, feelings, and desires openly and directly. Your interaction style maintains both respect and integrity. You are able to convey how the other person's behavior affects you. Your intent is to resolve problems without creating defensiveness. The outcome is dignity, confidence, and trusting relationships.

Total Points _____

81–95 points: Your interaction style is very similar to the people who score 96–110. The challenge for you is to maintain this responsible interaction style while you are angry or stressed. When you communicate differently, you begin to erode your relationships. Often this builds resentment and breaks down trust.

61–80 points: Your interaction style works for you in many situations. When you are irritated, frustrated, or angry you communicate in one of three different styles: passive, passive aggressive, and/or aggressive. These different behaviors destroy trusting relationships.

continued on page 62

- *Passive:* You don't communicate your ideas, opinions, feelings, or desires in a responsible way when they occur. Your intention is to not create conflict. By keeping things to yourself, it is difficult to build a relationship. The outcome is resentment for you and the other person involved.
- *Passive Aggressive:* Your comments are condescending or sarcastic. This behavior is confusing to others. Even though others may laugh, they usually ask themselves, does she really mean it or not? You may feel better in the moment, but you're still not expressing hidden feelings about judgment or fear. This makes it impossible to have a healthy relationship.
- *Aggressive:* Your interactions are dictatorial and controlling. You think you need to tell others what to do to get results. Most people react to your orders. They don't feel appreciated or heard. These behaviors undermine healthy and trusting relationships.

59 points or less: You are probably feeling very overwhelmed and angry. There is a strong possibility you are heading toward "flame out." The result is you aren't feeling appreciated or heard. You may react by venting your rage or you may withdraw and become depressed. At this time, it is very difficult to have healthy relationships with yourself or others.

Susan E. Greene, international coach and speaker, wrote "The Most Important Conversation Is the One You're Not Having" ISBN 1-9321961-0-2. To learn more about Susan's work and her books, go to www. communicatingworks.com *or* Amazon.com

✔ *You can use techniques to improve your communication skills.*

There are several ways to improve your communication skills. You can:
- Learn more about how people communicate
- Practice sending clear messages
- Practice listening to messages from others
- Learn about how to communicate with people who have special needs
- Ask your friends and teachers to provide constructive criticism

COMPONENTS OF COMMUNICATION

✔ *Communication has verbal, vocal, and nonverbal components.*

Dr. Albert Mehrabian identified the components of the communication process as being verbal, vocal, and nonverbal. The verbal part of the communication process is the words; the vocal part of the process is the tone of voice; and the nonverbal part is the gestures and expressions accompanying the verbal and vocal parts of the communication process. From his research, Dr. Mehrabian estimates that 7% of communication is verbal, 38% is vocal, and 55% is nonverbal.

Verbal Communication

Verbal communication is language expressed in speaking and in writing, in English or any other language. It is generally agreed that verbal communication has seven parts:
1. A source or sender (the person sending the message)
2. An encoder (eardrum, electrical wires, etc., convert the message into codes)
3. A message (what is being communicated)
4. A channel (face-to-face or over wires or cables)
5. A decoder (brain, television, radio, etc., convert codes into the message)
6. A receiver (the person who is the recipient of the message)
7. Feedback (the recipient responds in some way to the message)

Talking on the telephone to a friend would be one example. The source is you, the encoder is the mouthpiece of the telephone, the message is the words you speak, the channel is the wire along which the electrical impulses travel, the decoder is the earpiece of the telephone, and the receiver is the mind of your friend. To complete the process, your friend responds in some way (feedback) to what you said.

Verbal communication can be a one-way, two-way, or multidirectional process. An example of one-way communication is a news broadcast. The source is the news announcer, the message is the news, and the receiver is the person receiving the message. Two-way communication occurs when the sender of the message and the receiver can both send and receive messages. An example of two-way communication is a simple conversation between two people. Multidirectional communication involves more than two people. Several different people send messages to and receive messages from several different people who also send and receive messages. An example of multidirectional communication is a conversation about a patient that occurs among nurses, aides, doctors, and clerks.

Vocal Communication

How you speak can be as important as what you say because the sound of your voice and the style of your delivery can communicate hints of hidden meaning. Important messages lose their impact when delivered in a wishy-washy way, and distracting characteristics of speech, such as whining, shouting, or slurring words, detract from what is being said.

✔ *Vocal communication is the sound and tone of your voice.*

Self-consciousness is a big obstacle to clear speaking. If you are uncomfortable when talking, now is the time to analyze your speech habits. Learn which habits are reducing your effectiveness as a speaker and replace them with new ones. Practice your new behaviors alone at first and then with a friend or classmate.

When you begin to feel secure, try them out on strangers. Clear speaking is a skill that can be learned, just as poor speech habits can be unlearned. In a vocation where you will be "on stage" when you work, the sooner you improve your techniques, the more effective you will be.

To improve your vocal communication skills, study the way you speak. For example, you can use a tape recorder to hear how you sound to others, and speaking in front of a mirror will show you how you look when you are talking.

When you are speaking, face the person you are addressing. Keep eye contact and state your words clearly without skipping syllables or slurring their pronunciation. Use words you are comfortable with to avoid using terms that sound out of place, even though you understand their meaning. Your words, tone, rhythm, inflection, and posture should work together when you communicate. The failure of any one aspect of communication will detract from what you are saying and may create a wrong impression.

Nonverbal Communication

Nonverbal communication is found in all cultures. It includes signs, signals, and symbols. A sign could be a picture, drawing, or traffic sign. An example of a sign is a traffic stop sign; an example of a signal is a wave of the hand. Symbols are deeply embedded in culture and examples include things such as wedding rings and the caduceus, the symbol of the medical profession. Serious misunderstandings often occur when we are unaware of the signs, signals, and symbols of cultures other than our own.

✔ *Nonverbal communication is made up of signs, signals, and symbols.*

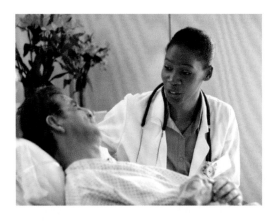

FIGURE 3-1. ● The nurse uses touch to communicate caring.

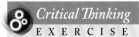
Critical Thinking
EXERCISE

As you enter Mr. Callahan's room, you ask him how he is feeling. He replies in a pinched voice saying, "I am feeling fine, thank you." You notice that his hand is clutching his side, he has a grimace on his face, and his skin is flushed. Use appropriate Characteristics of Critical Thinkers in Box 1-2 on pages 18–19 to develop your response to this question.

Nonverbal communication also includes body language, such as facial expressions, posture, body position, and other actions that do not use words. Examples include averting your eyes when speaking or being spoken to, tapping a foot, frowning, yawning, putting your hand on your hip, gently touching a patient (Fig. 3-1), smiling when entering a room, looking in the eyes of your patient, and presenting a clean and neat personal appearance. As you can see, nonverbal communication can be both positive and negative.

THE PROCESS OF COMMUNICATING

Verbal, vocal, and nonverbal communications are fairly simple when studied individually. However, when all three parts are put together, as happens in almost any face-to-face exchange of information, the results are not predictable. Many factors influence the communication process, as shown in Figure 3-2. With so many factors influencing communication, it's no wonder

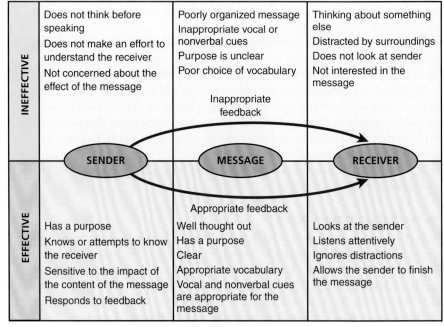

	SENDER	MESSAGE	RECEIVER
INEFFECTIVE	Does not think before speaking Does not make an effort to understand the receiver Not concerned about the effect of the message	Poorly organized message Inappropriate vocal or nonverbal cues Purpose is unclear Poor choice of vocabulary Inappropriate feedback	Thinking about something else Distracted by surroundings Does not look at sender Not interested in the message
EFFECTIVE	Has a purpose Knows or attempts to know the receiver Sensitive to the impact of the content of the message Responds to feedback	Appropriate feedback Well thought out Has a purpose Clear Appropriate vocabulary Vocal and nonverbal cues are appropriate for the message	Looks at the sender Listens attentively Ignores distractions Allows the sender to finish the message

FIGURE 3-2. ● Graphic organizer depicting the process of sending a message.

that learning the skills that can help us effectively communicate with others is so important.

✔ *Communication is a complex process.*

Sending the Message

The message is information that is communicated either from you or to you. Technology has given us so many ways of sending messages. We send (and receive) messages by talking to each other in person and by e-mail, cell phone, landline, voice mail, text message, Skype, Facebook, Twitter, online discussion groups, and personal blog pages, to name a few.

Be aware that electronic communications, except for voice and video connections, generally lack the vocal and nonverbal clues that accompany face-to-face communication. It is important to carefully think through your electronic message to avoid misunderstandings and misinterpretations.

✔ *The message is the idea you want to communicate to others.*

Be aware of your choices and use the method of sending a message that is most appropriate to the situation. For example, you might not want to send a message about a family tragedy by e-mail. It may be more appropriate to either deliver the message in person if possible or use the telephone, so there can be both verbal and vocal communication.

Speaking

When sending messages, it's important that you use correct vocabulary, grammar, medical terminology, and abbreviations when speaking. Speaking clearly (using good vocal skills) in a pleasant voice, using good judgment in what you say, giving simple and straightforward answers to questions, expressing confidence in what you say, listening without interrupting, and using accurate descriptions all contribute to presenting an effective message. It is important to use words in your message that the receiver can understand. Nursing team members will understand medical terminology, but your patients may not.

✔ *Before speaking, develop a clear message in your mind.*

In general, you should follow these guidelines to improve the quality of what you say, so that you can be understood easily:

- Organize your thoughts before speaking.
- Avoid set speeches that sound memorized.
- Keep your listener in mind when you're speaking.
- Keep your personal opinions and values out of communications where they don't belong.
- Use proper technical terms when speaking with colleagues.
- Give complete explanations in words your patients and their families will understand.
- Restate or repeat in your own words the questions or statements of others to make sure you understand what they've said.
- Ask your listener for an opinion or other response.
- Address people appropriately, as Mr., Mrs., Miss, or Ms., according to their wishes.
- Avoid trite terms of endearment, such as honey, dear, or grandpa, when addressing patients and families.
- Avoid teasing, even if your intention is to raise spirits.
- Never be sarcastic.
- Avoid giving false reassurances to anyone about your patient's condition.
- Do your best to sound cheerful, even when you don't feel it.

Presenting a clear, well-thought-out message will go a long way toward improving your ability to communicate effectively with others.

Writing

Sending written messages can be considered a part of verbal communication. Writing something down may be less threatening to you than telling someone directly, but writing requires the same attention as speaking. Writing is also a significant way of communicating information in health care.

✔ *Much communication in health care is in writing.*

You are already learning the importance of good writing from taking your class notes. Neatness, legibility, and expressing precise meaning in as few words as possible are the basics of good writing. Write clear, legible notes and highlight information so that you can retrieve it whenever it's needed and not have to dig it out. Muddled, scribbled, and erratic notes take more time and work to translate than re-reading the original material from which they were taken.

Nursing documentation is a special kind of writing skill that has a direct influence on patient care. Much of what you will "write" about a patient will be entered into the patient's electronic nursing record using a computer terminal, a tablet, a smartphone, a remote computer, or a yet-to-be released gadget. It is still essential that the information be precise, accurate, and legible. Long, vague, or meaningless observations do not communicate the hard information required to manage patient care. Use specific, concise terms and phrases that tell the facts, not opinions. Think about what you have observed, what you want to say, and how you are going to say it before writing anything. This process will become habit with time, but developing the habit requires thought and effort at the start.

✔ *Entering information on a patient's chart requires close attention to details and facts.*

You may use abbreviations when charting, but the abbreviations must be those that are approved for use in your clinical agencies. Do not use shorthand that nobody else can understand.

Receiving the Message

Reading

Although reading is not considered to be a direct communication skill, it is an important vehicle for conveying information and ideas you need to perform your job well. Your education from now on will depend heavily on how well and what you read. Reading is and will be required in your education and work. Developing good reading habits now will help you throughout your program and career.

How fast you read and how well you understand what you read are the essentials of effective reading. Both can be improved with practice.

How fast you read depends on what kind of material you are reading and how efficiently your eyes travel over the page. A textbook or nursing manual goes slower than a mystery story or a general-interest magazine article because their purposes are different. Technical reading requires more concentration than recreational reading, but it does not have to be difficult.

Your reading speed is also affected by how many words you read in a single glance, by whether you read each word, and by distractions, such as mouthing each word or reading aloud.

Observe how you read. Do you mouth or speak the words? Do you keep your place by running your finger along sentences as you read? Do you read each word separately? Do you go back over what you have read again and again? Your reading speed and comprehension will suffer if you do. If you have reading problems, ask for help. Changing poor reading habits will make learning easier.

How well you understand what you have read depends a great deal on the extent of your vocabulary. If you know the words, you will generally understand what is said; not knowing a key word may make the rest of a sentence meaningless.

Building a good vocabulary is an excellent way to improve comprehension. Nurses require two vocabularies, each having its own dictionary: one for common language and the other for medical terms.

When you find an unfamiliar word, look it up immediately, read the definition and the correct pronunciation, repeat the word, and define it in your own words. Online dictionaries available on the computer provide a definition as well as an audio pronunciation of the word. Then, go back and read the sentence where it was found. To increase word retention and make new words a part of your active vocabulary, use them soon and frequently.

✔ *Understanding what you read requires a good vocabulary.*

You will use medical terms extensively in much of your reading and in communications with colleagues and patients. Medical terminology has its own special rules, particularly regarding root words, suffixes, and prefixes. If you learn those rules well now, you can figure out the meanings of new words on your own and then look them up to verify your definition.

Listening

Your role as a receiver is to listen to the message being sent. Hearing and listening are two distinct activities. Hearing is biophysical and occurs when sound waves strike the structures in the inner ear. Listening is an active process requiring concentration and attention to the components of verbal, vocal, and nonverbal messages.

Effective listening skills can make a major difference in your expertise as a nurse. How good a listener you are affects communication between yourself and others. It can also influence how well you do your work. By listening closely and attentively, you will focus your attention on the information being communicated to you. When you are given directions to do something, knowing exactly what your instructor or supervisor is telling you will help you work with confidence.

✔ *A nurse must have excellent listening skills.*

A good listener also gains the confidence of the speaker. When instructors and supervisors are involved, this translates into approval of you and your performance. Establishing confidence with patients makes working with them easier and, equally important, is therapeutic for them as well.

Good listening skills don't come naturally for everyone, but they can be learned. In conversation or at other times when listening is important, some people focus their attention on what they themselves are saying or thinking and not on the speaker. This normal egocentricity (focus on the self) conflicts with the need for nurses to be exceptional listeners. There are three steps to good listening:
1. Focus your attention on the speaker and what is being said.
2. Interpret what is said to understand what to do.
3. Restate what you thought you heard to be sure you understood the message.

Throughout your nursing career, patients will turn to you to express their hopes, fears, opinions, and personal concerns. By listening closely to what they say, you will provide an outlet for feelings that they might otherwise keep bottled up. By listening between the lines (e.g., paying attention to the vocal and nonverbal components), you will know what they really need or want to say. This exchange can help to relieve their stress, which is often a component of illness.

✔ *Sometimes, a patient just needs someone to listen.*

Being a good listener does not mean inserting yourself or your opinions into your patients' lives as you might do in daily social conversation. It also does not mean you have the right to pry. Accept what they tell you without judging what they say. Treat information with total confidentiality. Remember that you are not the patient's only audience, but only one of many people in his or her life at the moment. You should be receptive and open, but it's not your role to be an adviser.

Sharing experiences is a normal part of ordinary conversation, but a patient who relates a significant life event is not looking for a similar story from you, and you should not offer any. Nod, smile, and acknowledge that you are listening. Be there for your patients without interrupting. Ask questions as a way to show your interest, but don't ask questions that are not related to what has been said or questions that can be construed as prying. Don't let boredom or lack of interest show. Be courteous, interested, and nonjudgmental in your conversations with patients.

✔ Ineffective communication skills can lead to errors in patient care.

Effective communication skills improve the quality of care; ineffective communication skills are the root of many errors in patient care. Thinking about and practicing to improve verbal, vocal, nonverbal, and listening skills are as important to you as a nurse as they are to you as a person.

COMMUNICATING WITH PATIENTS

Much of your time as a nurse will be spent communicating with your patients. This is how you will learn what they want, need, and expect from you and from the health care facility. Communicating with the patient will be important as you develop the plan of care and as you evaluate the effectiveness of nursing care and medical treatment.

✔ People who are ill and uncomfortable may need assistance in communicating their needs.

It is important to understand that people who are not feeling well or who are in severe pain can't always clearly express their thoughts. To compensate, you must continually work to improve your skills in communicating effectively.

Practicing Effective Communication

To communicate effectively with your patients requires paying close attention not only to what they say but also to how they say it. You may need to ask carefully worded questions to determine exactly what the patient is trying to say.

Suppose you have a patient who says that the sleeping pill he took last night didn't work. As the receiver of this message, you probably realize that this statement needs to be clarified for effective communication to occur. Is the patient trying to say he didn't sleep at all, that he slept only for a little while, that he has many things on his mind that kept him from sleeping, or that he was in pain? The nurse in this case must ask some clarifying questions to better understand the patient's message. The best questions to ask are those that need more than a simple yes or no answer. Asking, "Were you in pain last night?" might result in a yes or no answer. Asking, "Why do you say the sleeping pill didn't work?" might get responses such as "I took the same pill at home and it never worked" or "I was in so much pain that a sleeping pill would never work" or "I was too worried about the tests I am having today." Statements such as these will give you an opportunity to continue to communicate effectively with the patient.

✔ Ask clarifying questions to be sure you know what the patient wants or needs.

When you communicate with patients, you should use several techniques that will help keep the channels of communication open:

- Avoid frivolous conversation and joking.
- Show respect when speaking or listening.
- Be honest in your relationships with patients.
- Ask questions that cannot be answered with a yes or no.
- Restate what you thought you heard the patient say.
- Use clarifying phrases.
- Identify the purpose of your conversations.
- Keep confidential information confidential.
- Write down important facts or instructions.
- Sit down to indicate that you have time to listen.

✔ Use techniques that keep the channels of communication open.

People who are ill often benefit from a good sense of humor, but that is not to say that people who are ill appreciate frivolous conversations. Nurses should take their lead from the patient and should not initiate joke-telling or long conversations about the merits of local sports teams.

Nurses must show respect to their patients. Addressing the patient as Mr., Ms., or Mrs. is fitting unless the patient prefers otherwise. Calling an older patient "Grandpa" or addressing a middle-aged man as "Mister Good Looking" is inappropriate. It's also important to listen without interrupting. Save your questions or comments until the person has finished speaking.

Being honest with patients develops a trusting relationship. Telling a patient that an uncomfortable and lengthy procedure is relatively simple and takes only a few minutes is not honest even if the intent was to ally fear and apprehension. There are some situations in which you might not be legally or ethically permitted to give an honest response to questions about medical conditions, but you can be honest by saying that you are not permitted to provide that information but that you will find someone who can answer their questions.

Ask questions that cannot be answered with a yes or a no. Doing so will take practice, but it's well worth it. Asking these kinds of questions will, after practice, also carry over to your personal life. You will find that your relationships with others will improve because your attitude indicates that you really do want to know how the other person is thinking or feeling. "Do you feel better today?" will probably result in a yes or no answer; "Tell me about how you're feeling today" will probably result in more useful information.

✔ *Avoid asking questions that can be answered with a yes or no.*

Restating what you thought you heard is important to effective communication. All of us leave out important details when we speak, and it's at this point in communication that many errors occur. Restating what you thought the person said will clarify misunderstandings before they lead to serious consequences. Your patient says, "I am so depressed. I just don't know what to do. I feel like just giving up." You might restate what you thought you heard by saying, "I think I just heard you say that you feel like giving up. What does 'giving up' mean?"

Using clarifying phrases will help make communication more effective by making sure you understand what the sender was trying to communicate. A patient might say that someone will be with him when he goes home from the hospital. A clarifying phrase might be "Are you saying that your wife will be with you 24 hours a day for at least 2 weeks after you're discharged?"

Your communication with patients should have a purpose, and you should state that purpose to the patient. When entering a patient's room to explain a diagnostic test that has been scheduled, you should tell the patient why you are there. "I'm here to tell you about the CT scan that is scheduled for you tomorrow and to answer any questions you might have." This will help the patient focus on the purpose of the conversation.

✔ *Communication should have a purpose.*

You should, through what and how you communicate, establish a trusting relationship with your patients. You are required to keep confidential information confidential. If you are concerned about something a patient tells you and you are not sure what to do with the information, ask your instructor or charge nurse for advice. Remember to never discuss things of a personal nature that have been communicated to you with family, friends, neighbors, or others who have no need to know this information.

Communication can be improved by writing down important facts and instructions. You will be given information about procedures to perform, medications to administer, tests to complete, and observations to make for several different patients. Writing down instructions will help you avoid errors in care.

When a patient expresses the need to discuss something of importance, you can create an environment that encourages communication by pulling up a chair and sitting down. By sitting, your nonverbal communication indicates that you have time and want to listen to their concerns,

Using these techniques will help you to build effective communication skills. This requires continuous practice, and it will take some time for you to become a skilled communicator. Good communication skills will result in fewer misunderstandings and will lead to greater satisfaction in your professional as well as personal life.

✔ *The things you learn about patients and their families are confidential.*

Communicating Empathy

As a nurse, you are in a position that requires providing emotional support, encouragement, and understanding to your patients and their families. Meeting these needs can be emotionally draining for you. Early in your career, you must learn to provide compassionate care without emotionally exhausting yourself.

Emotions and feelings require energy, and energy is a resource you cannot afford to waste. At times, just meeting the physical demands of your work will take more energy than you think you have. Add to that the emotional strain of working with patients who depend on you for many of their needs, and you will quickly see how the conservation of physical and emotional energy is the only way to avoid exhaustion and loss of interest.

The way to provide emotional support to your patients and not deplete your own emotional reserves is to avoid becoming emotionally involved while still sharing with them their thoughts, feelings, and fears. The term used to describe this relationship is *empathy*.

✔ *Empathy is similar to sympathy but does not include self-involvement.*

To empathize is to be able to intellectually (not emotionally) identify with the feelings, thoughts, or attitudes of another person. You can understand and respect what a person is experiencing without experiencing it yourself. For example, you may have a patient who has just been diagnosed as having a life-threatening disease. You can intellectually understand that this patient and the family are probably having many different feelings, including anger, fear of the future, despair, and maybe even hope. You are able to understand the patient's and family's feelings without having them yourself. You can communicate empathy by acknowledging how the situation is affecting those who are involved.

Sympathy goes beyond empathy in that sympathy involves an emotional response from the person who is feeling sympathetic. When something bad or unpleasant happens to someone close to you, you may feel angry, sad, or distraught. You have an emotional response to the situation. From your own personal experiences, you know how emotionally exhausting it can be to have feelings of sympathy.

Being empathic is not callous or hard-hearted. It helps you keep the distance you need from the patient's problems so that you can think and act in his or her best interest. It also helps you conserve your emotional energy so that you can be of help to yourself and to your family and others who depend on you.

Blocks to Effective Communication

Many things we do, either consciously or unconsciously, can block communication. We can change the subject, avoid the person, or deny that an issue exists, or we can be so opinionated that others don't pursue a conversation.

These communication approaches do not lead to an understanding of what another person is trying to tell us. These techniques have no place in health care. We depend on the patient to participate in his or her plan of treatment, and we need to avoid using techniques that prevent us from knowing what and how the patient feels and thinks.

✔ *Avoid using techniques that block effective communication.*

Some of the blocks to effective communication are as follows:

- Nonverbal barriers
- Changing the subject
- Stereotyped responses
- Personal bias
- Asking questions that can be answered with a yes or no response
- Asking personal questions
- Belittling the patient's feelings
- Expressing disapproval

Different cultures interpret nonverbal communication differently; however, universal nonverbal barriers include yawning, sneering, entering information on the chart when the patient is talking, not looking directly at the patient, and looking as though you are "a million miles away."

✔ *When certain techniques do not lead to effective communication, try others.*

Nurses who feel uncomfortable when talking about certain subjects (e.g., death, euthanasia, abortion) will often try to change the subject. Stereotyped responses include statements such as "Everybody feels that way," or "You will be just fine," or "Don't worry, your doctor is very good."

Expressing your personal bias about a subject may prevent patients from expressing their own feelings about that subject. If you say that abortion is wrong and no one should have one, you may prevent the patient from feeling she can discuss this difficult decision with you—her nurse.

One of the best ways to block communication is to ask questions that can be answered with yes or no. It's easy for a patient who feels ill to answer the question "Do you want to get a bath today?" with a no. This leaves you little choice other than to respect the patient's wishes even though you know that bathing is important to infection control, skin condition, and feeling more comfortable. A better way to handle this situation is to say, "I know you aren't feeling so well today, but I'll be back in 15 minutes to give you a bath and change your bed. I'll try not to exhaust you, and I'll be sure you get your pain medication within the next few minutes." This statement doesn't require a response, but most likely the patient will give some indication that this is acceptable.

Be sure the questions you ask are necessary and do not pry into a patient's personal affairs. If a patient tells you he is concerned about the cost of the hospital bill and doesn't know how he will ever be able to pay it, it's not your duty to delve into his financial circumstances. The better response would be to ask the charge nurse to have a social worker talk with the patient to determine his financial situation.

A nurse has no right to belittle a patient's feelings or to deny a patient the right to those feelings. A patient scheduled for a magnetic resonance imaging test may tell you that she is afraid of the test and is thinking about canceling it. Statements such as "You can't be serious," "People in worse conditions than you have this test and they don't complain," and "I can't imagine why you're making such a big deal out of such a simple test" are belittling to the patient and will certainly prevent you from ever finding out why the patient is afraid.

Expressing disapproval of a patient's decision is not a therapeutic response. If a patient chooses to try an experimental form of treatment, that is his or her choice. The nurse does not have to personally approve of the patient's choice, but the patient does have the right to be supported in the decision.

Using techniques that block effective communication contributes to poor patient care. Nurses must do everything they can to avoid creating and using these blocks when caring for their patients.

COMMUNICATING WITH TEAM MEMBERS

✔ *Apply the same techniques to establish good communication with team members as you do with patients.*

The health care team is composed of a great number of people. Being able to communicate effectively with team members as well as with patients will provide a pleasant and productive working environment. The same techniques for ensuring effective communication with patients and avoiding blocks to communication also apply to working with health care team members.

Physicians

When communicating with physicians, be sure you have carefully collected all of the information you need to describe a particular situation. Everyone is busy, and having your information readily available will go a long way toward establishing effective relationships.

Be sure you don't cloud the facts with personal opinion, and don't offer your personal opinion unless it is requested. Use tact when necessary to clarify written or verbal communication that you don't understand. Calling a physician and saying, "Your writing is impossible to read. What did you order for Mr. Jones?" will most likely produce a negative response. Asking the physician to clarify the frequency of the dosage of carbamazepine ordered for Mr. Jones will probably result in a more positive response.

Supervisors

✔ *Communicating with physicians, supervisors, and team members must include respect for others.*

Your supervisor is in a position of legal liability for your actions. Assuming that you are functioning within the limits of your education and experience, your supervisor is the person who must be sure that your nursing performance is acceptable.

In this relationship, you have a responsibility to establish very good communications with your supervisor. You must incorporate all of the techniques that enhance communication in your day-to-day relationships. You need to clarify and restate instructions given by your supervisor to be sure you understand what is expected of you. You need to show respect in your verbal and nonverbal communication, and you must keep confidential information confidential.

While you are a student, your supervisor will probably be your clinical instructor. All of the rules for good communication apply equally to this relationship. Your instructor will not appreciate joking and frivolity on the clinical unit. You will be expected to follow directions, rules, regulations, and policies that will be communicated to you throughout your nursing education program.

Nursing Team Members

✔ *Good communication skills may help reduce misunderstandings.*

Developing good communication skills with the people you work with every day is critical to your success in nursing. Using good communication skills as a matter of routine will certainly reduce the frequency of misunderstandings and conflicts that can easily occur in the hectic health care environment.

Effective communication among team members is important in planning and implementing nursing care. Many people and departments are involved in meeting the needs of patients, and poor communication skills can lead to poor patient care as well as to poor interpersonal relationships.

When working closely with others, remember to think about what you are going to say before you speak. Maintain a professional attitude and show respect for the opinions of others. When in doubt about the intent of what someone says or asks you to do, ask for clarification. If you offend someone by what you say, apologize.

COMMUNICATING IN SPECIAL SITUATIONS

Using effective communication skills requires constant attention in ordinary and comfortable circumstances. When the circumstances are no longer familiar to us and the situations are unusual, we need to develop additional skills to effectively communicate with others.

Communicating With Culturally Diverse People

Working with patients and team members from backgrounds and cultures that are different from yours offers challenges as well as opportunities. The challenge is to avoid confusing or offending another person by what you say or do, and the opportunity is a chance to learn about other cultures and people who are different from yourself.

Cultural competence is the term used to describe the process of working effectively within the cultural context of another person. You need to learn about the cultural heritage of your patients so that you and your team members can incorporate that knowledge into each patient's plan of care.

It is impossible to know everything about all of the different cultures and subcultures you will encounter during the course of your career. Some general rules, however, will help you improve your cross-cultural communication skills:

- Understand your own cultural values and biases.
- Respect the culture of others.
- Have an interest in learning about others.
- Have an ability to avoid judging the behavior of others.

If you have not already done so, you should make a sincere effort to understand your own feelings and biases. Examining the reasons for your own feelings and biases forces you to realize that other people have reasons for their feelings and biases that are just as legitimate as yours. This knowledge helps you become more accepting and tolerant of those who are different from you. When communicating with people from different cultures, you will find that in some cultures, people do not look directly at the person to whom they are speaking. Doing so indicates a lack of respect. In other cultures, not looking at someone when speaking to them is considered disrespectful.

Personal space is also important in communication. Members of some cultures tend to move very close to the people with whom they are speaking, and others tend to keep much farther away. As a nurse, you will often have a need to be in what is called a person's "intimate space" or "personal space." Members of some cultures are comfortable with close physical proximity, whereas others are extremely uncomfortable.

✔ *Getting to know people from different cultures gives us an opportunity to learn more about the world in which we live.*

✔ *Know your feelings about people who are different from you.*

✔ *Learn as much as you can about the practices of people from different cultures.*

Critical Thinking
E X E R C I S E

You have a patient of the opposite sex who has, for the past 3 days, refused to allow you to bathe him or her. The patient has had a high fever and is unable to get out of bed, and the skin condition is deteriorating. You know that in the patient's culture, most people bathe no more than once a week. You also think that the patient might have a cultural code that forbids him or her from being alone with a member of the opposite sex. How could you resolve this situation? Use appropriate Characteristics of Critical Thinkers in Box 1-2 on pages 18–19 to develop your responses to this situation.

✔ *You can communicate caring and compassion without the use of words.*

Physical responses can be misinterpreted if you are unfamiliar with a patient's cultural background. Certain cultures value harmony, and members of these cultures may appear to agree with something you say, when in fact they are nodding merely to maintain harmony.

If you find that your health care facility frequently provides care for members of one, two, or even three cultures, it is your responsibility to learn as much as you can about each of those cultures. A number of nursing textbooks discuss cultural diversity, including how different cultures communicate with one another. If you have an interest in a particular culture or cultures, refer to one of the books from the "Read More About It" list. There are a number of Web sites maintained by specific cultural groups that describe social and health care practices. Your effectiveness as a health care provider will be greatly enhanced by taking the time to learn about your patients.

Communicating with Non–English-Speaking People

Nearly 61 million people in the United States speak a language other than English at home. This number is up from 47 million people in 2000. And the number is increasing every year. Chances are good that you will be providing nursing care for some patients and families who do not speak English. When your patient does not speak a language you understand, communicating is extremely difficult.

Many health care facilities provide printed information in a number of different languages (Fig. 3-3), some broadcast informational television in a language spoken by a large number of their patients, and some provide interpreters to help patients and their families understand their illness and treatments.

When using an interpreter, be sure you know his or her educational level so you can choose words that will be understood. Watch for nonverbal cues as information is communicated from you to the interpreter, then to the patient, and back to you. Here are some general guidelines to follow when an interpreter is not available.

- Don't shout; the person is probably not hard of hearing.
- Greet the person using his or her name and give your own name as you point to yourself.
- Pantomime actions or procedures that you need to perform.
- Use a preprinted list of phrases in the patient's language.
- Determine what words or other language the patient might understand.
- Use simple words and phrases if the patient has a limited vocabulary.

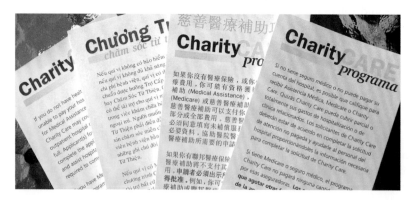

FIGURE 3-3. ● Multilanguage brochures provide important information to patients and their families.

If a significant number of your patients speak another language, you may find it necessary to learn that language or learn to use technology that can quickly translate printed or spoken words. Just remember—you can always communicate caring, compassion, and concern without the use of words.

Communicating with Hearing-Impaired People

When communicating with a person who is totally deaf, it will do you no good to shout. Even people with moderate hearing impairment don't comprehend very well when the speaker shouts. When talking with someone who has difficulty hearing, follow these guidelines:

- Speak slowly, one phrase at a time.
- Face the person directly.
- Don't move your head.
- Don't position yourself too far away.
- Repeat the information to clarify.
- Use bright lighting to help the person see your mouth and face.
- Eliminate as much background noise (radios, televisions, other conversations) as possible.

Computer technology, e-mail, text messaging, hearing aids, and telecommunications devices for the deaf all help hearing-impaired people communicate with others. If your patients use one or more of these devices, do all that you can to learn about how to use them. If your patient uses a sign language interpreter, be sure to use terminology and descriptions that the interpreter can accurately translate.

✔ *Make use of technology to assist in communication.*

Communicating With Vision-Impaired People

Box 3-1 gives some excellent rules of courtesy to apply when you are in the company of a blind person. Being honest and thoughtful will go a long way toward establishing good relationships and providing a safe environment.

When a blind or partially sighted person is your patient, there are a few additional rules you should follow.

✔ *Speak in a normal tone of voice.*

- Always announce yourself as you enter the room.
- State your name and the person's name. For example, "Good morning Mr. Thomas, my name is Mr. Watson, and I am here to give you your insulin."
- Continue talking as you are working. This will help the patient know where you are in relation to him.
- Say what you are going to do before you do it.
- Tell the patient you are going to touch him before you actually do.
- Tell him what foods are on his tray and where they are located.
- Put things he will need (e.g., call bell, tissues, telephone) within his reach and tell him where they are.
- Keep the room free of clutter.
- Don't move furniture in the room without telling him where it is.
- Ask the patient what he needs to make him most comfortable in the unusual surroundings of a health care facility.

Blind people can't pick up many of the nonverbal behaviors associated with communication. Therefore, it's important that you use vocal tones to convey feelings associated with conversation. Your concern for a patient's fears can be conveyed by your tone of voice probably better than by the words you choose.

BOX 3-1

The Courtesy Rules of Blindness

When you meet me don't be ill at ease. It will help both of us if you remember these simple points of courtesy:

1. I'm an ordinary person, just blind. You don't need to raise your voice or address me as if I were a child. Don't ask my spouse what I want—"Cream in the coffee?"—ask me.
2. I may use a long white cane or a guide dog to walk independently, or I may ask to take your arm. Let me decide, and please don't grab my arm; let me take yours. I'll keep a half-step behind to anticipate curbs and steps.
3. I want to know who's in the room with me. Speak when you enter. Introduce me to the others, including children, and tell me if there's a cat or dog.
4. The door to a room or cabinet or to a car that is left partially open is a hazard to me.
5. At dinner I will not have trouble with ordinary table skills.
6. Don't avoid words like "see." I use them too. I'm always glad to see you.
7. I don't want pity, but don't talk about the "wonderful compensations" of blindness. My sense of smell, taste, touch, or hearing did not improve when I became blind; I rely on them more and, therefore, may get more information through those senses than you do—that's all.
8. If I'm your houseguest, show me the bathroom, closet, dresser, window—the light switch too. I like to know whether the lights are on or off.
9. I'll discuss blindness with you if you're curious, but it's an old story to me. I have as many other interests as you do.
10. Don't think of me as just a blind person. I'm just a person who happens to be blind.
11. You don't need to remember some "politically correct" term, "visually impaired," "sight challenged," etc. Keep it simple and honest, just say blind.

In all 50 states the law requires drivers to yield the right of way when they see my extended white cane. Only the blind may carry white canes. You see more blind persons walking alone today, not because there are more of us, but because we have learned to make our own way.

*For more information about blindness contact the **National Federation of the Blind**, 200 East Wells Street at Jernigan Place, Baltimore, MD 21230 (410) 659–9314, www.nfb.org. This list is reprinted from A Blind Net, www blind.net, and may be reprinted as long as the text is not altered in any way, there is no fee charged, and this notice, in full, is included.*

Providing additional information verbally is also helpful. For example, saying "My name is Mr. Watson" only lets the patient know your name, whereas saying "My name is Mr. Watson and I am 5 feet 10 inches tall and have a medium build" will help the patient to better know who you are.

Communicating With Speech-Impaired People

✔ *Exercise patience when working with speech-impaired patients.*

People may have difficulty speaking as a result of a brain hemorrhage, brain injury, surgical removal of the vocal cords, or trauma. You will need to exercise a great deal of patience when communicating with people who have difficulty speaking because it can take a long time for them to express a simple thought.

Although most patients who can't speak are able to write, some are not. For those who can write, the following guidelines will aid in communication:

- Provide paper and pencil or a computer with which to write.
- Look at the patient as she writes the message.
- Don't allow interruptions during your conversation with the patient.
- Don't allow yourself to be distracted while the patient is writing (communicating).
- Encourage the patient to pantomime her thoughts.
- Ask for clarification of what the patient wrote to be sure you understand her intent.
- Don't shout. The patient probably does not have difficulty hearing.

Some patients who have had a brain hemorrhage or brain injury have a difficult time finding and saying the words they want to use. Although they can't speak the words, they can often understand what you are saying and what they read. You can ask these patients yes or no questions. For example, if a patient is pointing to his head and trying to tell you something, ask about possible reasons. Does he have a headache? Is the light hurting his eyes? Does he want his glasses? Does he want to shave? You may have to ask a number of questions to find out what he wants. This can be frustrating for both of you. Reassure the patient that you are not frustrated, encourage him to relax, and take as much time as necessary to determine what he needs.

Some patients are able to use picture cards to communicate some of their basic needs. The patient selects the card that will show the nurse what she wants or needs. The card can communicate only the most elementary thoughts. The nurse should try to fill in the details by asking the patient questions that can be answered with a simple yes or no.

✔ *Share tips and techniques that improve communication with patients with other team members.*

Communicating with people who have hearing, vision, or speech impairments can be difficult and often a time-consuming endeavor. It is wise to ask other members of the nursing and health care team for specific tips and techniques that will help you communicate better with your patients. Experienced nurses, family members, physicians, occupational therapists, and speech therapists are all resources you can ask for help.

Communicating with people who have sensory impairments or who come from a culture that is significantly different is a true challenge for nurses. How well you are able to work with people who are different from you will depend on how comfortable and secure you are with yourself and how willing you are to learn about the needs of others.

SUMMARY

It is important to continually assess and evaluate the effectiveness of your verbal, vocal, and nonverbal communication skills. When you notice that your skills are weak in some areas, you should work to improve them. This requires an effort on your part and is a process that takes practice and time. The result of learning to be a better communicator will positively affect relationships with patients, their families, with your coworkers, and in your relationships outside of your work.

APPLY

Critical Thinking Skills

1. In the opening story at the beginning of this chapter, John believes that the chaos on his clinical unit is due to the charge nurse's poor communication skills. Can you think of one or two things that John, a student practical nurse, might do to improve his situation on 6 West?

2. Demonstrate messages that you can give by different postures, appearances, and body language. Practice in front of a mirror or with a classmate. Does your classmate get the same message you think you are sending?

3. Using forms other than verbal communication, try getting a message across to a friend or a classmate. For example, try asking for a drink of water.

4. Analyze a recent conversation that was less than pleasant. Why did you feel uncomfortable and what could you do the next time to create a better outcome?

5. Participate in the following simulations in which you are the nurse and your partner is the patient. After you finish the three exercises, reverse roles and do them again.

SITUATION: Your patient is hearing-impaired and does not read English. Your task as the nurse is to explain to the patient that he is scheduled to have a CT scan at 8:00 tomorrow morning.

SITUATION: A patient who is blind was just admitted to room 608. She has been blind since birth and is fairly independent. Your task as the nurse is to explain what the room looks like and where things are in the room.

SITUATION: Your patient had a laryngectomy (removal of vocal cords) 2 days ago. The patient is frowning, sweating, and restless, and he appears to be apprehensive about something. Your task as the nurse is to find out what is bothering him.

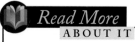

Read More

ABOUT IT

Andrews MM, Boyle JS: Transcultural Concepts in Nursing Care, 7th ed. Philadelphia, PA: Lippincott Williams & Wilkins, 2015.

Arnold E, Boggs KU: Interpersonal Relationships: Professional Communication Skills for Nurses, 7th ed. St. Louis, MO: WB Saunders, 2015.

Balzar-Riley J: Communication in Nursing, 7th ed. St. Louis, MO: Mosby, 2012.

Callahan M, Kelley P: Final Gifts: Understanding the Special Awareness, Needs, and Communications of the Dying. New York, NY: Simon & Schuster, 2012.

Dahlkemper TR: Anderson's Nursing Leadership, Management, and Professional Practice for the LPN/LVN, 5th ed. Philadelphia, PA: FA Davis, 2013.

McFarland MR, Wahbe-Alamah HB: Leininger's Culture Care Diversity and Universality: A Worldwide Nursing Theory, 3rd ed. Sudbury, MA: Jones and Bartlett, 2014.

Mehrabian A: Silent Messages: Implicit Communication of Emotions and Attitudes, 2nd ed. Belmont, CA: Wadsworth, 1980.

CHAPTER 4

Education for Nursing

LEARNING OBJECTIVES

When you complete this chapter, you will be able to:

1. Explain the difference between professional and nonprofessional in terms of education.

2. Give examples of duties included in the scope of practice of various members of the nursing team.

3. Describe the educational preparation for registered nurses.

4. Describe the educational preparation for practical/vocational nurses.

5. Describe the educational preparation for certified nursing assistants.

6. List at least three types of institutions that can sponsor practical/vocational nursing programs.

7. Explain the difference between the terms "program approval" and "program accreditation."

LEARNING OBJECTIVES *continued*

8. Explain the purpose of student organizations.

9. Paraphrase the major points of either the NFLPN or the NAPNES Standards for Practical/Vocational Nurses.

10. Describe the procedure for obtaining a license as a practical/vocational nurse.

11. List some of the reasons why a nursing license can be suspended or revoked.

It was Rose's first visit to her high school since her graduation a few years earlier. She breathed deeply as she opened the door of the red brick building. The familiar smells of books and lockers and disinfecting cleaners struck her nostrils. The long rows of lockers still lined the hallway. Even the paint on the walls was the same color. Nothing had changed.

Suddenly, the hall was filled with girls and boys rushing to their classes. She watched them hurry by. Then, the familiar buzz sounded, and, as if by magic, the long hall became deserted. Rose walked slowly down the hall. She knew exactly where she was going. "Locker 213," she said aloud. There was her old locker, nestled against the wall in a line of others that had seemed a mile long when she used to run to it between classes.

"Rose?"

A woman in a flowered smock with a stethoscope around her neck threw her arms around Rose. "Terri!" laughed Rose. She hugged the woman tightly. They had been classmates in this very school.

"Come to my office," Terri said, "so we can talk."

Rose looked around the tidy office. A student lay on a cot with a damp cloth on her forehead. A boy was weighing himself on a scale in the corner. A woman in a brightly colored smock was talking to the boy. Rose turned to Terri. "Remember how I wanted to be a nurse when we were in school?" she said. "Now it's too late. I've got two kids …" Terri smiled. "So do I," she said. "And I've been a nurse for only 2 years. I went back to school 3 years ago and…" Rose rubbed her eyes. "It only takes 1 year to be a nurse?" she asked.

"One year of hard work," Terri said. "I'm a licensed practical nurse," she added proudly. "And you can be too, if you really want to be."

"I do!" Rose said excitedly. "But how? Tell me all about it."

✔ *Practical/vocational nursing education has changed a lot over the past nearly 125 years.*

It would take more than a short meeting in a busy nurse's schedule to describe practical/vocational nursing today. The vocation has come a long way since the first school of practical nursing in the United States opened in 1892. The YWCA program at the Ballard School in New York was a mere 3-month course.

Other programs to educate practical/vocational nurses and nurse's assistants, such as those developed to train Red Cross nurse's aides in World Wars I and II, were also short. For example, the World War II practical nursing program consisted of only 35 hours of lecture and 45 hours of supervised clinical experience.

It was already clear that there was a permanent place for practical nurses in American health care. A number of schools were in operation, but before 1941, they operated with minimal educational planning and supervision. With the establishment of a practical nurse association, the National Association for Practical Nurse Education (NAPNE), in 1941 to regulate education and practice, programs for training practical/vocational nurses became more uniform. Laws for certification and licensure were also established, so that today, virtually every program in every state is governed by regulating agencies.

DEFINING PROFESSIONAL AND NONPROFESSIONAL

The term *professional* generally implies that someone is competent and qualified to perform a specific occupation. Examples include a professional electrician, a professional secretary, and a professional painter. In this context, professional refers to someone who is an expert in a particular occupation. When someone refers to a person as "a real professional," it means that the person approaches the occupation with seriousness, has a high level of integrity, and can be trusted to maintain high personal standards when performing that occupation.

When the term *professional* is used in education, it has a somewhat different meaning. A professional education requires a minimum of 4 years of college; more often, a total of 6–8 years of formal study beyond high school is required. A person who studies theory and its application in a specific occupation subscribes to an occupational code of ethics, participates in the development of the occupation through organizational activities and research, and works independently of others is a professional.

The term *nonprofessional*, therefore, refers only to a nurse's educational preparation. All nurses should approach their responsibilities with a professional attitude. Any nurse, regardless of educational preparation, should be serious about the occupation, have a high level of integrity, be trustworthy, and maintain high standards.

NURSING EDUCATION STATISTICS

The U.S. Bureau of Labor Statistics predicts that the increase in employment for licensed practical/vocational nurses (LP/VNs) from 2012 to 2022 will be 25% as compared to the 11% growth rate for all occupations. In 2012, there were approximately 738,400 jobs for LP/VNs, so unless unpredictable events occur in the next few years, the employment outlook for the LP/VNs is good.

The figures in Table 4-1 illustrate recent trends in the number of nursing education programs and the number of people who passed the NCLEX examination. The number of people passing the NCLEX is a good indicator of how many new nurses are entering the profession in the United States. Knowing the number of nursing programs provides information on the potential for people to become nurses. Understanding trends in nursing education will be important to you as you plan your career in nursing.

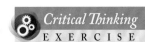

Critical Thinking EXERCISE

The licensed practical nurses (LPNs) in the agency where you work are referred to as nonprofessional staff. Your LPN friends don't like being called nonprofessionals, and they want you to join them in demanding that they be called professionals. How will you handle this situation? Use appropriate Characteristics of Critical Thinkers in Box 1-2 on pages 18–19 to develop your response to this situation.

✔ *The term professional can be used in more than one way.*

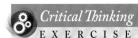

Critical Thinking EXERCISE

What trends in the statistics in Table 4-1 are important to you and to practical/vocational nursing? Use appropriate Characteristics of Critical Thinkers in Box 1-2 on pages 18–19 to develop your response to this situation.

TABLE 4-1	Number of Nursing Education Programs and Number Passing the NCLEX Exam		
	2006	2010	2014
Number of RN programs	1,694	1,812	1,839 (2012)
Number passing NCLEX-RN (First time US educated taking the NCLEX)	97,545	123,158	157,372
Number of P/VN programs	1,297	1,321	1,297 (2012)
Number passing NCLEX-PN (first time US educated taking the NCLEX)	55,843	64,432	55,489

Source: National Council of State Boards of Nursing: NCLEX Pass Rate 2014. Retrieved from http://www.ncsbn.org

National League for Nursing (2003–2012): Number of Basic Programs by Program Type, NLN Data Review™. Retrieved from http://www.nln.org

SCOPE OF PRACTICE

There are a number of educational pathways to become a nurse. Each pathway leads to a certain kind of license and to what is called a scope of practice. Scope of practice is a phrase that is used to describe what tasks and duties members of a particular occupation are legally permitted to perform. State laws, employer rules and regulations, and professional standards all contribute to defining the scope of practice of nurses. Table 4-2 offers a comparison of how levels of preparation affect selected nursing functions. You should note that the duties a nurse is permitted to perform are regulated by state law; therefore, the scope of practice (sometimes called "functions") varies significantly around the country.

✔ *It is essential that you understand your scope of practice.*

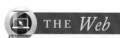
THE *Web*

Visit your State Board of Nursing Web site and read the description of the LPN scope of practice in your state.

TYPES OF NURSING PROGRAMS

Certified Nurse Aide Programs

✔ *OBRA regulations require that NAs complete training prior to employment.*

On December 22, 1987, the federal government passed the Omnibus Budget Reconciliation Act (OBRA). This act and subsequent revisions require states to establish specific educational programs for nurse aides (NAs) working in Medicare-funded long-term care facilities and for homemaker-home health aides.

In addition to the OBRA-mandated minimum 75-hour training program, each state is required to develop a mechanism for measuring competency. To do this, most states require that those NAs who have completed an approved course of study also pass a written and practical examination. The names of those who successfully pass the written and practical examination are placed on the state NA registry. To remain on the registry, each NA must document completion of a minimum of 12 hours of continuing education each year.

Educational programs for NAs are offered by a number of agencies including long-term care facilities, hospitals, vocational schools, community colleges, and private and governmental agencies. The U.S. Department of Labor estimates that 1,534,400 NAs, orderlies, and attendants were working in the United States in 2012. That number is expected to increase to 1,855,600 by the year 2022.

A NA whose name appears on a state registry can request to be placed on the registry in another state. Provided the original educational program, competency evaluation procedures, and work history meet the state requirements, the

TABLE 4-2 Comparison of Nursing Educational Preparation with Selected Functions

Education	Credential/ Examination	Health Care Setting	Level of Illness	Assessing[a]	Diagnosing[a]	Planning[a]	Implementing[a]	Evaluating[a]
4 years in college	BSN/NCLEX-RN	Structured and unstructured settings	Critically ill and unstable patients to those seeking health maintenance	Performs admission and periodic complete physical assessments. Also assesses other aspects of a patient's, client's, or resident's human needs	Analyzes and interprets data to select and revise nursing diagnoses; contributes to research on nursing diagnoses	Determines, in collaboration with others, individualized plans of care for groups of patients, clients, or residents	May directly provide care or may supervise others who provide care. Often directly supervises the work of other RNs plus LPNs, LVNs, and NAs[b]	Consults with peers and others to evaluate the effectiveness of care and to propose alternate strategies
2 years in a community, junior, or technical college	ADN/NCLEX-RN	Structured and supervised unstructured settings	Somewhat unstable patients, clients, and residents to those seeking health maintenance	Participates in an extensive data collection process related to the patient's, client's, or resident's degree of illness. Evaluates data to identify changes in health status	Analyzes and interprets data to select appropriate nursing diagnoses for individual patients, clients, and residents	Develops client-centered nursing care plans	Directly provides care and makes adjustments as needed; supervises the work of LPNs, LVNs, and NAs	Using data, collaborates with immediate team members to evaluate the plan and quality of care
2–3 years in a hospital-sponsored school of nursing	RN/NCLEX-RN	Structured and supervised unstructured settings	Somewhat unstable patients, clients, and residents to those seeking health maintenance	Participates in an extensive data collection process related to the patient's, client's, or resident's degree of illness. Evaluates data to identify changes in health status	Analyzes and interprets data to select appropriate nursing diagnoses for individual patients, clients, and residents	Develops patient-centered nursing care plans	Directly provides care and makes adjustments as needed; supervises the work of LPNs, LVNs, and NAs	Using data, collaborates with immediate team members to evaluate the plan and quality of care

continued on page 84

TABLE 4-2 Comparison of Nursing Educational Preparation with Selected Functions *continued*

Education	Credential/ Examination	Health Care Setting	Level of Illness	Assessing[a]	Diagnosing[a]	Planning[a]	Implementing[a]	Evaluating[a]
10–18 months in a high school, hospital, vocational, or technical school, or 2-year college	LPN or LVN/ NCLEX-PN	Structured settings	Stable patients, clients, and residents with common well-defined health problems	Collects a wide range of physical data and identifies and reports deviations from the normal	Not usually within the LPN/LVN scope of practice, although the LPN/LVN may contribute information to assist RNs in determining diagnoses	Contributes to the development and revision of the nursing care plan	Provides bedside care, teaches health maintenance, and works as a team member	Seeks guidance in developing and modifying nursing care approaches
Minimum of 75 hours of instruction in a course approved by the state in which it is offered	NA[b] written and performance exam	Any setting where supervision is adequate	Limited duties with any level of illness provided supervision is adequate	Collects specific data (e.g., vital signs, food and fluid intake and output, physical appearance) and reports deviations from the normal	Not within the scope of practice of an NA	In collaborative teams, the NA is often asked to contribute his or her observations when planning care.	Implements the NA portion of the plan of care outlined in the nursing care plan	Follows directions to modify approaches to patient care

[a]Assessing, diagnosing, planning, implementing, and evaluating are the five steps of the nursing process. For a better understanding of the nursing process, please refer to Chapter 9.
[b]NAs, nurse's assistants.

NA requesting permission to work in a different state may be exempted from additional educational and testing requirements.

Depending on individual state laws, professional and practical/vocational nursing students who have completed specific course work may be eligible to apply for placement on the NA registry. Professional and practical/vocational nursing students often find that working part-time as an NA is an excellent way to earn valuable experience in nursing as well as supplemental income while in school.

Practical/Vocational Nursing Programs

A practical/vocational nurse is prepared to take the licensing examination in practical nursing in approximately 1 year. The emphasis in practical/vocational nursing education is on learning nursing skills that can be applied to patients in a variety of health care settings. The LP/VN, in most health care situations, functions under the supervision and direction of an RN, physician, dentist, or nurse practitioner.

✔ *In 2012, there were 1,297 practical/vocational (LPN or LVN) programs in the United States (excluding US territories).*

Program Overview

The philosophy, objectives, and curriculum of a practical/vocational nursing program are developed by the faculty. This basic framework of your educational program is periodically reviewed, evaluated, and revised by the faculty to ensure a program of instruction that will prepare students for their first positions as LP/VNs.

Most adult programs are between 10 and 18 months in length. Practical/vocational nursing programs are classified as adult programs if the program is for adults and is not part of a high school curriculum. High school practical/vocational nursing programs are those offered to high school students.

✔ *A variety of agencies sponsor practical/vocational nursing education programs.*

A variety of agencies sponsor practical/vocational nursing programs. They include trade, technical, and vocational schools, colleges and universities, junior and community colleges, hospitals, and private or government agencies.

Curriculum and Objectives

Generally, the early practical/vocational nursing programs were combined courses of theoretical (classroom) and clinical (practical) instruction that took about 2,000 hours, or 1 year, to complete. The classroom phase took about one third of that time and consisted of lecture and laboratory classes. The remainder of the course was given to the clinical phase, with supervised experience in approved hospitals and institutions, in combination with some homecare nursing experience.

It is no longer believed that classroom instruction, followed by clinical instruction, is educationally sound. The trend today is to relate classroom theory, laboratory practice, and clinical experience by offering integrated sections over the length of the entire program. However, there is considerable variety in the actual organization of individual programs around the country in this regard, just as there is in the specific courses that are offered.

A typical program consists of 1,200–1,800 hours of instruction and starts in the fall (or first semester) with an introduction to basic nursing. Subjects covered through the year include fundamentals of nursing, communication skills, anatomy and physiology, nutrition, mental health, microbiology, maternity nursing, medical and surgical nursing of adults and children, diet therapy, pharmacology and math for medication administration, and geriatrics. Elective courses in the humanities and the behavioral sciences may also be offered.

✔ *Nursing education programs are organized so that students learn through hands-on experiences.*

On successful completion of a practical/vocational nursing course, a graduate should
- Have the education and experience needed to qualify for and pass the licensing exam in practical/vocational nursing
- Have the knowledge and skills to perform entry-level tasks under appropriate supervision
- Have the knowledge and skills to help to meet patients' physical, emotional, social, and spiritual needs
- Have up-to-date information about health and disease prevention to teach the community
- Be familiar with the effects of social, medical, health, and technologic change on health care
- Be an active member of local and national nursing associations
- Possess a desire to continue the process of learning and growing in the field

Diploma Nursing Programs

Nursing education programs sponsored by hospitals are called diploma nursing programs. These programs vary in length from 2 to 3 years. Graduates of these programs who pass the RN licensure examination are sometimes called diploma nurses. The programs of study vary greatly; however, the emphasis is on developing skills in clinical nursing practice. Many diploma programs are affiliated with colleges and universities so that students in these programs have accumulated 40 or more college credits upon graduation.

✔ *In 2012, there were 59 diploma (RN) programs in the United States (excluding US territories).*

Two-Year Associate Degree Programs

The nurse who prepares for the occupation of nursing in 2 years and passes the RN licensure examination is sometimes called an associate degree (AD) nurse. These 2-year programs are sponsored by community, technical, and junior colleges. The development of 2-year nursing programs has grown rapidly since Mildred Montag established the first programs in 1952.

✔ *In 2012, there were 1084AD programs in the United States (excluding US territories).*

Four-Year Professional Nursing Programs

A professional nurse is one who has completed at least 4 years of college and has passed the registered nurse (RN) licensure examination. The individual has studied nursing theory and its application to practice, performs responsibilities according to a strict code of ethics, and participates in the development of nursing through membership in nursing organizations. In addition, the professional nurse engages in nursing research and often works independently, without direct supervision. Many RNs who have completed a professional nursing education program have advanced to positions of leadership in nursing education and nursing service.

✔ *In 2012, there were 696 Bachelor of Science in Nursing (BSN) programs in the United States (excluding US territories).*

Combination Programs

All of the types of nursing programs previously discussed are "stand-alone" programs. In other words, a student enters the program, completes the classroom and clinical requirements, and then takes a licensing or certifying examination. If a person wants to advance to the next level of nursing education, he or she applies to the next school and is considered a "new" student. There is little, if any, consideration of previous education or experience.

More and more nursing education programs recognize the value of previous nursing education and experience. These schools have developed career ladder programs and articulated (joined) programs.

A *career ladder program* is one in which the pathway to a bachelor's or master's degree in nursing is clearly defined. The sequence of courses, where the courses are taken, the length of each course, and academic and attendance requirements are published by the schools that participate in the career ladder program. Career ladder programs are specifically designed to provide a sequence of instruction that begins at the NA or LP/VN level and progresses through the associate, baccalaureate, and sometimes the Master's degree levels. Most programs allow students to exit and enter at certain points on the ladder.

✔ *Career ladder programs help students efficiently progress from one level to the next.*

For example, a student in a career ladder program might complete a nursing assistant course in high school and then enter a practical or vocational nursing program immediately upon graduation. At the end of the nursing program, the person takes the licensing examination and works as an LP/VN for a few years. After several years, he or she decides to continue his or her education in nursing. This person could return to the career ladder program and begin the nursing education at the point where he or she left the program.

Articulated (joined) programs usually involve only two levels of nursing education and one or two schools. These programs are designed to avoid duplication of education content from one level to the next. The most common articulation programs are between practical/vocational nursing and AD nursing programs. All articulated programs have academic and clinical requirements that must be met to progress from one level to the next.

✔ *Articulated programs generally include an agreement between two schools or programs.*

External degree programs are programs in which students work independently and at their own pace. Students are usually given a schedule of assignments that they complete and then submit to the faculty. There is usually little interaction among other students. There are no lectures to attend, and the college does not supervise clinical practice. Students develop clinical skills by working with a mentor; they develop academic skills through independent study. At prescribed points in the program, the student must travel to the college and demonstrate proficiency in nursing skills to the nursing faculty. Academic examinations are conducted electronically.

✔ *Students can earn a degree through independent work.*

Students who are considering an external degree program should be certain that the program is accredited by an accrediting agency such as the Accreditation Commission for Education in Nursing (ACEN) (formerly the National League for Nursing Accrediting Commission) or by the Commission on Collegiate Nursing Education (CCNE) and approved by the state board of nursing of the state in which the school operates (see the section "Approval and Accreditation").

For some of the cautions and considerations related to these types of programs, see Chapter 14.

Distance Learning

Technology (computers, television, and the Internet) is being used to make many of the required courses in nursing education programs available to students in their own homes, 24 hours a day, 7 days a week. Distance learning is the term used for this kind of instruction. Students can register for a course by e-mail, participate in lectures on a personal computer, submit assignments electronically, and meet with their classmates and instructors in a computer chat room.

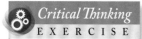

E X E R C I S E

Do you think you would ever consider continuing your formal education in nursing? If yes, what programs would you consider and why, and how can you begin planning now for your future? Use appropriate Characteristics of Critical Thinkers in Box 1-2 on pages 18–19 develop your response to this situation.

The actual campus may be hundreds or thousands of miles away, or it may exist only in cyberspace.

Students who are considering enrolling in distance learning courses must be prepared to participate in meeting the requirements of this type of instruction. Complete the self-assessment "Are You Ready for Distance Learning?" on page 89 to see if you would be ready to enroll in distance learning courses. The idea of being able to earn credits at home and at times that are convenient for you is very tempting. However, distance learning requires an ability to use and maintain your computer, good keyboarding skills, and strong independent learning skills.

Students who are taking distance learning classes should be certain that the credits they earn could be transferred to other schools. They should also make sure that any nursing program offered through distance learning is approved by the ACEN or the CCNE. Programs must be approved by the board of nursing of the state in which the school is located (see the following section).

APPROVAL AND ACCREDITATION

Each state has a board of nursing composed of nurses, consumers, and others interested in health care. As part of their responsibility for safeguarding the well-being of their constituents, the various state boards of nursing evaluate and approve nursing education programs within their state. Schools or organizations offering nursing programs must have the approval of the state board of nursing to operate nursing education programs. Part of the approval process includes meeting specific regulations governing the length (in hours) of nursing education programs. Graduation from a state-approved nursing school is one of the prerequisites for taking the nurse licensing examinations.

✔ *Program approval is mandatory; accreditation is voluntary.*

In addition to mandatory approval by the state board of nursing, many practical/vocational nursing schools voluntarily seek accreditation from the ACEN. The key words "approval" and "accreditation" are essential to understanding the difference between the purpose of the state board of nursing and the purpose of the ACEN. Approval by the state board of nursing is mandatory; accreditation is voluntary.

The ACEN maintains a list of accredited practical/vocational nursing schools on their Web site; each state board of nursing maintains a list of approved practical/vocational nursing schools on their Web sites.

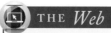 THE *Web*

The Accreditation Commission for Education in Nursing Web site provides a list of ACEN-accredited nursing schools.

Accreditation of a practical/vocational nursing program by the ACEN is often an indication that a particular educational program exceeds minimum requirements. This doesn't imply, however, that programs not accredited by the ACEN don't exceed minimum standards established by a state board of nursing. Because the accreditation process is voluntary, some schools, for their own unique reasons, don't seek ACEN accreditation. The nonaccredited program may

ASSESS YOURSELF	**Are You Ready for Distance Learning?**

To help you decide if you are ready to take a distance learning course, answer the following questions about your computer skills and learning style. Be honest with yourself. Enrolling in a course that is not right for you can be a costly mistake.

PART I		**Computer-Related Questions**
Yes ☐	No ☐	Can you install software on your computer?
Yes ☐	No ☐	Do you have access to the World Wide Web (www)?
Yes ☐	No ☐	Do you know the monthly cost to you for accessing the www?
Yes ☐	No ☐	Can you send and receive e-mail?
Yes ☐	No ☐	Can you create, save, and move files on your computer?
Yes ☐	No ☐	Can you attach a file to an e-mail message?
Yes ☐	No ☐	Can you open a file sent to you by e-mail?
Yes ☐	No ☐	Can you copy and paste text from a word processing application into an e-mail message?
Yes ☐	No ☐	Can you run the applications required in the courses you are registering for?
Yes ☐	No ☐	Can you use video conferencing on your computer?

If you answered "No" to any of these questions, you should learn how to perform all these functions before enrolling in a distance learning course.

PART II		**Learning Style Questions**
Yes ☐	No ☐	Are you able to follow written instructions?
Yes ☐	No ☐	Are you able to learn best from reading books, journals, and Web site documents?
Yes ☐	No ☐	Are you able to manage your time and meet deadlines on your own?
Yes ☐	No ☐	Are you able to list learning priorities and stick to the list?
Yes ☐	No ☐	Are you able to complete work without direct supervision?
Yes ☐	No ☐	Are you able to find answers to most questions on your own?
Yes ☐	No ☐	Are you a self-directed and fairly independent learner?

If you answered "Yes" to all of the questions in Part I and "Yes" to at least five of the questions in Part II, you will probably do well in a distance learning course. If you answered "Yes" to all of the questions in Part I and "No" to three or more questions in Part II, you should probably enroll in a course that meets with a teacher on a regular basis.

exceed minimum standards by far and may offer an outstanding educational program. One must be careful when using the term *approval*, which is required, and the term *accreditation*, which is voluntary, when discussing nursing education programs.

Your school may be scheduled for a program review by the state board of nursing or the ACEN during the time you're enrolled. Having an approval or accreditation visit is an important process and one in which your participation will be expected.

ORGANIZATIONS

Organizations are groups created for a specific purpose. You can probably think of many examples.

Organizations require bylaws and procedural rules (rules of order) if their stated purpose is to be met. Meetings also follow established procedures or run the risk of accomplishing nothing. Meetings generally follow recognized rules of order, the most familiar being Robert's Rules of Order (see "Read More About It" at the end of this chapter). These rules define the duties and responsibilities of the officers and organize discussion, vote taking, and other procedures. Minutes, which are detailed notes of the business conducted in a meeting, become a permanent record of an organization's meetings.

Two types of organizations are important to you as a nursing student: student organizations and nursing organizations. Nursing organizations are discussed in Chapter 14.

Student Organizations

Your nursing program may be an integral part of a larger institution, or it may be small and independent. The type, complexity, and size of its student government will reflect the nature of its affiliation. A program that is a part of a college, for example, must consider the regulations that apply to living on campus, whereas a vocational school program with only day students need not. The bylaws of the student governments of each will be either complex or simple, according to the needs and purposes of the group.

A student council is the most common form of student organization. It is a group made up of student and faculty members who serve as representatives of the student body to the sponsoring organization. Student members are elected by the student body. A faculty member elected by the student body serves as adviser to the student council.

The student council's function is to make recommendations to the sponsoring organization on matters affecting students, such as the rules that govern students; their social, recreational, and extracurricular activities; and student discipline. The council also serves as a disciplinary board for infractions of school regulations. The precise manner in which each council operates is set by its bylaws. Secure a copy of your student council's bylaws and read them, because they relate directly to your student life.

Involvement with your student council or government is an opportunity for you to have a voice in the daily affairs of your education and a chance to learn and exercise leadership skills. Involvement doesn't mean that you must be on the council. It means participating as an active, interested member of a student body with a common goal. It can also mean volunteering to be on special committees.

✔ *HOSA is a national organization for students enrolled in health occupations programs.*

Nursing students in programs sponsored by larger organizations may have an opportunity to join other student organizations. These other organizations may emphasize politics, photography, journalism, or drama, to name a few possibilities.

One student organization of interest to practical/vocational nursing students is Health Occupations Students of America (HOSA). HOSA is a national organization with state affiliations and local chapters in secondary and postsecondary schools that offer courses in the field of health care and related services.

The purpose of this organization, which held its first convention in 1976, is to assist students in developing vocational understanding, an awareness of social intelligence, civic consciousness, and leadership skills. HOSA chapter members participate in local, state, and national competitions in health-related areas.

If your school doesn't have a HOSA chapter, you might want to ask your faculty to consider sponsoring this worthwhile activity. Details on how to begin your own chapter are available from the national HOSA office.

Alumni Associations

If your program or school has an alumni (graduates) association, you and your classmates will have the opportunity to join other graduates of your program or school after graduation. By becoming active, you can keep in touch with one another and with the activities, programs, and progress of the school. Your experience will become valuable to those who follow you, just as the suggestions and help of those who have gone before you have been of benefit to your education.

Keeping in touch with your school and classmates can also provide you with networking opportunities and access to continuing education programs, job opportunities, information on advances and changes in practical/vocational nursing, and other developments of special interest to you.

Professional Organizations

The National Federation of Licensed Practical Nurses, Inc. (NFLPN) is a national professional membership organization for student and graduate practical and vocational nurses. This organization fosters high standards of nursing care and promotes continued competence through education and certification NFLPN sponsors student chapters as well as the NFLPN Student Honor Society Achievement Awards program.

The National Association for Practical Nurse Education and Service (NAPNES) is a national professional organization that admits to membership anyone interested in promoting practical/ vocational nursing. The Education division provides resources for practical/vocational nurse educators, it provides resources for continuing education, and it publishes educational standards.

A number of states as well as several Canadian provinces have LP/VN organizations that include students. Additional organizations to consider are the National League for Nursing, the American Assembly for Men in Nursing, the National Association of Hispanic Nurses, the Nurses Christian Fellowship, the National Black Nurses Association, and many, many more.

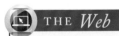 THE *Web*

> Use the search phrase—*list of professional nursing organizations*—to find several sites that list national nursing organizations.

The organization(s) that you choose to join should help you create relationships that will assist you in achieving your professional goals. Membership usually provides career resources, networking opportunities, and access to career-oriented workshops and conferences. It also provides opportunities for you to develop leadership skills through committee activities. Take advantage of all of the benefits of membership in whatever organization you choose.

STANDARDS FOR THE LICENSED PRACTICAL/ VOCATIONAL NURSE

Two national organizations are primarily concerned with the practice of practical nursing. Membership in the National Federation of Licensed Practical Nurses (NFLPN) is open only to licensed and student practical/vocational nurses. The National Association for Practical Nurse Education and Service (NAPNES) accepts for membership anyone interested in promoting the practice of practical/ vocational nursing. Both NFLPN and NAPNES have issued statements defining the standard of nursing that the public can expect from an LP/VN.

✔ *Practice standards outline what is expected from members of an occupation.*

In 1970, the NFLPN approved the "Statement of Functions and Qualifications of the Licensed Practical Nurse," which was written to help clarify the responsibilities of an LP/VN. It was revised in 1972 and again in 1979. In 1987, that statement was replaced by a new statement titled "Nursing Practice Standards for the Licensed Practical/Vocational Nurse."

The most recently revised NFLPN statement defining LP/VN nursing practice standards was published in 1991. This document basically outlines the standards of performance expected of LP/VNs in the areas of education, legal and ethical status, practice, continuing education, and specialized nursing practice. The full text of this statement appears in Appendix B.

NAPNES has set the standards for nursing practice of LP/VNs since 1941. The most recently revised "Standards of Practice and Educational Competencies of Graduates of Practical/Vocational Nursing Programs" was issued in 2007. The full text of the NAPNES Standards appears in Appendix C. The NAPNES Standards outline the professional behaviors and competencies in communication, assessment, planning, caring interventions, and managing that are expected of graduates of LP/VN programs.

JOB RESPONSIBILITIES OF THE LICENSED PRACTICAL/ VOCATIONAL NURSE

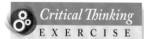

Critical Thinking
E X E R C I S E

Why is it important to know about these standards, and what is their relationship to your practice as a practical or vocational nurse? Use appropriate Characteristics of Critical Thinkers in Box 1-2 on pages 18–19 to develop your response to this situation.

The broad objective of a practical/vocational nursing education is to prepare students to pass the practical/vocational nursing licensing examination and to become competent nurses who possess certain entry or beginning nursing knowledge and skills. As graduates gain experience and acquire new skills, job responsibilities increase. Whereas job responsibilities change and increase, there are limits on what the LP/VN is permitted to do.

Each state has nurse practice acts and laws governing the practice of nursing. Based on these acts or laws, state boards of nursing issue guidelines or administrative rules that further define the role and function and job responsibilities of an LP/VN in that state. Some state associations of education also define entry-level nursing competencies.

✔ *Job responsibilities vary widely across employers and across the country.*

Within the limits of the law, job responsibilities vary according to employer or institution policies regarding the LP/VN's role. Some institutions permit LP/VNs to start intravenous therapy; others do not. Some permit LP/VNs to care for critically ill patients; others do not. It is important for the LP/VNs to know the skills they are expected to perform (Fig. 4-1).

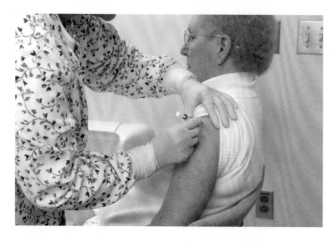

FIGURE 4-1. ● Giving injections is one of the skills performed by LP/VNs.

BOX 4-1 Partial List of Procedures Performed by Beginning LP/VNs

Admit patients.
Assist in transferring and discharging patients.
Help patients with bathing.
Help patients ambulate.
Assist adults, children, and infants with feedings and meals.
Perform range-of-motion exercises.
Maintain traction.
Assist in positioning patients in bed.
Care for dying patients and their families.
Provide skin care.
Care for ostomy sites.
Give enemas.
Perform urinary catheterizations.
Monitor oxygen therapy.
Supervise coughing and deep breathing exercises.
Teach and supervise postural drainage.
Perform nasopharyngeal and endotracheal suctioning.
Obtain specimens.
Perform cardiopulmonary resuscitation.
Administer compresses, sitz baths, and therapeutic baths.
Measure temperature, pulse, respiration, and blood pressure.
Provide preoperative and postoperative care.
Administer oral, injectable, and intravenous medications.
Care for patients with infectious diseases.
Assist patients in elimination needs.
Assess neurologic status.
Document nursing care on patients' records.
Contribute to patient care conferences and nursing care plans.
Check emergency equipment and supplies.
Initiate, administer, and monitor intravenous therapy.
Administer skin tests.
Collect venous blood samples.
Use the nursing process to administer care.
Apply sterile dressings.

Some of the procedures that a newly licensed LP/VN may be expected to perform are listed in Box 4-1. With experience and continuing education, the number and complexity of nursing procedures increase.

The range of specific nursing services and job responsibilities provided by practical/vocational nurses is extensive and continues to grow as the increasingly sophisticated and specialized field of health care keeps up with discoveries in science and technology and the needs of an ever-changing population.

 THE *Web*

Go to the NCSBN Web site and use the search term "Nurse Practice Acts" to get the latest information on LP/VN beginning skills.

The National Council of State Boards of Nursing (NCSBN) collects information about the beginning skills required of newly LP/LNs every 3 years. In addition to publishing these findings on their Web site, they use the information to develop the National Council Licensure Examination for Practical Nurses (NCLEX-PN) licensing examination.

LICENSING

One of the major goals of your practical/vocational nursing program is to prepare you to pass the licensing examination. This examination measures your knowledge of nursing practice in a number of areas and requires that you retain information you were taught during your entire educational program. Many graduates spend some time reviewing their textbooks and notes before taking the licensing examination. Even though the examination can be taken more than once, you and your faculty expect that you will pass the licensure examination on your first attempt.

The laws governing who qualifies to be licensed as an LP/VN are set by each state, but the trend is toward uniformity in all states. Most states require that an applicant be a graduate of a state-approved practical/vocational nursing program. The director of the school of practical/vocational nursing may be required to sign an application for licensure for each graduate who has met all of the objectives of the school's program. The director's signature on the application indicates to the state board of nursing that the candidate for licensure has met the theoretical and clinical requirements of that school and is considered to be ready to enter the practice of practical/vocational nursing. In some states, an official transcript must be submitted with the application. State boards of nursing charge a licensure application fee that in most cases must be paid by the applicant.

Originally, each state had its own licensing exam. Today, however, there is one licensing examination for practical/vocational nurses in all states. This examination is developed by the NCSBN and is called the NCLEX-PN. The NCLEX-PN is discussed in detail in Chapter 5.

The testing agency provides each state board of nursing with a list of people who have passed or failed the NCLEX-PN. The state board of nursing then determines who will be issued a license as a practical or vocational nurse. In general, state boards of nursing will not issue a nursing license to a person who has been convicted of certain crimes, is mentally ill, or is addicted to drugs or alcohol.

Legal Title

The legal title granted when a person successfully passes the licensing examination is either an LPN or, in California and Texas, an LVN. The words practical and vocational have the same meaning in this context, but California and Texas chose to use the word vocational in their original Nurse Practice Acts, whereas all the other states chose to use the word "practical." A license entitles the holder to enter the practice of practical/vocational nursing as described by the state. Persons holding a license have demonstrated to the issuing authority (state board) that they have the knowledge and ability to provide the minimal safe practices required to fulfill the duties of a practical or vocational nurse in that state.

A license belongs only to the person it is issued to. It can't be transferred to anyone else for any reason. The unqualified use of a license can lead to legal prosecution. Reporting anyone known to be practicing without a license preserves the integrity of the license and the licensing procedure, protects the investment of the license holder, and guards unknowing consumers from potentially dangerous care. Fifty boards of nursing mandate reporting of nurse practice act/administrative rules violations.

✔ *State laws determine who will be issued a nursing license.*

✔ *The NCLEX-PN is the name of the practical/ vocational nurse licensing examination.*

✔ *Report fraudulent use of a nursing license to your state board of nursing.*

All states require practical/vocational nurses to be licensed before they can practice. Called mandatory licensing, this requirement helps to keep unqualified persons out of the health care system. Mandatory licensing protects the public from untrained people and upholds nursing standards set by law and nursing organizations.

✔ *It is illegal to practice nursing without a license.*

Boards of Nursing

Laws that govern nursing, including nurse licensing, are called nurse practice acts or administrative rules. The nurse practice acts or administrative rules of each state are administered by boards called by various names, such as Board of Nursing, Board of Nurse Examiners, or Nurse Registration Board.

The Boards of Nursing have the authority to issue licenses and the right to revoke or suspend them for a variety of reasons. This authority protects patients and nurses alike by eliminating those who are incompetent or unfit for practice. The standing of practical/vocational nurses is upheld when all members of the group must meet the same high standards.

✔ *The nursing license is issued by the state in which the nurse practices nursing.*

The license gives legal authorization to perform (permission to practice) the skills learned in the practical/vocational nursing program. A license must be kept current. It is a violation of the nurse practice act or administrative rules to continue to practice after a license has expired or been revoked.

A nursing license must be renewed periodically as required by that state's regulations. Four states require renewal every year, while most states require renewal every 2 years. Two states require renewal every 3 years, and Arizona requires renewal every 4 years. At least 44 states require licensees to provide proof of acceptable continuing education before a license can be renewed.

✔ *State boards of nursing are responsible for protecting the safety and welfare of people who receive nursing service in their state.*

There are 59 boards of nursing in the United States; there are boards in each state, one in the District of Columbia, and four in US territories (the Virgin Islands, American Samoa, Guam, and the Northern Mariana Islands). The three states that have two boards, one for RNs and one for PN/VNs, are California, Louisiana, and West Virginia. One state, Nebraska, has both the board of nursing and the board for advanced practices nurses.

Board members include experienced nurses as well as consumers. The primary way to become a board member is to be appointed by an elected official, an elected body, or both. For example, state governors appoint the members of 33 nursing boards. Governors, with the confirmation of their Senates, appoint the members of 18 nursing boards. The board members of the District of Columbia nursing board are appointed by the mayor with the advice and consent of city council, whereas members of the North Carolina nursing board are elected by nurses in a general election. The number of members on each board varies from 7 in Georgia, New Mexico, West Virginia, Iowa, Guam, Wyoming, and Nevada to a maximum of 25 in New York. The average number of board members is 14.

These boards of nursing operate under their own state laws but cooperate with one another and belong to the NCSBN—the organization that develops the licensure examinations. State boards of nursing are authorized to perform certain duties. Some of these duties include evaluating nursing program curricula and developing nursing standards; approving nursing schools; issuing, renewing, and endorsing licenses; and initiating disciplinary actions, such as license suspension or revocation. Anyone found in violation of the state's nurse practice act is subject to investigation and prosecution by the state board. You can learn more about your state board of nursing on their Web site.

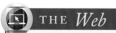

THE *Web*

To learn more about licensing, visit the National Council of State Boards of Nursing and your own state board of nursing Web sites.

Licensure by Endorsement

All LP/VNs must be licensed by the state in which they practice. Licensed nurses who move to or want to work in a state in which they aren't licensed must apply for a license in that state. Obtaining a license in another state without taking the licensing exam again is termed *licensure by endorsement*. In most cases, this process must be completed before the nurse can work in that state. You can obtain the information you need on how to apply for licensure in another state through the Web site or by writing to the state board of nursing in the state in which you want to work.

Nurse Licensure Compact

✔ *Proponents of the NLC believe multistate licensure for nurses would help resolve licensing issues for those who work in neighboring states or are involved in interstate work.*

In a special session of the Delegate Assembly of the NCSBN held in Chicago in December 1998, the delegates approved the proposed language for the Nurse Licensure Compact (NLC). The NLC refers to the legal agreement or compact between states to recognize a nurse's license in another state. This compact between states is referred to as mutual recognition, interstate practice, or multi-state licensure.

The nurse whose primary state of residence is a compact state will be issued a license by that state and will no longer need an additional license to practice in another compact state. The licensee is granted multistate privileges to practice nursing in other compact states. A nursing license issued by a noncompact state is valid only in the state in which it was issued.

The RN and LP/VN compact to allow multistate licensure began in January 1, 2000, in Maryland, Texas, Utah, and Wisconsin. Since then, 20 more states have enacted compact legislation. Connecticut, Massachusetts. Minnesota, Illinois, Montana, New York, Georgia, and New Jersey either submitted or have pending legislation to join the NLC but are not yet members. If you reside in a state that has not passed compact legislation, you might want to get involved in the process of getting legislation through your state board of nursing and your state legislators. The NCSBN Web site provides a list of states that are partici-pating in the NLC.

People who support this action say that it will reduce many of the real or perceived barriers to health care while continuing to protect the public health, safety, and welfare. The number of nurses involved in interstate telemedicine has increased, many nurses travel across state lines to work, many nurses move from one state to another in relatively short periods of time, and there are travel nurses who relocate every few months. Proponents say that a national nursing license would benefit both consumers and nurses.

✔ *Opponents of multistate licensing believe that it may be difficult to discover disciplinary sanctions on a licensee.*

Opponents of the NLC say that the compact requires states to uncondition-ally accept the licensure standards of other states, which include educational preparation, clinical experience, and licensing examination scores. Continuing education and practice requirements for license renewal vary widely from state to state. State laws also vary with regard to treatment of various offenses, so there are disciplinary jurisdiction issues. The ability to oversee standards of practice, and therefore protect consumers, could be reduced by not being the state that issued the original nursing license.

The NLC is an issue that could have an impact on you at some time in the future. You should keep informed of the pros and cons of this issue so you are prepared to support or oppose the participation of your state in this licensing arrangement.

Disciplinary Sanctions

State boards of nursing, through nursing practice acts, have the authority to suspend or revoke nursing licenses for just cause. A nursing license can be revoked or suspended when the board of nursing finds a licensee guilty of an offense. Examples of offenses include the following:

- Certain mental or physical illnesses
- Conviction of a felony
- Fraud or deceit in obtaining a license
- Conviction of a crime involving moral turpitude or gross immorality
- Willful neglect of a patient
- Negligence
- Habitual use of or chemical dependence on drugs or alcohol
- Violations of the nurse practice laws of the state
- Suspended or revoked license in another state

A nurse whose right to practice is being questioned must first be notified of the charges by the state board and must be given a hearing in which to enter a defense, either in person or through an attorney, before his or her license can be revoked or suspended.

In addition to revoking and suspending practical/vocational nursing licenses, the state board of nursing can also, for just cause, issue letters of reprimand, refuse to issue or renew a license, or place a licensee on probation.

Almost all state boards of nursing have a formal rehabilitation program for nurses who risk losing their licenses. These programs, often called *Impaired Nurse Programs*, are individually prescribed programs for recovery. If the nurse successfully completes all program requirements, he or she will be permitted to retain his or her license. If he or she does not comply with all of the requirements for rehabilitation, then the license will be revoked.

Licensees should be aware that federal law requires state licensing boards to comply with various reporting requirements of the Health Insurance Portability and Accountability Act of 1996. That law established the National Practitioner Data Bank and the Healthcare Integrity and Protection Data Bank (HIPDA). Those two agencies merged in May 2013 and became the National Practitioner Data Bank. This national health care fraud and abuse data collection agency is one to which all state health licensing boards are required to report final adverse actions imposed on health care providers, suppliers, or practitioners. You can explore the functions of the NPDB on their Web site.

SUMMARY

Your educational program will prepare you to take and pass the practical/vocational nursing licensing examination. After you pass this exam, you will be legally permitted to use the letters "LPN" or "LVN" after your name. Your license to practice practical/vocational nursing is a valuable document. Always conduct yourself in a manner consistent with the standards and ethics of your profession; doing so will ensure you a long and rewarding career as an LP/VN.

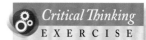

Critical Thinking
EXERCISE

You have been asked to give a 2-minute presentation on why you do (or do not) support the NLC. How would you respond? And why? Use appropriate Characteristics of Critical Thinkers in Box 1-2 on pages 18–19 to develop your response to this question.

✔ *Nursing licenses can be suspended or revoked.*

✔ *Protect the integrity of your nursing license by actively participating in organizations that support the practice of practical/ vocational nursing.*

APPLY
Critical Thinking Skills

1. In the opening story at the beginning of this chapter, Terri is a school nurse. Do school districts in your state hire LP/VNs to work as school nurses? (Hint: Most school districts have Web sites and post job opportunities on these sites.)

2. What is the name of the agency that approves your practical/vocational nursing program?

3. What is the name of the agency that accredits your practical/vocational nursing program?

4. Go to your state board of nursing Web site and read the rules and regulations governing the practice of practical/vocational nursing.

5. Review the bylaws of your student organization if you have one. Do they clearly state the purpose of the organization and its rules of operation? Should the bylaws be revised?

6. Discuss with your classmates how the standards published by the NFLPN or NAPNES may affect your nursing practice.

7. How do you think you might handle a situation in which you're asked to complete nursing tasks you're not legally permitted to perform?

8. How might you handle a situation in which you observe a nurse (either an RN or an LP/VN) working while obviously chemically impaired? Does your state board of nursing offer anonymous reporting of impaired nurses?

9. You have read in the local newspaper that a nurse has been convicted of child abuse. Do you inform your state board of nursing? Give the reasons for your answer.

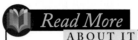

Read More
ABOUT IT

Boards of Nursing: Available at https://www.ncsbn.org. Chicago, IL; National Council of State Boards of Nursing, 2015.

Department of Labor: Bureau of Labor Statistics. Available at: http://www.bls.gov/home.htm

deWit SC: Saunders Student Nurse Planner: A Guide to Success in Nursing School, 10th ed. Philadelphia, PA: Saunders, 2014.

Ellis JR, Hartley CL: Nursing in Today's World: Trends, Issues, and Management, 10th ed. Philadelphia, PA: Lippincott Williams & Wilkins, 2012.

Harrington N, et al.: LPN to RN Transitions: Achieving Success in Your New Role, 4th ed. Philadelphia, PA: Lippincott Williams & Wilkins, 2012.

Kalisch PA, Kalisch BJ: The Advance of American Nursing, 3rd ed. Philadelphia, PA: Lippincott Williams & Wilkins, 1995.

NLN Data Review™: Available at http://www.nln.org. New York, NY: National League for Nursing, 2015.

Nursing 2015 Journal. Philadelphia, PA: Lippincott Williams & Wilkins, 2014.

Robert HM: Robert's Rules of Order: Document. Available at: http://www.robertsrules.org

Watkins R, Corry M: E-Learning Companion: Student's Guide to On-line Success, 4th ed. Florence, KY: Cengage, 2013.

The NCLEX-PN®

CHAPTER CONTENTS

LEARNING OBJECTIVES

When you complete this chapter, you will be able to:

1. Explain the concept of computerized adaptive testing (CAT).

2. Describe the function of NCLEX item writers and item reviewers.

3. Outline the NCLEX-PN® test plan.

4. Follow NCLEX-PN® application procedures.

5. Comply with test center regulations.

6. Assess your level of test anxiety.

7. Evaluate the quality of NCLEX-PN® review materials.

It was a bright, sunny day, and Sharon was looking forward to getting to her practical nursing classes. She had just finished 3 weeks of school, and so far, she was doing quite well. The bus arrived at her bus stop on time, and she reviewed her notes on the way to class. There was so much to remember; she often wondered if she would be able to remember everything.

Sharon arrived at her Issues and Trends class a few minutes before it was scheduled to begin, so she started talking with some of her classmates. "Did you know that the examination we have to take to get our license covers everything we're going to learn this year?" she asked Rodney.

"No," he said, "who told you that?"

"I was reading about the exam last night in one of our textbooks. And, we take the test on a computer."

"I'm not very good with the computer," said Monica. "I'll never be able to pass a test on the computer."

Karen joined in the conversation. "I was reading about the test too and it makes me very nervous. I just know that I'll never get my license."

With that, Mr. Carlson, the teacher, entered the room. "Why don't you all take your seats so we can get started. I think I can make you feel better about the exam."

It is probably fair to say that all students who are enrolled in a nursing program expect to obtain a nursing license after graduation. You might say that it's too early in your education to be thinking about something that is not going to happen for many months. But now is the time to begin preparing for the exam. If you wait until the end of your nursing program, it will be too late. The more you know now about the exam and the procedures for taking it, the better you can prepare yourself every day for what is possibly the most significant test you will ever take. Going to your state board of nursing Web site or opening your mailbox and getting the letter that says that you passed the licensing examination will be a moment in your life that you will never forget.

✔ *Finding out that you passed the licensing exam is a moment you will never forget.*

The licensing examination for practical and vocational nurses is called the National Council Licensure Examination for Practical/Vocational Nurses (NCLEX-PN). Before April 1994, the NCLEX-PN® written examination was given only in April and October. Since April 1, 1994, the NCLEX for licensure as a registered nurse or a practical/vocational nurse has been administered by computer at a local test center.

COMPUTERIZED ADAPTIVE TESTING

✔ *CAT testing is more reliable, and results are available much quicker than paper-and-pencil tests.*

Computerized adaptive testing (CAT) is a term used to describe not only the technology (the computer) used to give an examination but also the theory that is used to make sure the test is accurate and measures what it is supposed to measure.

A CAT exam is administered at a computer terminal. Students begin testing at different times, and students in the testing room may be taking entirely different tests on totally different subjects. Some tests have a time limit, and others have a number-of-questions limit. Some tests have both limits.

The NCLEX-PN® has a limit on both. A practical/vocational nursing school graduate taking the NCLEX-PN® has 5 hours in which to answer a maximum of 205 questions. At the end of 5 hours and/or 205 questions, the computer will shut off. The developers of the test suggest that students spend 1–2 minutes on each question.

When taking a CAT exam, you must answer every question you are given, even if you have to guess on some of the answers. You can't go back to review previous questions or change answers. The way the CAT exam works is as follows: You are given the first question. If you choose the correct answer, you get a slightly more difficult question. If you choose an incorrect answer, you get a slightly less difficult question. Whether you pass the test depends not on how many questions you answer correctly, but on how many of the more difficult questions you answer correctly.

✔ You must answer every question you are given on the NCLEX-PN® exam.

After you have answered the minimum number of questions, which is 85, the computer compares your performance to the passing standard and makes one of three decisions. In the first case, if you're clearly above the passing standard, you pass the exam and the computer shuts off. In the second case, if you're clearly below the passing standard, the computer shuts off and you fail the examination. In the third case, you're close to the passing standard but it's not clear whether you pass or fail. In this case, the computer continues to give you questions until it's clear that your knowledge is sufficient for you to pass the test or insufficient and you fail the test.

Items are selected from a very large pool of questions based on the NCLEX-PN® Test Plan. The computer will select questions for you based on your performance on the previous question. For you to pass the exam and be eligible for a license, about half of the questions you answer correctly must be in the "difficult" category.

Each person completes a different examination with different questions and different numbers of questions. Computer programming permits incorporating measurement theory and statistical analysis during the examination, making the test fair to everyone who takes it.

Each NCLEX-PN® examination candidate will be given a tutorial before starting the examination. The tutorial explains how to use the computer, how to use the mouse, and how to use the on-screen optional calculator.

✔ Each person gets different questions on the NCLEX-PN®.

Test items are presented in a variety of formats. There are multiple-choice items that require one response, and there are multiple-choice items that require more than one response. There are items that require you to fill in the blank with correctly calculated answers, and there are test items that require you to identify a hot spot on a drawing or diagram. There are items that use a chart or exhibit that contains information to be used in selecting an answer. There are audio items in which headphones are used to listen to an audio clip that is used to select an answer. There are graphic answer options where you select the correct answer from a graphic. There are also drag-and-drop or ordered response questions that require you to put responses in a specific order. The National Council of State Boards of Nursing (NCSBN) Web site provides detailed information, including sample test questions, in the Examination Candidate Bulletin.

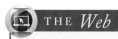 THE *Web*

Both the National Council of State Boards of Nursing and Pearson VUE (the exam administrators) provide samples of the format of the NCLEX-PN® questions on the Web sites.

DEVELOPMENT OF THE NCLEX-PN®

The NCSBN is the organization that is responsible for the development of actual test questions and the procedures associated with taking the examination. The National Council Examination Committee, the Item Review Subcommittee, the National Council staff, and a commercial testing service are all involved in developing and administering the examination.

The NCSBN Examination Committee, composed of at least nine members, oversees the development and administration of the exam. The committee is composed of representatives from different state boards of nursing. One or more of the members of this committee must be a licensed practical or vocational nurse.

The Item Development Panel is part of the Examination Committee and is composed of hundreds of volunteer nurses. These Panel members meet for 3 or 4 days each year and spend their time writing hundreds of test questions. This panel includes practical and vocational nurses as item writers and item reviewers. After you get your license and work for at least a year, you might want to apply for a position on the Item Development Panel. You can get further information at the NCSBN Web site or by writing to the NCSBN. This is a worthwhile activity as well as an outstanding learning opportunity.

✔ *Licensed vocational nurses and licensed practical nurses help write the actual NCLEX-PN® test questions.*

The NCLEX Sensitivity Panel looks for wording of questions that could be considered elitist or stereotypical or have different meaning for different ethnic, gender, or geographic groups or have inappropriate tone. The Differential Item Functioning (DIF) statistical data are used to assess potential testing bias of every test item. If a question is found to be biased through a Sensitivity Panel review or the sophisticated DIF statistical analysis, that question is removed from the pool of NCLEX questions.

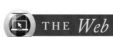
THE *Web*

Visit the National Council of State Boards of Nursing Web site to learn more about how to become a NCLEX-PN® item writer.

The Item Review Subcommittee reviews all of the questions written by the Item Development Panels. This Committee also evaluates actual candidate examinations in relation to a variety of criteria.

The National Council staff is composed of a number of people who work every day on tasks related to the development of the examination. These people are specialists in testing and research, nursing content, and administrative details. These experts make sure the examination conforms to all accepted procedures.

The NCSBN contracts with a commercial testing service to administer the computer-based NCLEX examinations. This testing service manages test-site security, test-site monitors, computers, and networks, and it sends reports of test scores to the NCSBN.

THE NCLEX-PN® TEST PLAN

The questions for the NCLEX-PN® examination are based on the NCLEX-PN® Test Plan, which is developed with an understanding of what a beginning practical or vocational nurse needs to know to be a competent and safe practitioner. This knowledge is accumulated through a survey of entry-level job skills that is conducted every 3 years. The survey is sent to recent practical or vocational

TABLE 5-1 NCLEX-PN® Test Plan Effective April 1, 2014 Through March 31, 2017	
Categories of Client Needs	**Percentage of Questions**
A. Safe, effective care environment	
1. Coordinated care	16%–22%
2. Safety and infection control	10%–16%
B. Health promotion and maintenance	7%–13%
C. Psychosocial integrity	8%–14%
D. Physiologic integrity	
1. Basic care and comfort	7%–13%
2. Pharmacological therapies	11%–17%
3. Reduction of risk potential	10%–16%
4. Physiologic adaptation	7%–13%

nurse graduates, so if you receive one in the mail, it is important for you to complete it to the best of your ability. The results of this survey are used to revise the Test Plan.

✔ *The NCLEX-PN® Test Plan is a must-have document.*

The NCLEX-PN® Test Plan is like a blueprint. It outlines what percentage of questions will be asked for each Category of Client Needs. Table 5-1 lists the percentage of questions that will be asked for each category. The nursing process (clinical problem solving), caring, communication and documentation, and teaching and learning are integrated within all questions throughout the examination. A publication titled NCLEX-PN® Test Plan provides valuable details about the content of the examination. This document is updated every 3 years and

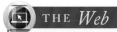 **THE** *Web*

> The National Council of State Boards of Nursing provides the Test Plan for the NCLEX-PN® examination on their Web site.

✔ *Use the NCLEX-PN® Test Plan to guide your studies.*

is available from the NCSBN Web site under the heading NCLEX Examinations.

After reviewing the Categories of Client Needs and the content areas on the NCLEX-PN®, you are probably beginning to see why knowing all of this information about the licensing examination now is so important. You will be expected to retain information you are learning now for many months and years to come.

✔ *Now is the time to begin preparing for the NCLEX-PN® licensing exam.*

The best way to retain what you are learning is to avoid cramming for an exam. Retention of information occurs best through repetition. When you learn something, use it in as many settings and situations as you can. Connect classroom learning with clinical assignments and specific patients. Welcome questions from your instructors; get together with classmates to question and think about what you are learning. Ask questions, discover relationships between concepts, memorize what must be memorized, and then apply it in appropriate situations. Preparation for a licensing examination begins long before you are scheduled for the test.

REVIEWING FOR THE NCLEX-PN®

Your teachers know what you need to learn in your nursing program, and they will do everything they can to be sure you are prepared for the examination. Now is the time early in your nursing program to develop sound learning habits. Avoid cramming for examinations and practice applying classroom knowledge in the clinical setting.

✔ *Take the exam as soon as possible after you complete your nursing program.*

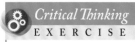

Critical Thinking
E X E R C I S E

You have always gotten by in school by cramming the night before a test and then promptly forgetting the information right after the exam. Now that you know you have to remember a lot of information for a long period of time, you are feeling very concerned. What can you do about your concerns? Use appropriate Characteristics of Critical Thinkers in Box 1-2 on pages 18–19 to develop your response to this question.

You are most likely to pass the NCLEX-PN® on your first attempt. You can increase your chances of passing the exam the first time by taking it as soon as possible after you complete the nursing program requirements. If you were a good student and if you were able to connect what you learned in class to the care of your patients in the clinical setting, you should do well on the NCLEX-PN® examination.

If you decide you should participate in a formal review program, discuss your plans with your teachers. They should be able to give you good advice on the quality of various books, courses, and mock tests.

Review Books

If you decide to prepare for the exam by using a review book, here are some guidelines that will help you avoid wasting time and money on materials that are inappropriate for your needs.

- The book should explain how the most recent NCLEX-PN® Test Plan is incorporated in the review content and questions.
- The test questions in the book should be based on the most recent NCLEX-PN® Test Plan.
- The book should contain questions in a variety of formats similar to those used in the actual NCLEX-PN® examination.
- Each question should provide an explanation of why the correct answer is correct and why incorrect answers are incorrect.
- The book should be published by a reputable nursing publishing company.
- The review book should be cross-referenced to popular practical nursing textbooks.
- The book should not have errors on the answer keys.

✔ *Choose review books carefully.*

You should be aware that Web sites with interactive questions that come with many of the review books are simply multiple-choice questions. They will help you feel comfortable with the computer. The NCLEX-PN® questions are highly confidential; therefore, you can't purchase a book that contains NCLEX-PN® questions. You can, however, purchase review books that feature NCLEX-PN-*style* questions and those books could assist you in preparing for the actual examination.

Review Courses

Review courses vary in length and quality, and they may be offered locally or online. When looking for a review course, be sure it's a review course and not additional lectures on the content you have already covered during your nursing program. Also, be sure the person who is teaching the course has experience in teaching in a practical nursing program and has advanced preparation in test construction.

✔ *Review courses can be costly.*

If you decide to enroll in a review course, here are some guidelines.

- Be sure you will get your money back if you aren't satisfied with the instruction or if you don't pass the exam.
- Don't pay excessive fees or buy more textbooks.
- Be sure you have direct contact with an instructor.
- Avoid courses taught through audiotapes. Most students don't do well with this type of instruction.

- Review the course outline before enrolling. Does the outline include what you think you need to review?
- The course should include homework and written assignments.
- The course should be able to meet your individual needs.
- Ask the opinion of someone who took the course.
- Ask the sponsor of the course to provide letters of recommendation from former schools and students.

The course that would help you most would be one in which you take a series of diagnostic tests. The teacher would then prescribe an individual plan of study and review.

Mock Examinations

Mock examinations that simulate the NCLEX-PN® are also available. Most don't achieve the level of sophistication of the NCLEX-PN®, but they do provide good practice. You will need a computer and, for some exams, access to the Internet.

If you decide to purchase a mock examination, here are some guidelines.
- The examination should not be extremely expensive.
- The examination should follow the current NCLEX-PN® Test Plan.
- A list of people who developed the exam, their educational credentials, and their types of employment should be provided by the publisher of the test.
- Be sure your computer system can run the software (mock examination).
- The publisher should describe how the mock examination simulates the NCLEX-PN®.
- You should get a diagnostic profile after you finish the examination.

Whatever materials you choose for your review—books, courses, or mock examinations—be sure they incorporate the most recent NCLEX-PN® Test Plan. Also be aware that a number of Web sites appear to be affiliated with the National Council of State Boards of Nursing when in fact they are not. If in doubt, look at the bottom of the page for "Contact Us" information for ownership of the site.

TEST ANXIETY

Almost all students experience some nervousness and anxiety when confronted with an examination. Because the NCLEX-PN® is such an important examination, you will probably feel more anxious than usual. A little anxiety improves performance; too much causes poor performance. The self-assessment test "How Serious Is Your Test Anxiety?" will help you learn more about your level of test anxiety.

If your score on the self-assessment is high or you believe you get overly anxious when taking a test, the following tips might help reduce your test anxiety.
- Develop a daily study schedule so you can **review**—not learn materials the night before the test.
- Know the areas that will be covered on the test.
- Know how many and what type of questions will be on the test.
- Study previous tests when possible.
- Take practice tests to get comfortable in timing yourself and sitting for a period of time.

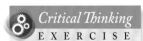

Critical Thinking
E X E R C I S E

It is near the end of your nursing program, and your friends are talking about taking an NCLEX-PN® review course at the local community college. The class meets two evenings a week from 6:00 pm to 9:00 pm for 8 weeks, and it costs $300. Your friends are telling you that you should register for the class because you will do better on the NCLEX-PN®. What is your decision and why? Use appropriate Characteristics of Critical Thinkers in Box 1-2 on pages 18–19 to develop your responses to this question.

✔ *Mock examinations do not reach the level of sophistication of the NCLEX-PN®.*

✔ *Some test anxiety is good; too much prevents you from showing what you know.*

ASSESS YOURSELF   How Serious Is Your Test Anxiety?

Read through each statement and reflect on past testing experiences. You may wish to consider all testing experiences or focus on one particular subject (history, science, math, etc.) at a time. Indicate how often each statement describes you by choosing a number from 1 (never) to 5 (always) as outlined below.

Never	Rarely	Sometimes	Often	Always
1	2	3	4	5

1. _____ I have visible signs of nervousness, such as sweaty palms and shaky hands, right before a test.
2. _____ I have "butterflies" in my stomach before a test.
3. _____ I feel nauseated before a test.
4. _____ I read through the test and feel that I do not know any of the answers.
5. _____ I panic before and during a test.
6. _____ My mind goes blank during a test.
7. _____ I remember answers that I blanked on once I get out of the testing situation.
8. _____ I have trouble sleeping the night before a test.
9. _____ I make mistakes on easy questions or put answers in the wrong places.
10. _____ I have difficulty choosing answers and read information into answers.
_____ **Total** (add your score.) Range is 10–50 points.

SCORING

10–19 points: You do not suffer from test anxiety. In fact, if your score was extremely low (close to 10), a little more anxiety may be healthy to keep you focused and to get your blood flowing during exams.

20–35 points: Although you do exhibit some of the characteristics of test anxiety, the level of stress and tension is probably healthy.

More than 35 points: You may be experiencing an unhealthy level of test anxiety. You should evaluate the reasons for the distress and identify strategies for compensating.

Adapted with permission from the Academic Learning Center, St. Cloud State University.

- Think positive thoughts about your knowledge of the material and your ability to take tests.
- Practice relaxation techniques such as deep breathing and alternating muscle contraction and relaxation during exams.
- Eat a light meal and avoid sugary drinks, caffeine, and other stimulants or depressants.
- Get plenty of regular sleep including the night before an exam.
- Arrive at the test site early enough to avoid the stress of possibly being late.
- Avoid talking with other students about what they "guess" will be on the test.
- Remember: You will not know the answer to some questions so don't let that destroy your confidence.
- The more you practice these techniques, the less anxious you will feel.

If you become overly anxious in testing situations and nothing seems to help you get the exam in perspective, you might want to consider professional counseling. Many psychologists specialize in helping students overcome serious test anxiety.

APPLICATION PROCEDURES

In order to take the NCLEX-PN® exam, you must complete an application. Near the end of your nursing education program, you will receive information on how to apply for the NCLEX-PN® in your state. The procedures and costs for applying for the NCLEX-PN® are very specific and exact, and they vary somewhat from state to state. The best advice is to follow the instructions from your school and your state board of nursing or to ask your teachers if you don't understand what you must do to apply for the examination.

THE *Web*

Details about the NCLEX-PN® examination, including a candidate hand-book, can be found at the National Council of State Boards of Nursing Web site.

It is critical that you use the same form of your name on all applications and that this name matches the photo identification (driver's license or passport) you intend to use for admission to the test center. In other words, if the name on your driver's license is Mary Elizabeth Connor, but everyone calls you Beth Connor, you must use your full name (Mary Elizabeth Connor) on your applications for licensure. Spelling, middle initial, date of birth, and address on your photo identification must exactly match what you put on your applications. If you need to correct your photo identification, now is the time to do it.

✔ *Use the same form of your name on all applications.*

Assuming that your applications are in order and accepted, you will receive an Authorization to Test card by e-mail. After you receive this card, you must follow the procedures for scheduling an appointment to take the test at the test center. First-time applicants must be scheduled for the NCLEX-PN® examination within 30 days from when they call to schedule a test. Repeat applicants must be scheduled for the exam within 45 days from when they call to schedule it. The Authorization to Test card has a range of validity dates; if the test is not taken within the validity dates, the candidate must submit another application and pay another fee.

If you need special accommodations because of a disability, you must request information from your state board of nursing about how to file a request. You should then file the completed request as soon as possible so the board can make a determination. The board will let you know what accommodations have been approved.

✔ *To get special testing accommodations, you must file a request with your state board of nursing.*

TEST CENTER REGULATIONS

Test center regulations are very strict and are designed to provide an appropriate testing environment as well as security for examination content. People who don't comply with test center regulations will not be admitted to the center or, if already admitted, will be removed (Fig. 5-1).

✔ *Test center regulations are strictly enforced.*

You will be required to present a valid acceptable ID. You will be asked to provide your digital signature, a palm vein scan, and you will have your photograph taken. You will be monitored by a video camera, an audio recording, and test center monitors.

You will be given note boards and pens that will be collected and counted when you finish the exam. The first optional break will be offered after 2 hours of testing; the second optional break will be offered after 3.5 hours of testing.

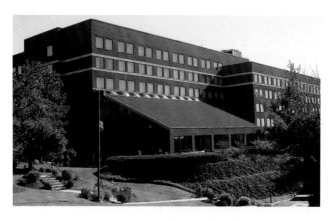

FIGURE 5-1. ● Knowing the exact location of the test center reduces test day stress.

✔ *Read all information you receive about testing procedures and rules.*

All breaks count against testing time. If you take one or both of these breaks, you must leave the testing room. A palm vein scan will be completed when you leave the room and again when you return. Test center staff will assist you with technical questions related to the computer; they can't assist you with answering examination questions.

The booklet you receive with your Authorization to Test card provides addresses to the Web sites that will tell you what you will need to know about testing procedures and about test center regulations. You should read the regulations carefully, so you feel comfortable about what to expect and what your responsibilities and rights are during the examination.

GETTING YOUR RESULTS

During the examination, the network to which your computer is connected scores your test. Your exam and score are then electronically transmitted to the commercial test service, where the results are verified. The test service then transmits your scores to your state board of nursing. The state board of nursing is the only agency that provides official examination results to candidates. Figure 5-2 illustrates the exam results process. It may take up to 6 weeks to after the examination to get your results from your board of nursing. Many state boards of nursing post information about licensed nurses within hours of receiving test results. Graduates often go to this Web site to find out if they were issued a license number. You can get "unofficial" results for a fee after 48 business hours through the quick results service available on the NCLEX Candidate Web site at www.pearsonvue.com/nclex.

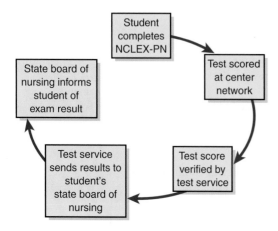

FIGURE 5-2. ● The process of getting NCLEX-PN® results.

RETAKING THE EXAMINATION

Just over 82% of all practical/vocational nursing school graduates passed the examination on the first attempt in 2014. However, if you don't pass on the first attempt, don't give up. Many things happen that prevent us from doing our best, and sometimes experience is a good teacher.

If you don't pass the examination, you will receive an NCLEX Candidate Performance Report (CPR). This is an individualized report that describes your performance on the content areas of the examination. Your performance is described as (1) above the passing standard, (2) near the passing standard, or (3) below the passing standard.

✔ *If you don't pass the NCLEX-PN®, use the CPR to determine where you need to improve.*

If you need to take the exam again, here are some things you can do to prepare for the next time.

- Ask one of your teachers to help you understand your CPR.
- Make a review plan based on your identified weaknesses.
- Read textbooks and review notes related to the content you need to review.
- Ask one of your teachers to recommend a review course or a review book.
- Practice answering questions similar to those on the NCLEX-PN®.

The NCSBN policy is that candidates must wait a minimum of 45 days between each examination. While boards of nursing comply with the 45-day rule, some boards require that candidates wait for as many as 90 days or more before being permitted to take a reexam.

SUMMARY

You will work hard during your nursing program to learn what you need to know to provide safe and compassionate nursing care. You will also work hard to acquire the knowledge you will need to pass the NCLEX-PN® licensing examination. Receiving your license will be the ultimate reward for all of your study and hard work.

APPLY

Critical Thinking Skills

1. In the opening story at the beginning of this chapter, Monica says she will never be able to pass the NCLEX-PN® exam on the computer because she is not very good with computers. What steps can she take to become better with computers?

2. Although it may be too early in your education to answer many of the questions on an NCLEX-PN® review test, go online or get a recently published review book and read some of the questions to get a feel for the kinds of questions you will be expected to answer.

3. Attempt to write test questions similar to those that you might find on the NCLEX-PN®. If you can't think of a topic, try writing questions that ask about infection control that also include something about cultural awareness.

4. Visit the Web site that describes the NCLEX-PN® examinations (www.ncsbn.org). Find information on how to become an NCLEX examination item developer.

5. Ask to see the actual application forms you will need to complete at the end of your program. Do you need to clarify your name or other important information with your school or state to properly complete the applications?

6. Talk with your classmates about test anxiety. What helps them relax before and during an exam? What kinds of things make your classmates feel more anxious?

7. Examine Web sites describing review books or review courses. What information is missing? Does it provide enough information for you to make a decision about its value?

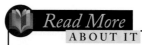
Read More
ABOUT IT

Anderson J: How to Cure Test Anxiety: Simple and Effective Strategies for Test-Stress Relief and Overcoming Exam Anxiety for Life [Kindle Edition]. Amazon Digital Services, Inc., 2013.

Elsevier: Elsevier Adaptive Quizzing for the NCLEX-PN Exam. St. Louis, MO: Elsevier, 2014.

Eyles MO: Mosby's Comprehensive Review of Practical Nursing for the NCLEX-PN® Examination, 17th ed. St. Louis, MO: Elsevier, 2014.

Lippincott: Lippincott's NCLEX-PN PassPoint: Powered by PrepU. Philadelphia, PA: Lippincott Williams & Wilkins, 2014.

National Council of State Boards of Nursing: NCLEX Candidate Bulletin. Chicago, IL: National Council of State Boards of Nursing, 2015. Available online at: http://www.ncsbn.org, then NCLEX Examinations.

National Council of State Boards of Nursing: NCLEX-PN Test Plan. Chicago, IL: National Council of State Boards of Nursing, 2014. Available online at: http://www.ncsbn.org, then NCLEX Examinations.

Orman, D: The Test Anxiety Cure: How to Overcome Exam Anxiety, Fear and Self Defeating Habits (Stress Relief) [Kindle Edition]. Sparks, MD: TRO Publishing, LLC, 2014.

Rupert, DL: Lippincott's NCLEX-PN Alternate Format Questions, 3rd ed. Philadelphia, PA: Lippincott Williams & Wilkins, 2014.

Silvestri LA: Evolve Resources for Saunders 2014-2015 Strategies for Test Success, 3rd ed. St. Louis, MO: Elsevier, 2014.

Silvestri LA: Saunders Comprehensive Review for NCLEX-PN, 6th ed. St. Louis, MO: Elsevier, 2014.

Timby BK, Rupert DL: Lippincott's Review for NCLEX-PN, 10th ed. Philadelphia, PA: Lippincott Williams & Wilkins, 2014.

UNDERSTANDING *Your Profession*

Nursing From Past to Present

LEARNING OBJECTIVES

When you complete this chapter, you will be able to:

1. Give the dates of the major historical periods and identify a significant event in each period.

2. Describe the contributions of Florence Nightingale to the development of modern nursing.

3. Construct a time line that includes four major events in the history of nursing in the United States.

4. Name at least three nursing leaders and their major contribution(s) to nursing.

5. Trace the development of practical nursing from the late 1800s to the present time.

6. Name the two organizations primarily concerned with practical/vocational nursing education and practical/vocational nursing practice.

October 1854
The British Light Brigade was under attack at Balaclava, Turkey, by Russian troops. It was a bloody war, this war in the Crimea. Cannons blazed under the heavy gray skies of late autumn. Muskets cracked, spitting fire and sudden death. Many soldiers would die in the Crimean War.

The British field hospital in Scutari smelled of dirt, blood, and death. Thousands of sick and wounded soldiers, many still in their blood-caked uniforms, lay helpless and cold on filthy straw beds. The hospital was under-staffed and short of supplies. Hunger and disease added to the soldiers' suffering. The death rate soared. In London, 2,000 miles and many days' travel away from the battle, the London Times told the awful story of misery at the war front. The public was outraged but felt helpless. No organized care for British victims of war yet existed.

A brave young woman offered her services. She was a nurse. Although she had been raised in comfortable surroundings, the woman gave no thought to her own well-being or safety in volunteering to go to Turkey to care for the sick and dying. Her offer was accepted immediately.

A group of 38 women accompanied the nurse to Scutari. They were appalled by what they found. Suffering was widespread. Wounds festered for lack of soap and clean dressings. Rats, mice, bedbugs, and lice crawled amid the moaning men, adding to their torment. To many, death was a relief—and death came to many. More than half the men were dying.

Every night, the nurse walked the cold corridors to comfort the sick men. They could hear her footsteps, softly at first and then growing louder. But only when the flickering glow of her lamp brightened the darkness did they know that the kind lady with the lamp was not a dream.

The next months were a miracle. Using her own money, the nurse bought supplies and food. The small group of dedicated women scoured the dingy hospital. The kitchen prepared hot, nutritious meals for the patients. There were organized activities for the men. The death rate decreased with astonishing speed. Six months after the women's arrival, only 2% of the patients were dying.

The courageous young nurse who volunteered her services in the Crimean War was Florence Nightingale. Her lamp, still burning brightly after more than 175 years, is the beacon of modern nursing.

✔ *"A people without knowledge of its past has no present and a people without knowledge of its past will never have much of a future." Marie O. Pitts Mosley, RN, EdD, PNP*

Nursing is deeply rooted in history, even though it's relatively new as a career. Learning about the history of nursing will not only provide you with a better understanding of the rich heritage of your chosen career but also help you put in perspective the continually growing contributions that nurses make to improve the health of people throughout the modern world.

Nursing today is a rapidly growing, highly skilled service that is as technically sophisticated as the latest discoveries in science and medicine. But people have practiced nursing for ages, and the tradition of serving people in need can be traced far into the past.

The historical record of nursing in very early times is vague, but the conditions for nursing have always existed. New babies, illness, injury, aging, and the need for personal care are facts of life. One can assume that people have always needed what today is called nursing.

There is also no clear record of who in a group, tribe, or society performed the functions of nursing. Modern medicine can trace its primitive origins to the skills and wisdom of witch doctors, shamans, and medicine men. They performed healing rituals and administered herbs and roots that were known for their medicinal value. Their knowledge of the natural world came from tens of thousands of years of observation and experience passed down from generation to generation. That knowledge evolved into the traditions and tools of health care as it is practiced today. Your role in nursing has been defined by long experience.

✔ *Conditions that required "nursing care" have always existed.*

ANCIENT CIVILIZATIONS (3000 BCE–0)

Before Common Era (BCE)			Common Era (CE)									
3000	2000	1000	0	500	1000	1500	1600	1700	1800	1900	2000	2010

[3000–0]

As cultures developed and the civilizations based on them flourished, guidelines for behavior were made into rules. The rules were intended to protect people and guarantee group survival. They governed sanitation, hygiene, diet, sexual relations, fitness and disease, and other areas of life.

Like many early civilizations, ancient Egypt developed on the banks of a river. Waterways such as the Nile were a source of life. But when large numbers of people lived together and used the river for drinking, washing, and sanitation, the need for personal hygiene and public sanitation became evident. Rules—early versions of community health laws—were made.

Egyptian physicians were skilled in treating fractures, filling teeth, and classifying drugs. Midwives practiced obstetrics, and friends or attendants served as nurses at births.

In ancient Babylonia, illness was seen as punishment for displeasing the gods. It was believed that atonement was possible through purifying the body with herbs and chants. Purification was performed in special temples that, in a sense, were care centers.

The Old Testament refers to many dietary, hygienic, and health laws. For example, it was forbidden to eat meat after the 3rd day because in a hot climate without refrigeration, the meat would spoil. People with communicable diseases were isolated in sick houses. Provisions were made for the aged. Variations of those laws are still practiced today. Health, healing, and a tradition of caring for the sick and homeless are parts of an ancient heritage that continues in present times.

✔ *The Egyptians had many health-related rules that are similar to those we practice today.*

Other early cultures practiced health and healing principles that were also forerunners of today's medicine and nursing. Over 3,000 years ago, the Vedas (sacred Hindu books of India's earliest cultures) told of major and minor surgery, nervous afflictions, and urinary system diseases. Later, in India, advances were made in medicine, surgery, prenatal care, hygiene, and sanitation. They included public hospitals that were staffed by male nurses who would be qualified by today's standards to be practical nurses.

In ancient China, acupuncture, medical diagnosis by a complex pulse theory, and a vast knowledge of medicine and drugs were well known. This knowledge has survived and, in various forms, is still practiced today.

A Greek physician named Hippocrates (460–370 BCE) was referred to by early Greek writers as the Father of Medicine. He is still called by that name today. He taught at a medical school on Kos, a small Greek island (Fig. 6-1). Little is known of his ideas and discoveries, and much of his life is unknown, as well. The Hippocratic Oath, which is taken by medical school graduates today, is attributed to Hippocrates.

✔ *Hippocrates is known as the Father of Medicine.*

As the teachings of the school at Kos and another at Cnidus gained acceptance, the dominance that magic held in early medicine declined. The study of medicine shifted to a more scientific course. The followers of Hippocrates believed diseases always had specific causes that could be discovered by examination and analysis. The causes they sought were often wrong in that they blamed disease on "humors" in the body, such as blood, phlegm, and yellow and black bile.

The idea that it isn't magic or wrongdoing that causes illness was a big step forward. Diagnosis (the process of identifying a disease or medical condition scientifically) and prognosis (predicting the probable outcome of a patient's disease), rather than cure (restoration to health), were the foundations of Hippocratic medicine. It would be more than 2,000 years later that scientists would discover the germ theory of disease.

The healing method taught by Hippocrates' followers was to help nature do its work. This way of thinking was similar to what Florence Nightingale would write about nursing in her *Notes on Nursing: What It Is and What It Is Not* in 1859, more than 2,000 years later. She said that nursing should "put the patient in the best condition for nature to act upon."

Practitioners of Hippocratic medicine were men who did not train nurses to provide the care that their method ("helping nature do its work") suggested. They did it themselves. Women in Greek society were subordinate to men. It was

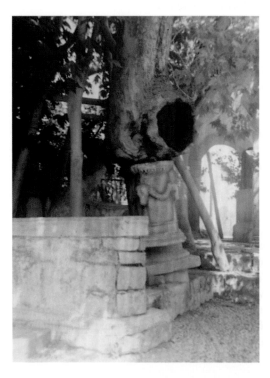

FIGURE 6-1. ● Legend says that Hippocrates taught medicine from this location on Kos.

believed that women were not worthy of medical or nursing education. Greek nurses were little more than household servants, usually slaves, who took care of the children and family.

✔ *Men provided medical and nursing care: Women were subordinate to men.*

The rise of the vast Roman Empire (753 BCE–476 CE) was based on military might. Military hospitals were established to care for wounded soldiers, but Roman medicine was still based on superstition. This was a setback from advances made earlier by the Greeks. The Romans held their women in greater esteem than did the Greeks. Roman women enjoyed a liberated position for the times, but organized nursing care was not yet established.

THE EARLY CHRISTIAN ERA (1–476 CE)

Before Common Era (BCE)	Common Era (CE)										
3000 2000 1000	0 500	1000	1500	1600	1700	1800	1900	2000	2010		

[1–476]

Nursing by women who were dedicated to its practice began with the rise of Christianity, which taught caring for others. Deacons and deaconesses—men and women with equal rank in the church—served the sick, the poor, the aged, orphans, widows, slaves, and prisoners. They fed and clothed the needy, cared for the sick, visited prisoners, sheltered the homeless, and buried the dead. All were works of mercy.

✔ *Deacons and deaconesses cared for the sick.*

Deaconesses were frequently well-bred, cultured widows or daughters of Roman officials. They performed services similar to today's community health or visiting nurses, carrying baskets of food and medicine to needy homes. Phoebe, a friend of St. Paul, who lived around the year 55, is considered to be the first deaconess and visiting nurse. She is mentioned in the New Testament.

Two other women's groups, the Order of Widows and the Order of Virgins, were also dedicated to the principle of merciful care for those in need. Like the deaconesses, they lived in humble, selfless service to others. They are sometimes called the first organized public health service nurses.

✔ *The church had a great influence on the development of charitable acts, which included nursing.*

The deaconess movement reached its peak at about 400 in Constantinople (today's Istanbul, Turkey), which was an important center of the early Christian church. The movement diminished when the church took away the role of the deaconesses, but not before spreading as far west as present-day France and Ireland.

In 380 in Rome, a beautiful and wealthy woman named Fabiola founded the first public hospital. She had divorced her first husband and was remarried when she converted to Christianity. Her second husband died. Because remarriage after divorce was considered a sin, Fabiola atoned by dedicating her life to charity. To the dismay of others, she personally cared for the sick and injured, often cleaning and dressing sores and wounds with her own hands.

THE EARLY MIDDLE AGES (476–1000)

Before Common Era (BCE)	Common Era (CE)										
3000 2000 1000	0 500	1000	1500	1600	1700	1800	1900	2000	2010		

[476–1000]

The influence of the Roman Empire peaked at the time of the birth of Jesus. It ended in 476 after hundreds of years of attacks by barbarians. Europe was split into many separate kingdoms. The next 500 years are called the Dark Ages because intellectual progress nearly halted. Christians retreated to walled monasteries while the world was plunged into war, rivalry, and ignorance. The teachings of the early Greek Classical period were saved by the dedication of monks who lived in relative safety in monasteries. They kept learning alive and preserved the record of the past in handwritten books.

✔ *Medicine and health care became associated with religious groups.*

The idea of caring for people in need was also preserved. The emphasis in medicine shifted from a scientific interest in anatomy, physiology, and the healing effects of nature's drugs to personal care and comfort, which is the foundation of nursing. Monks and nuns performed nursing tasks in the monasteries under the direction of the Catholic Church.

Hospitals were founded at monasteries in Lyon in 542 and Paris in 650. Santo Spirito Hospital was founded in Rome in 717. The first nursing order of nuns, the Augustinian Sisters, staffed the hospital in Paris.

THE HIGH MIDDLE AGES (1000–1475)

Before Common Era (BCE)		Common Era (CE)									
3000	2000	1000	0	500	1000	1500	1600	1700	1800	1900	2000	2010

[1000–1475]

The small states that emerged from the Early Middle Ages were dominated by the Catholic Church, which had slowly filled the vacuum left by the collapse of the Roman Empire. Almost all aspects of life, from philosophy, politics, art, and architecture to everyday activity, were deeply influenced by the church.

✔ *The church continued to have an enormous influence on people's lives.*

During this time, huge cathedrals were built and universities were founded. Some of the universities are still in existence today. A lengthy series of religious wars, the Crusades, began. The early Middle Ages had closed off much of Western civilization for almost 500 years; the Crusades reopened it.

The Crusades (1095–1291)

The military orders of the Knights Hospitallers and the Knights Templars were priests, brothers, and knights who sought to reclaim the Holy Land from the Moslems. At the same time, they established a hospital to care for pilgrims of Jerusalem.

✔ *The symbol for the International Red Cross originated with the Knights Hospitallers.*

The Moslems used organized facilities for the care of their sick and wounded. The Crusaders saw this method of treatment and adopted it to care for their own casualties. They built hospitals near the battlefields. While some knights fought on the battlefield, others cared for the injured in the hospitals. The insignia of the Knights Hospitallers of St. John of Jerusalem, also known as Knights Hospitallers, was a bright red cross. It is now the symbol of the International Red Cross.

The Knights Hospitallers' strict principles of discipline, obedience, and devotion became an important part of organized nursing for hundreds of years. Knights who returned home from the wars in the Holy Land created a new version of society based on a middle class. The deaconess movement vanished and was replaced by monastic nursing orders, such as the Franciscans, the Alexians, the Brothers of Mercy, and the Knights of St. John, a military order that was formed to fight the Crusades.

Hospices

Monasteries continued to play an important role in nursing during the Middle Ages. Hospices were established within their walls. As refuges of safety from the outside world, hospices welcomed travelers, the poor, and the sick. The idea of separate hospitals for the sick came into being later. They were based on the hospitals of the Persians and Arabs, whose ideas had been brought back to Europe by the Crusaders. The hospitals were staffed by both secular and religious orders.

✔ *Secular orders began providing services in hospitals and hospices.*

Two of these early religious orders are still active. The First Order of St. Francis and the Second Order of St. Francis were regular monastic orders. Order members lived secluded lives under strict vows of poverty and chastity. The First Order of St. Francis was founded by Saint Francis of Assisi. The Second Order, now called the Poor Clares, was founded by his disciple, St. Clare. St. Francis also founded the Third Order of St. Francis for laypersons who wanted to follow his teachings but did not want to give up normal life for the strict discipline of the monastery. The Poor Clares continue to serve the poor and the aged today, but they don't perform nursing functions.

Nursing Orders and Church Influence

Nursing during the Middle Ages was an important way of life to its practitioners and a valuable service to those in need. Its practice reinforced its place in the slowly growing science of medicine. Its strict organization according to church rules was also important. When new members joined nursing orders, they first had to spend a probationary period before they could wear the white robe that symbolized their work. After an additional novitiate period, they were allowed to wear the hood of the order. A nursing director, called a maîtresse, supervised their activities. Order members were expected to be obedient, unselfish, and totally devoted to the performance of their duties. These and other regulations are the roots of traditional nursing.

✔ *The Catholic Church encouraged the development of nursing orders.*

During this time, the power of the Catholic Church grew. Because the nursing orders were sponsored by the church, their strength and status also grew. The numbers of women entering nursing increased. Nursing was a popular and acceptable occupation for women.

At the same time, medicine as an occupation declined. The church did not favor medicine in the way it did nursing. The church, not medicine, held authority over nursing. What a nurse could and could not do was dictated by the church. For example, because it was believed that the human body was basically unclean, procedures such as perineal care, enemas, and douches were not performed. A nurse's priority was to serve her patients' spiritual needs. However, her duties included feeding, bathing, and washing patients; administering medications; changing dressing and linens; and all-around cleaning. The nurse, not the physician, provided most health care in hospitals, even though the care was more custodial and centered on reducing discomfort rather than on treatment.

✔ *The bubonic plague killed one fourth of the population in Europe.*

The church's authority and dominance eventually began to decline. The kingdoms that were formed after the end of the Roman Empire grew in power. Traveling merchants returned to Europe with ideas from the Arab and Byzantine worlds. They also brought the deadly bubonic plague ("black death"), a highly contagious, epidemic disease that swept Europe from 1347 to 1351. One fourth of the entire population died, while famine and war killed many more people and economies faltered. With such chaos raging, people's religious fervor turned to cynicism and hope was lost. The times were ripe for change.

THE RENAISSANCE THROUGH THE 17TH CENTURY (1300–1700): THE DECLINE OF NURSING

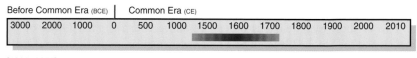

Before Common Era (BCE)				Common Era (CE)									
3000	2000	1000	0	500	1000	1500	1600	1700	1800	1900	2000	2010	

[1300–1700]

The Renaissance (1300s–1600s)

The disruption of society by plague and famine meant that there were more sick and poor persons than ever. The early Greeks and Romans had developed wonderful ideas, but these ideas had been lost for centuries. Now, they were replanted.

In a burst of collective creative genius known as the Renaissance (meaning rebirth) that lasted into the 17th century, classical thought was raised to near perfection. The idea that the world could be studied became the foundation of a new science of discovery and exploration. That idea is still alive today.

Medicine took a lead among the sciences. Anatomy, physiology, and the scientific basis of healing were studied. Nursing went into a decline. Nursing had been neglected during the Greek era, when Hippocratic medicine prevailed. It rose to dominate medicine during the monastic period. Now, during the Renaissance, it fell once again.

The Reformation (1500s–1600s)

An Augustinian monk named Martin Luther opposed many of the teachings of the Catholic Church. His protests led to the beginning of the Reformation in 1517 and the foundation of a new view of religion, Protestantism, which ended the absolute domination of the Catholic Church. It also opened the way for new ideas in areas other than religion, some of which had a dramatic effect on nursing.

✔ *Protestantism ended the dominance of the Catholic Church.*

Monasteries were closed and the religious orders that ran them were disbanded. Nursing work once performed by women in hospitals virtually stopped. Women's role in society changed dramatically. Under the influence of the Catholic Church, women had been revered. They were encouraged to do charitable work outside the home. Women from Europe's finest families had become nuns who taught and nursed.

Under Protestantism, women were considered to be subordinate to men. They were expected to stay at home to bear and raise children and to care for the home. Respectable women did not work in hospitals. Instead, nursing was done by "wayward" women of low status, such as prostitutes and alcoholic women who were given the work instead of being sent to jail. Nursing fell to a low state, and its practitioners were reduced to poorly paid servants. Except for the efforts of dedicated people such as St. Vincent de Paul, a French priest who, with follower Louise de Marillac, founded the Sisters of Charity in 1633, nursing remained dormant until the early 1820s.

THE 18TH, 19TH, AND EARLY 20TH CENTURIES (1700–1940)

Before Common Era (BCE)	Common Era (CE)											
3000	2000	1000	0	500	1000	1500	1600	1700	1800	1900	2000	2010

[1700–1940]

Social conditions deteriorated sharply by the end of the 1700s. Industrialization was replacing familiar agricultural society. Cities with large populations were breeding grounds for poverty, poor hygiene, and disease. Societies treated their members badly. The sick, insane, poor, and homeless were put into hospitals, jails, asylums, and poorhouses that were little more than warehouses for the needy. Living, health, and sanitary conditions were deplorable. Change was desperately needed, setting the stage for social reform. All that was needed were people with social vision.

Early Reformers

A Londoner, John Howard (1726–1790), fought for reforms in public health. He had visited many foreign countries and had seen firsthand how prisoners were treated. He pushed for prison reforms that resulted in dramatic improvements in prison conditions and increased public awareness.

Howard's work was carried on by a London philanthropist, Elizabeth Fry (1780–1845). She organized a group called the Protestant Sisters of Charity, later called the Institute of Nursing Sisters, to provide nursing care for London's poor.

In Germany, a minister in Kaiserswerth was concerned with the problems of poverty faced by his parishioners. Pastor Theodor Fliedner (1800–1864) visited England, where he was impressed by Elizabeth Fry's work in British prisons. With his wife, Friederike, Fliedner opened a school in Germany to train deaconesses, the Kaiserswerth Deaconess Institution. It marked a revival of the deaconess movement that had ended 400 years earlier. It was the first real nursing school.

✔ *The Kaiserswerth Deaconess Institution was the first nursing school.*

Pastor Fliedner opened his hospital in Kaiserswerth in 1836. Its first deaconess was Gertrude Reichardt. Many women were trained as deaconesses at the school. They became the core of the movement that would lead to modern nursing. Graduates of the Kaiserswerth Deaconess Institution founded similar programs to train women around the world. One of them, Florence Nightingale, opened the way to the new age of nursing (Fig. 6-2).

Florence Nightingale

Florence Nightingale was the younger of two sisters. She was born on May 12, 1820, in Florence, Italy, and was named after that city. Her parents were visiting there from their native England. She returned to England with her family when she was 1 year old. As a daughter of wealthy parents, she was given an excellent classical education in languages, history, mathematics, and philosophy. She was taught the social manners and customs of the privileged class and grew up to be a cultured, attractive young lady. Her family expected her to become the wife of an equally eminent gentleman and live a life of comfort and plenty. Her own goals were decidedly different.

✔ *National Nurses Week is celebrated annually from May 6 through May 12, the birthday of Florence Nightingale, who is considered the founder of modern nursing.*

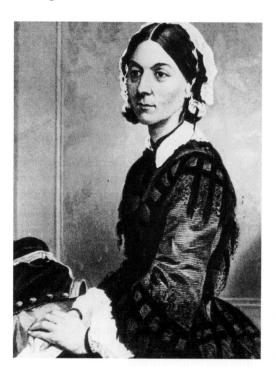

FIGURE 6-2. ● Modern nursing began with Florence Nightingale. (Photo courtesy of the Center for the Study of the History of Nursing, University of Pennsylvania.)

From childhood on, Nightingale was a sympathetic and sensitive girl with a great affection for animals and people. As a youngster, she visited the sick and poor. Her visits were a hint of her growing ambition to serve humanity. She began to think of a career as a nurse. She declared her intentions in 1844, when she was 24 years old.

The idea astounded her parents. Not only did such work not fit her social rank, but also at that time women in nursing were often disreputable. The more her family objected to her calling, as she believed it to be, the more determined she became.

✔ *Nightingale attended nursing school at the Kaiserswerth Deaconess Institution.*

Nightingale traveled to foreign countries. She visited hospitals and orphanages where she observed how nursing was performed by untrained individuals. She became an authority on public health and hospitals.

Dr. Elizabeth Blackwell, a close friend who was also America's first woman physician, encouraged Florence Nightingale to pursue her ambition to be a nurse. In 1851, at 31 years of age, Nightingale went to the Kaiserswerth Deaconess Institution, which she had heard about from friends. She studied there for 3 months. After her training, she worked in Paris with the Sisters of Charity. She also observed skilled French surgeons operate. Although she was pleased with her training, she knew it was not enough for the kind of nurse she wanted to be.

Florence returned to London, where she became superintendent of a small institution, the Establishment for Gentlewomen During Illness. Her family had still not accepted her independent attitude. Then, in 1854, the Crimean War broke out. This dark moment of history would certify her behavior. It would also help her leave her mark on the world.

British newspapers told of appalling conditions in the Crimea, where England, France, and Turkey were fighting against Russia. Ill and injured British soldiers lay neglected, while both allied and enemy soldiers were treated and cared for by organized groups of nurses. French casualties were taken care of by the Sisters of Charity. The Russians were cared for by the Sisters of Mercy. The English public was outraged. Nightingale volunteered to take a group of nurses to the Crimea to care for English and Turkish soldiers. Her friend Sidney Herbert, Britain's Secretary of War, had already written to her requesting her services.

On October 21, 1854, Florence Nightingale left for the front with 38 women. Some were trained as nurses and others were not. They took with them a stock of badly needed supplies. Conditions at the front were disgusting. Wounded soldiers, still in bloody uniforms, lay crowded into filthy wards on dirty straw. Sanitation was poor to nonexistent. There was no soap, clean linen, or even tables and chairs. The food was often inedible.

Adding to the horror, the reception the women received from army medical officers was characterized by resentment. Nightingale took matters into her own hands. With her nurses, she tended to ill and injured soldiers. She fought red tape to obtain supplies and hired people to clean the hospitals. She set up laundries, organized kitchens to turn out nutritious meals, and personally made endless rounds to comfort wounded and sick soldiers. She even used her own money to purchase supplies.

✔ *Many nursing practices suggested by Nightingale are still appropriate for today's nurses.*

Within 6 months, Nightingale's labors paid off. Deaths dropped dramatically, from 420/1,000 to 22/1,000. Discipline and organization took over from neglect and disorder. She had become the "Lady with the Lamp" to her patients. It was an endearing reference to the nightly rounds she made with a lamp in hand to see to their comfort and care.

Florence Nightingale returned to England in July 1856. She was the unchallenged heroine of the war. But her strength was sapped by sickness and exhaustion. She remained a semi-invalid for the remaining 54 years of her life. Nightingale did not stop her work, however. Her powerful influence was felt in civilian and military hospitals and in nurse training. She also wrote books. Her best-known work is *Notes on Nursing: What It Is and What It Is Not*. She was awarded medals and jewels by grateful admirers who included England's Queen Victoria and the sultan of Turkey. A fund contributed by soldiers and citizens alike was used to establish a training school for nurses, the Nightingale School, which opened in 1860. The school became the model for modern nursing schools. Florence Nightingale died in 1910 at 90 years of age.

✔ *Florence Nightingale transformed nursing from a profession for poor women into a noble occupation.*

Nursing was changed forever by Florence Nightingale and the methods she introduced. The old practices fell away as major advances in nursing were made around the world.

In her memory and as a tribute to all nurses, National Nurses Week (May 6–12) was established in 1990 by the American Nurses Association (ANA). The International Council of Nurses designated May 12 as International Nurses Day.

International Red Cross

J. H. Dunant was instrumental in founding the International Red Cross in Switzerland in 1864. Like Nightingale, Dunant had been horrified by the almost complete lack of care for the sick and wounded in wartime. Until that time, there was no neutral international health organization that nations could turn to in time of war or after natural disasters. One of the early accomplishments of the Red Cross was to make rules for the treatment of the wounded and for the protection of medical personnel and hospitals. Today, most countries have their own Red Cross organization that also belongs to the International Red Cross.

✔ *The International Red Cross makes rules for caring for those injured in war.*

Scientific Developments

During this time, science and medicine were making gigantic strides. Ignaz Philipp Semmelweis's conquest of puerperal sepsis (childbed fever) in 1847 reduced maternal death rates. Louis Pasteur's discoveries in 1862 in chemistry and microbiology created the pasteurization process that kills most harmful bacteria in liquids like milk. Joseph Lister's aseptic surgical techniques were initially used in 1865 and greatly reduced wound infections. The germ theory of disease developed in 1876 by Robert Koch, a German bacteriologist, was that bacteria, not "bad air," carry anthrax and other diseases. Scientific developments were changing humankind's ability to do something about its health. Nursing and nurses were deeply involved in improving the well-being of patients who were benefiting from scientific discoveries.

Nursing in the United States

In the United States, there were no formal programs to train nurses, and there were scarcely any trained nurses at all. War and other social conditions were major influences in the reform of the haphazard nursing practices that did exist. Government agencies became aware of the problem, and important changes were made. The Civil War (1861–1865) dramatized the need for skilled nurses. People realized that society was responsible for its own health.

The status of women was improving; Florence Nightingale's example led to advances in nursing education and practice. Women were beginning to assume new roles in public affairs, including nursing. The first nursing school in the United States was opened in 1872 at the New England Hospital for Women and Children in Boston. Bellevue Hospital's Training School, which opened in 1873, was organized along the lines of the Nightingale School model.

✔ Nursing schools began admitting students in the United States in the late 1800s.

Fifteen years later, the Mills School of Nursing, a school for training male nurses, was opened at Bellevue Hospital. Other schools were opened as the new nursing movement grew. Textbooks, uniforms for secular nurses, and a growing appreciation of nurses by a grateful public for their devotion to duty encouraged the growth.

The curricula of nursing education programs and the knowledge required to practice nursing in the United States have increased tremendously since the first schools opened in the late 1800s. Much of the progress in nursing is because of the emergence of nursing leaders who were dedicated to the improvement of the health and well-being of their patients.

Emergence of American Nursing Leaders

During this time, nurse leaders created and improved nursing education programs; addressed segregation in nursing education and in the workplace; emphasized equal health care for all; created organizations to improve the welfare of nurses and patients; contributed research; developed theories of nursing; began rural, public, and community health nursing; and established nursing as a respectable profession.

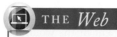

THE *Web*

The American Nurses Association maintains a nurse's "Hall of Fame" on their Web site.

Some of those who made significant contributions are recognized on the following pages: A multitude of others who are not included have made contributions that are equally significant.

Dorothea Lynde Dix (1802–1887) was concerned about the inhumane treatment of mentally ill persons. She traveled across the United States to encourage legislators to pass protective laws. As an untrained volunteer nurse in the Civil War, she was appointed superintendent of women nurses for all military hospitals. She was the first U.S. Army nurse.

Clara Barton (1821–1912) was a dedicated teacher at a time when few women held such jobs. She obtained permission from the US government to take volunteer nurses to field hospitals during the Civil War. She cared for the ill and wounded of both sides, North and South, and for black and white patients with equality. She was given the name Angel of the Battlefield. Miss Barton formed the American Association of the Red Cross in 1881 after seeing the awful conditions of soldiers on the battlefield.

Linda Richards (1841–1930) was the first nurse to be trained in the United States. Richards graduated from the New England Hospital for Women and Children in Boston after a 1-year training program. She developed a system for writing accurate patient reports that later became the basis for nursing and hospital recordkeeping. She was a lifelong student of nursing and taught its methods. She traveled extensively, studying, lecturing, consulting, and opening schools.

✔ *Hundreds of nurses have contributed to moving nursing to a position of importance in our contemporary health care system.*

Mary Eliza Mahoney (1845–1926) was the first African American graduate professional nurse in the United States. Her work for integration in nursing and improved working and health care conditions was a lifelong endeavor. The Mary Mahoney Award, first instituted in 1936, is given by the ANA to a contemporary nurse who has made significant contributions to integration, retention, and advancement of minorities in nursing.

Lavinia Dock (1858–1956) was instrumental in the beginning of what is now called the National League for Nursing. Her four-volume work, *History of Nursing*, coauthored with Mary Adelaide Nutting, is the classic text on nursing history.

Mary Adelaide Nutting (1858–1948) graduated from the first class of the Johns Hopkins School of Nursing. She founded the first college-level department of nursing at Columbia University Teacher's College and was instrumental in raising the standards of nursing education.

Isabel Hampton Robb (1860–1910) advocated nurses' rights, a 3-year training program, a 6-day work week, 8-hour instead of 12-hour workdays, and licensure to protect patients.

Lillian Wald (1867–1940) founded public health nursing in the United States when she opened the Henry Street Settlement in 1893 to provide free nursing care for the poor on the Lower East Side of New York City.

Adah Belle Samuel Thoms (circa 1870–1943) was a Crusader for equal opportunity for African American people in nursing. She felt a deep sense of responsibility to improve relationships between persons of all races. She became an acting director of nursing at a time when African American nurses rarely held high-level positions. During her 7-year term as president of the National Association of Colored Graduate Nurses, Thoms worked for acceptance of African American nurses as members of the American Red Cross and in the U.S. Army Nurse Corps. She wrote *Pathfinders: A History of the Progress of Colored Graduate Nurses.*

Annie W. Goodrich (1866–1955) was a strong-willed advocate of nursing training and the need to raise nursing to professional status. When World War I created the need for more nurses, she wrote plans for the Army School of Nursing.

Clara Maass (1876–1901) was a former volunteer contract nurse with the U.S. Army. She gave her life in an experiment to discover the cause of yellow fever. As a test subject, she was infected twice by mosquito bites and died at 25 years of age.

Margaret Sanger (1879–1966) opened the first birth control clinic in the United States. She was jailed in 1917 for "maintaining a public nuisance." She founded the American Birth Control League and organized the first World Population Conference and was the first president of the International Planned Parenthood Federation. She was an outspoken and controversial figure who is remembered for revolutionizing women's health.

Susie Walking Bear Yellowtail (1903–1981) helped to bring modern health care to her own people and to end abuses in the Native American health care system, such as the sterilization of women without their consent. From 1930 to 1960, this Montana nurse traveled throughout North American reservations to assess the health, social, and educational problems Native Americans faced. Through her work with the then Department of Health, Education and Welfare, the founder of the Native ANA was instrumental in winning tribal and government funding to help Native Americans enter the nursing profession. In 1962, Yellowtail received the President's Award for Outstanding Nursing Health Care.

Hildegard Peplau (1909–1999) is regarded as the "mother of psychiatric nursing" and was a pioneer in the development of the theory and practice of psychiatric and mental health nursing. Her achievements, including her revolutionary work in patient–nurse relationships, are valued by nurses around the world, and her ideas have been incorporated into virtually every nursing specialty and into the practices of other health care professionals.

Martha Elizabeth Rogers (1914–1994) is known for her discovery of the science of unitary human beings. She provided a framework for continued study and research and influenced the development of a variety of modalities, including therapeutic touch. Over a long and productive career, she demonstrated leadership skill and a futuristic vision that improved nursing education, practice, and research in the United States.

Mary Elizabeth Carnegie (1916–2008) exhibited courage, integrity, and commitment to the advancement of the nursing profession as well as to the advancement of African American and other minority nurses. She is the author of the award-winning *The Path We Tread: Blacks in Nursing Worldwide, 1854–1994*. She initiated the baccalaureate nursing program at the historically African American Hampton University in Virginia and served as dean and professor of the school of nursing at Florida A&M University (1945–1953).

Randolph Rasch (1952–Present) has a long history of firsts. He was the first African American man to graduate from the nursing program at Andrews University in Berrien Springs, Michigan. He then became the first African American male public health nurse in his native state of Michigan. He followed that by becoming the first African American man to complete an MSN as a family nurse practitioner at Vanderbilt in 1979. Finally, he became the first African American man to earn a PhD in nursing when he graduated from the University of Texas at Austin in 1988.

Ildaura Murillo-Rohde (1933–2010) was, in 1975, one of a very few Hispanic nurses working in academic settings, doing research on Hispanic health issues, and advising federal policy makers about the health care needs of Hispanic people. There was no unified voice to speak up in advocacy for the unique cultural concerns of Hispanic nurses. Deciding to do something to increase the representation of Latinos in the nursing profession led her to create the organization known today as the National Association of Hispanic Nurses, which currently represents the interests of more than 40,000 Hispanic nurses.

Rebecca Anderson (1957–1995) LPN died as a result of a head injury she received while trying to save victims involved in the April 19, 1995, Alfred P. Murrah Building (Oklahoma City, OK) bombing. Though all of the rescue workers risked their lives when they entered the crumbling hulk of mangled metal and shattered cement, she was the only one who died. She gave her life trying to save ordinary people like herself. Rebecca wasn't a victim of the bombing. She didn't have to be there. She went to help others in need, and it cost her life. Her actions epitomize the selfless acts that nurses commit every day.

History will someday include many contemporary nurses for their contributions to improving patient care and education, forming new health care systems, research, designing patient care models, informatics that support health care, and other unforeseen frontiers in nursing. These and other nurses like them are paving the way for you. Now is the time for you to think about what you will leave as a legacy to future nurses. Will your name be among those recognized for making the world a better place?

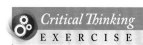

Critical Thinking
E X E R C I S E

Now that you have finished reading a very brief history of medicine and nursing, try to identify some of the characteristics of nurses that seem to be present throughout history. Use appropriate Characteristics of Critical Thinking in Box 1-2 on pages 18–19 to develop your response to question.

THE DEVELOPMENT OF PRACTICAL/ VOCATIONAL NURSING

Practical nursing has had a similar history, although formal practical nursing education programs came later than professional nursing education programs. Box 6-1 lists nurses' duties in 1887. Box 6-2 summarizes the history of practical/ vocational nursing. The Industrial Revolution of the mid-1800s began a population shift from rural to urban areas of the United States. Many of the people who left the farm for the city were untrained and often uneducated. The young women who arrived in the cities were particularly disadvantaged because there were few job opportunities. Men could find work in factories, but women were limited to domestic service.

Emergence of Practical Nursing Schools

To train women so that they could increase their opportunity to compete for jobs, the Young Women's Christian Association (YWCA), a church-affiliated organization that originated in Europe, gave classes in cooking and domestic chores. It is likely that simple home nursing skills and child care instructions were included.

✔ *Practical nursing as a separate career began over 120 years ago.*

In 1892, an informal, 3-month YWCA course in practical nursing was offered in Brooklyn, New York. Its objective was to teach women how to care for children, invalids, and the elderly. Women who completed this training were called practical nurses and were often in demand to fill nursing shortages. The Ballard School of Practical Nursing, named for its sponsor, Lucinda Ballard, opened in 1897. This school offered the first formal curriculum for educating practical nurses.

BOX 6-1	Nurses' Duties in 1887

The following job description was given to floor nurses in 1887: In addition to caring for your 50 patients, each nurse will follow these regulations:

1. Daily sweep and mop the floors of your ward, and dust the patient's furniture and window sills.
2. Maintain an even temperature in your ward by bringing in a scuttle of coal for the day's business.
3. Light is important to observe the patient's condition. Therefore, each day fill kerosene lamps, clean chimneys, and trim wicks. Wash the windows once a week.
4. The nurse's notes are important in aiding the physician's work. Make your pens carefully; you may whittle nibs to your individual taste.
5. Each nurse on day duty will report every day at 7 am and leave at 8 pm except on the Sabbath on which day you will be off from 12 to 2 pm.
6. Graduate nurses in good standing with the director of nurses will be given an evening off each week for courting purposes or two evenings a week if you go regularly to church.
7. Each nurse should lay aside from each pay day a goodly sum of her earnings for her benefits during her declining years so that she will not become a burden. For example, if you earn $30 a month, you should set aside $15.
8. Any nurse who smokes, uses liquor in any form, gets her hair done at a beauty shop, or frequents dance halls will give the director of nurses good reason to suspect her worth, intentions, and integrity.
9. The nurse who performs her labors and serves her patients and doctors without fault for 5 years will be given an increase of 5 cents a day, providing there are no hospital debts outstanding.

Fifteen years later, in 1907, the Thompson School in Brattleboro, Vermont, was opened. In 1918, the Household Nursing Association School of Attendant Nursing was founded in Boston. The objective of the programs at these schools was to train practical nurses in home nursing skills. The training emphasized cooking, cleaning, and other household duties. Some early practical nursing programs also provided hospital experience. If the program was affiliated with a hospital, it paid its students for their services.

✔ *The demand for the skills of practical nurses increased around the time of World War II.*

BOX 6-2	History and Practical Nursing

1892	YWCA opened a 3-month training program for practical nurses in Brooklyn, New York.
1897	Ballard School for practical nursing education was opened in New York. Funding was provided by Lucinda Ballard.
1907	Thompson School for practical nurses was opened in Brattleboro, Vermont.
1914	Mississippi passed the first law that provided practical nurses the option to be licensed.
1918	Household Association School of Attendant Nursing was opened in Boston.
1918	National League for Nursing Education was founded.

BOX
6-2   **History and Practical Nursing** *continued*

1938	New York was the only state to mandate the licensure of practical nurses.
1940	Six states had passed laws that provided practical nurses the option to be licensed.
1941	Association of Practical Nursing Schools (later known as the National Association for Practical Nurse Education and Service [NAPNES]) was founded.
1944	U.S. Department of Education, Division of Vocational Education studied and made a number of recommendations that resulted in a significant increase in the number of practical nursing programs.
1949	National Federation of Licensed Practical Nurses (NFLPN) was organized by Lillian Kuster.
1950	The National League for Nursing was created by combining the National League for Nursing Education, the National Organization of Public Health Nurses, and the Association of Collegiate Schools of Nursing.
1951	The *Journal of Practical Nursing* was first published by NAPNES.
1955	All states had licensure laws for practical nurses.
1957	The National League for Nursing established a Council of Practical Nursing Programs.
1961	The National League for Nursing began offering accrediting services for practical nursing schools.
1965	The ANA issued a position paper on nursing education. The ANA position was that professional nurses should be educated in colleges and universities and that technical nurses should be prepared in junior colleges. The ANA position proposed that practical nurses be replaced by the technical nurse. The ANA's position remains unchanged.
1965	Controversy surrounding the education of professional nurses and the role of the practical nurse began in earnest in 1965 and continues to be discussed by nursing organizations, nonnursing health care organizations, judicial bodies, state boards of nursing, health care providers, and individual nurses.
1976	Mary Eliza Mahoney, the first African American professional nurse, was inducted into the American Nurses Association Hall of Fame.
1979	NLN published the first edition of a document listing the competencies of graduates of practical/vocational nursing programs.
1984	NAPNES discontinued providing accrediting services for practical/vocational nursing schools.
1989	The American Medical Association proposed a 9-month training program for a Registered Care Technologist. This "new" worker would perform many professional and practical nurse functions. Opposition from the nursing community prevented the implementation of this training program.
Early 1990s	The nursing shortage decreased and the job market for all nurses declined.
1994	April—The first computerized adaptive test (NCLEX-PN) for licensing nurses was administered.

continued on page 130

BOX 6-2	History and Practical Nursing *continued*

1995	Economic pressures on hospitals changed the locus of care from hospitals to the community and the home. Hospitals implemented staffing patterns that reduced the number of full-time employees and the nurse/patient ratio.
1996	The National Council of State Boards of Nursing, along with NAPNES, began offering a certification examination in long-term care for licensed practical/vocational nurses.
1997	NAPNES formed the Multi-Skilled Nursing Care Certification Organization (MSNC CO) to administer its Long-Term Care Certification program. MSNC CO has an Administrative Board that serves the Long-Term Care Certification Board and the Pharmacology Certification Board.
2000	Multistate nurse licensure began in Maryland, Texas, Utah, and Wisconsin.
2001	Nursing leaders and federal government analysts predict a progressive nursing shortage that will reach a critical level by the year 2010.
2002	The ANA releases *Nursing's Agenda for the Future*, a document that outlines the desired future state of nursing in the year 2010.
2002	Susie Walking Bear Yellowtail, RN, was inducted in the ANA Hall of Fame for her work to improve the Indian health care system.
2002	President Bush signed the Nurse Reinvestment Act, which authorized the creation of programs to combat the nursing shortage.
2004	Texas combined the professional and vocational boards of nursing into one Texas Board of Nurse Examiners.
2007	Twenty-two states had joined the Nurse Licensure Compact.
2007	NAPNES issued revised educational and practice outcomes for new graduates.
2007	NAPNES continues to develop a national certification for infusion therapy for LP/VNs.
2010	The Patient Protection and Affordable Care Act was signed into law by President Obama on March 23, 2010. NAPNES offers the Allied Health Professional Certificate in Long-Term Care for unlicensed assistive personnel.
2011	Implementation of electronic medical records begins for most health care providers.
2013 May	The National Federation of Licensed Practical Nurses establishes the NFLPN Education Foundation to administer the IV Therapy and Gerontology Certification examinations.
2014 April	A new edition of the NCLEX-PN examination is administered.
2015 January	The NCLEX-RN exam becomes the licensing examination for 10 Canadian registered nurse regulatory bodies.

By 1930, there were 11 schools of practical nursing in the United States. Between 1930 and 1947, 25 more schools were opened. Probably as a result of World War II and the serious shortage of registered nurses, 260 more schools were opened between 1948 and 1954.

Rise of National Organizations

There were few controls, little educational planning, and minimum supervision of practical nursing schools before 1940. Standards were nonexistent and the programs varied widely. It was only after state agencies that were subject to legislation took over that controls were established. Although Mississippi offered licensing for practical nurses in 1914, it was not until 1938 that New York passed the first mandatory practical nurse licensing law. The Minneapolis Girls' Vocational High School offered the first high school vocational practical nurse program in 1919. It was not until 1941 that a national association for practical nursing was formed.

The Association of Practical Nurse Schools was organized in Chicago in 1941 to address the needs of practical nursing education. Hilda M. Torrop, director of the Ballard School; Etta Creech, director of the Family Health Association in Cleveland; and Katherine Shephard, executive director of the Household Nursing Association in Boston were the association's officers. Its name was changed to the National Association for Practical Nurse Education (NAPNE) in 1942 when membership was opened to practical nurses.

A service for accrediting practical nursing schools that was begun by NAPNE in 1945 ended in 1984 at which time the National League for Nursing became an accrediting agency for practical/vocational nursing education programs. In 1959, NAPNE organized a summer school and workshops for directors and instructors of practical nursing programs. Its journal, the first one for practical nursing and now called the Online Journal of Practical Nursing, was first published in 1951.

The Association changed its name in 1959 to the National Association for Practical Nurse Education and Service (NAPNES). By then, this organization was sponsoring summer courses at colleges and universities, was emphasizing continuing education for practical nurses, and had established a Department of Education and a Department of Service for State Practical Nursing Associations. Membership in NAPNES is open to anyone who is interested in promoting the interests, concerns, and occupation of practical nursing.

In 1949, Lillian Kuster organized and became executive director of the National Federation of Licensed Practical Nurses (NFLPN), the official membership organization for practical and vocational nurses. Membership in NFLPN is limited to licensed or student practical/vocational nurses.

These two organizations, NAPNES and NFLPN, set standards for practical/vocational nursing practice, generally promote and protect the interests of practical/vocational nurses, and educate and inform the general public about practical/vocational nursing.

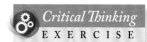

Critical Thinking EXERCISE

How would you answer if someone asks you to explain how practical or vocational nursing was started? Use appropriate Characteristics of Critical Thinking in Box 1-2 on pages 18–19 to develop your response to this question.

✔ *Two national organizations represent the interests of practical and vocational nurses: NAPNES and NFLPN.*

SUMMARY

Knowledge of nursing history will help you put your own nursing practice in the context of its evolution from the beginning of time to the current complex curriculum you are required to complete. You will recognize that change in nursing practice has been consistent over time. You will find that a study of nursing history will help you recognize patterns and avoid making mistakes that are detrimental to nursing. And you will learn that nursing and nurses have a heritage and an identity of which they can be proud. The future of nursing will profit from the strong historical foundation that has developed over many centuries.

APPLY

Critical Thinking Skills

1. Read the chapter on Personal Cleanliness from Nightingale's *Notes on Nursing*. Are there similarities between Nightingale's writings about personal hygiene and what you are learning about cleanliness and skin care in your Nursing Skills classes?

2. Discuss how the changing role and status of women may have influenced the development of nursing.

3. Identify some of the personal characteristics of the nurses who made important contributions to nursing between 1850 and 1950.

4. Use Internet resources to explore in detail the contributions of a particular nurse.

5. Write or go to NAPNES and NFLPN Web sites to obtain information on membership in these organizations.

6. Compare early practical nursing journal articles with articles in current journals. Try to identify changes in the articles in these journals that reflect changes in practical nursing.

7. Compare the duties in Box 6-1 with the duties in Box 4-1 on page 93. How many of the broad concepts in 1887 are still important today? For example, documentation was important in 1887, and it is still quite important today.

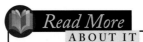

Read More

ABOUT IT

American Association for the History of Nursing Bulletin, Spring 2014. Wheat Ridge, CO: American Association for the History of Nursing, Inc. Available online at: http://www.aahn.org

Dolan JA, et al.: Nursing in Society: A Historical Perspective, 15th ed. Philadelphia, PA: WB Saunders, 1983.

Donahue MP: Nursing: The Finest Art: An Illustrated History, 3rd ed. St. Louis, MO: Mosby, 2010.

Hallett C, Lynaugh JE: Celebrating Nurses: A Visual History. Hauppauge, NY: Barron's Educational Series, 2010.

James J, Reverby S, (eds.): Lavinia Dock Reader (A History of American Nursing). New York, NY: Garland, 1985.

Jones C: The American Nurse. New York, NY: Welcome Books, 2012.

Judd D, Sitzman K, Davis GM: A History of American Nursing: Trends and Eras, 2nd ed. Sudbury, MA: Jones and Bartlett, 2013.

Kalish PA, Kalish BJ: American Nursing: A History. Philadelphia, PA: Lippincott Williams & Wilkins, 2003.

Mosby: Nursing Reflections: A Century of Caring. St. Louis, MO: Mosby, 2000.

Nightingale F: Notes on Nursing: What It Is and What It Is Not, Replica Edition. Philadelphia, PA: Lippincott Williams & Wilkins, 1992. (Originally published in 1859.)

Nursing History Review. New York, NY: Springer Publishing, 2015.

O'Lynn C, Tranbarger R: Men in Nursing: History, Challenges, and Opportunities. New York, NY: Springer Publishing, 2006.

Zwerdling M: Postcards of Nursing: A Worldwide Tribute. Philadelphia, PA: Lippincott Williams & Wilkins, 2003.

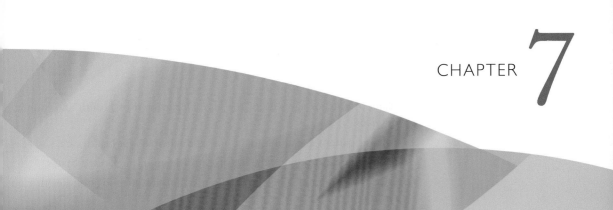

CHAPTER 7

The Health Care System

LEARNING OBJECTIVES

When you complete this chapter, you will be able to:

1. Define the terms health care provider, health care facility, health care service, health care regulation, health care financing, and health care system.

2. Describe the purpose of health care regulatory agencies.

3. Participate in quality assurance programs.

4. List the two major sources of health insurance.

5. Explain how diagnosis-related groups are used to control the cost of health care.

6. Discuss the role of the US government in health care.

LEARNING OBJECTIVES *continued*

7. Name the major agencies of the U.S. Department of Health and Human Services.

8. Answer patient questions about how and where to get health care.

9. Participate in improving the health care system in the United States.

10. Give three examples of current events that are affecting the health care system.

A hot shower always changed Mary Kelly's outlook on life. The shower she took one Saturday morning saved her life. Mary was 31 years old. She was married and had a son, Erik. Her husband was a successful automobile dealer. The young family had a bright future.

As Mary lathered herself, she touched a small lump in her right breast. She had never noticed it before. She felt it again. She had two choices. She could assume the lump was not serious and do nothing, or she could make an immediate appointment with her doctor for a breast examination. For a moment, Mary was undecided. Then, she laughed nervously, "Oh, it's nothing," she said. She finished her shower and quickly dressed. By midmorning, the lump was forgotten. But that afternoon, Mary remembered a pamphlet sent by the American Cancer Society. It told her how to do a breast self-examination. She located the pamphlet and followed its instructions. This time, she immediately called her doctor.

The discovery of the lump and taking appropriate action saved Mary's life. Her own and her family's future remain secure because she used the services of the health care system.

People who are seeking health care in the United States have many options and choices. While having many options and choices usually means that you will find something that is right for you, it also means that finding the option that is right for you and your family can be confusing and complicated. This chapter will help you understand where and how health care is provided, regulated, and financed. With this understanding, you'll be better able to influence legislation regarding health care, answer your patient's questions about health care, participate in approval and accreditation procedures, and influence the future of health care in the United States.

✔ *National health care expenditures in the United States were $2.9 trillion in 2013.*

THE HEALTH CARE SYSTEM

Some general descriptions will help you understand the present health care system and why Americans are so concerned about the future of one of the largest industries in this country.

Health care providers, health care facilities, health care services, health care regulation, and health care financing together comprise the health care system. The goal of the health care system is to improve the health of people in this society.

There are government (public) and nongovernment (private) components of the health care system. Some of the government components include veteran's hospitals and nursing homes, military hospitals, Medicare and Medicaid health insurance, and the Department of Health and Human Services (DHHS).

Some of the nongovernment components of the health care system include private providers (physicians, optometrists, dietitians, psychologists, nurse practitioners, etc.), private for-profit health care facilities, private nonprofit health care facilities, health clinics, private health insurance companies, preferred provider organizations (PPOs), health maintenance organizations (HMOs), and managed care systems.

A variety of health care providers who provide a wide range of services in a multitude of health care facilities that function under an array of regulations make it difficult for the public to know how to obtain the best treatment from the best provider at the least cost. An understanding of the components of the health care system will help you not only as a consumer but also as a patient advocate.

✔ *Patients often find the health care system to be complex and confusing.*

Health Care Providers

Health care providers include people, institutions, and organizations that make health care services available to those who want or need them. Physicians, dentists, optometrists, nurse practitioners, and podiatrists are examples of people who provide health care.

Primary health care providers are those whom people see first for health maintenance or treatment of illnesses. Primary health care providers are usually a person's initial contact with the health care system. Health care providers and members of the health care team are reviewed in more detail in Chapter 8.

✔ *Primary care physician visits are expected to exceed 565 million visits in the year 2025.*

Some of the institutions that provide health care include hospitals, long-term care facilities, ambulatory care facilities, walk-in clinics, community mental health centers, kidney dialysis centers, retail medical clinics, and state or local health department clinics. Institutions qualify as health care providers because they, through their employees, provide health care to their customers.

Organizations such as HMOs, PPOs, managed care organizations, and health insurance companies also qualify as health care providers. These organizations qualify as health care providers because they either hire or contract with individuals or groups of individuals to provide health care. These organizations usually charge a fee that allows members access to all necessary medical and hospital services. This fee is not increased, even for prolonged hospitalization, nor is it refunded if the member doesn't use any health care services.

Health Care Facilities

Health care facilities are the buildings or locations where health care is provided. Until the late 1800s, the traditional health care facility for treating illness, injury, and dying was the patient's home. Care was provided by the patient's family. If a patient could afford the services of a physician, these services were also provided in the patient's home.

The changes in hospitals and nursing begun by Florence Nightingale during the Crimean War (1854–1856) and by American reformers after the Civil War (1861–1865) started the trend toward improvement of health care facilities that is still going on today.

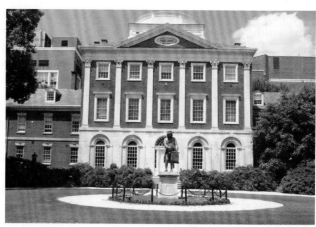

FIGURE 7-1. ● Pennsylvania Hospital, the nation's first hospital, is located in Philadelphia, PA.

From 1751, when Pennsylvania Hospital, the first hospital in the United States, was founded, to present time, the growth in the number of health care facilities has been amazing (Fig. 7-1). According to the Centers for Disease Control, in 2012, there were 5,815 hospitals, more than 3,700 hospice agencies, 15,700 nursing homes, 22,200 residential care communities, 4,800 adult day service centers, and 12,200 home health agencies.

Hospitals

A primary role of hospitals is to provide health care. In addition, hospitals are often medical education centers. They furnish training, seminars, and resources to physicians, nurses, technicians, social workers, dietitians, therapists, emergency medical technicians, many other health care workers, and patients and their families.

Some areas of education available at hospitals include disease prevention information, health maintenance instruction, childbirth classes, and behavior modification training. Hospitals also have clinics and laboratories for the treatment, analysis, and research of illness and injury. Many large hospitals have specialty divisions that provide specific types of care. For example, a large medical center may have a division devoted to research and treatment of patients who have cancer. That division may be located within the main hospital or it may be located in another geographic area and in its own buildings.

Types of Hospitals

Hospitals are classified by ownership, the kind of services they offer, their size, and the length of patient stay. Eligibility for funding, accrediting guidelines, staffing requirements, and allocation of medical equipment often depend on how a hospital is classified.

Ownership can be public or private. Public hospitals are those owned by federal, state, or local governments. Veterans Administration hospitals, U.S. Public Health Service hospitals, and military hospitals are examples of hospitals owned by the federal government. State university hospitals, state mental institutions, and state prison hospitals are examples of state-owned hospitals. County and municipal hospitals are owned by local governments.

Private hospitals, also called voluntary hospitals, are owned and operated by individuals, partnerships, corporations, religious groups, and labor unions.

✔ *Approximately 17.2 million people in the United States stayed overnight in a hospital in 2012.*

Private hospitals are called proprietary, investor-owned, or for-profit hospitals. Hospitals that don't make a profit are called nonprofit, nonproprietary, official, or not-for-profit hospitals. Public hospitals are not-for-profit hospitals. Private hospitals can be for-profit or not-for-profit hospitals, depending on their financial purpose.

In the past, a for-profit hospital was often owned by a group of local investors. The current trend is toward investor-owned corporations that may own hundreds of hospitals and other health care facilities across the country.

Hospitals can also be classified by the kinds of services they provide. General hospitals provide health care for most kinds of disorders to patients of most ages. Specialty hospitals provide health care only for specific disorders or conditions or for limited age groups. Psychiatric hospitals, children's hospitals, and rehabilitation hospitals are examples of specialty hospitals.

Hospitals can also be classified according to their size. The DHHS classifies urban hospitals as follows: 0–99 beds, 100–199 beds, 200–299 beds, 300–399 beds, 400–499 beds, and 500 or more beds.

The last way hospitals can be classified is by the average length of stay. Short-term care hospitals provide treatment for acute conditions requiring specialized personnel and sophisticated equipment and procedures for a short time. Short-term hospitals serve patients whose average stays are generally less than 30 days.

Long-term hospitals provide treatment, maintenance, and rehabilitation for patients with conditions that need extended care. Long-term acute care hospitals provide care for patients whose length of stay is greater than 30 days. They may be stand-alone hospitals or they may "rent" space within a general hospital. These hospitals provide important care services, but with a focus on rehabilitation.

Patient Care Units

An acute care general hospital serves a variety of patients with diverse medical and nursing needs. To provide competent and efficient care, a patient may be assigned to a patient care unit according to the primary diagnosis or by the amount of care required.

Units that specialize in specific types of care include coronary care, pediatric, medical, surgical, obstetric, and psychiatric units. Depending on the size of the facility, these units may fill a portion of a floor, a whole floor, or even a wing.

✔ *The number of special units in a hospital depends on the size and type of hospital.*

Patients can also be assigned to nursing units in which all the patients require the same relative amount of care. The overall management of patients by the amount of care needed is called *progressive care nursing*. Progressive care units include intensive care, intermediate care, self-care, and long-term care units.

Intensive care units are reserved for patients who are seriously or critically ill, who require total care and monitoring by means of specialized techniques and knowledge, and who require equipment that is immediately available in the unit. Personnel working in these units are highly skilled in using all available resources to assist the patient to recover from serious injury, disease, or major surgery.

Intensive care units include the following:
- Coronary care units
- Surgical intensive care units
- Medical intensive care units
- Neonatal intensive care units
- Pediatric intensive care units
- Burn intensive care units
- Postanesthesia and recovery units

✔ *In the United States, there are more than 15,700 nursing homes with beds for more than 1.4 million people.*

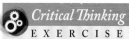

Critical Thinking
E X E R C I S E

There are many other types of health care facilities in addition to those discussed in the previous paragraphs. Walk or drive around your neighborhood or community and make a list of all of the health care facilities you can find. Don't forget to include those that are health related, such as Meals on Wheels, drug treatment centers, rehabilitation centers, and so forth. How many different types of health care agencies were you able to find? What does what you found say about access to adequate health care in your community or neighborhood? Is there a need in your neighborhood or community for additional health care facilities? Use appropriate Characteristics of Critical Thinking in Box 1-2 on pages 18–19 to develop your response to this situation.

Intermediate care units include the general medical and surgical units, the pediatric unit, the orthopedic unit, the newborn nursery, and the psychiatric unit.

Some or all of these units are found in a general short-term (acute) care hospital. Patients in these units are admitted for diagnosis or treatment of illness that cannot be treated on an outpatient basis. Patients admitted to these units are not critically ill; however, they do need the specialized medical and nursing care available in a hospital. During the early stages of rehabilitation, teaching patients how to care for their own health is an important activity in an intermediate care unit.

Self-care units are for patients with no or minimal limits on what they can do for themselves but who still need extensive rehabilitation and health care teaching or specialized therapy. These units are as homelike as possible. Patients eat in dining rooms, wear their own clothes, use recreational facilities, and keep their own appointments at other departments within the hospital.

Some short-term care hospitals have designated wings or floors for use as long-term care units. Patients in these units have needs similar to those of patients who are admitted to nursing homes. Long-term care is the care provided to patients who have an illness that may not be curable but whose condition may be improved through medical and nursing care.

Other Health Care Facilities

Among other types of health care facilities that provide health services are nursing homes, rehabilitation centers, free-standing surgical centers (surgicenters), dialysis centers, doctors' offices, neighborhood health centers, retail medical clinics, local health departments, industrial health centers, and community health centers.

A nursing home is a facility that provides care, generally to older people who can't care for themselves. Nursing homes are classified as either skilled nursing facilities (SNFs) or nursing facilities (NFs). SNFs provide skilled nursing services; residents in SNFs are too well to remain in a short-term care hospital but too ill to return to their home. Rehabilitation services are often an important part of an SNF. SNF residents often require the level of nursing service that is directed by licensed registered nurses (RNs) and licensed practical/vocational nurses (LP/VNs).

The NFs are designed to provide long-term care, usually to people over the age of 65 years who can't continue to live alone or with their families. Residents of NFs often have chronic medical problems, such as senility, Alzheimer's disease, paralysis resulting from a stroke, or a generalized weakness that makes it difficult for them to care for themselves or for their families to care for them. These residents often need assistance with activities of daily living such as bathing, dressing, eating, and walking.

Rehabilitation centers may be a division within a short-term care hospital, or they may be privately owned by physicians, physical therapists, or occupational therapists. These centers work with individual residents and their families to assist residents in attaining as much independence as possible (Fig. 7-2).

Surgicenters, usually not part of a hospital, provide minor surgical services for outpatients. The cost of procedures performed in these centers is less expensive than the same procedure performed in the hospital. Patients go home the same day that they have the surgery.

End-stage renal dialysis centers are often privately owned by physicians or other health care providers. They provide dialysis services to people whose

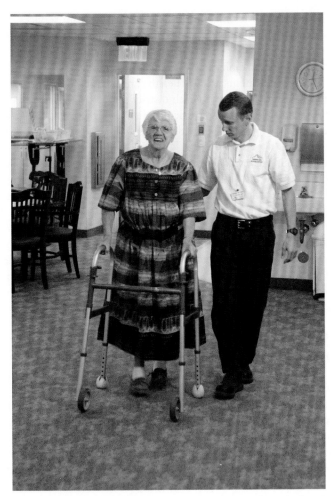

FIGURE 7-2. ● A patient in a rehabilitation center gains independence by learning to use a walker.

kidney function is inadequate. People report to the dialysis center three or more times a week for renal dialysis. The cost of renal dialysis is often covered through one of the federal government health insurance programs.

Doctor's offices can also be considered health care facilities. The major portion of health care is provided through them. There are many arrangements of doctor's offices. Some offices have only one doctor; others have many. When several doctors share patients and space, the term *group practice* is used to describe the office.

Neighborhood or community health centers usually serve a small geographic area. These facilities provide a range of health care services to people of all ages who live in the immediate area of the center. These centers depend on local, state, and federal funding to subsidize the cost of the medical care they provide.

Medical clinics operate in grocery stores, pharmacy chains, and mass merchandisers: urgent care clinics usually operate in stand-alone buildings. Both of these types of clinics are changing the way consumers can choose to obtain treatment for common illnesses such as strep throat and ear, eye, sinus, bladder, and bronchial infections. Patients see a physician, a nurse practitioner, or a physician's assistant. Appointments are not necessary and some of the stand-alone

✔ *More health care is provided in doctors' offices and health agencies located in the community than in hospitals.*

clinics offer x-rays, lab testing, and other basic health care services. Prices are usually posted on a menu board, and often, the patient just needs to make the co-payment required by her health plan. If the patient needs to have a prescription filled, there is often a pharmacy in the building.

Local health departments are also health care facilities. Larger cities are often divided into health districts, with each district served by an office that provides health care to residents of that particular district. In less populated areas, the county health department may provide the services to all residents of the county or parish.

Industrial health care facilities are found in business offices and industrial plants. These centers are staffed by a variety of health care personnel. Larger businesses and industries may employ physicians and nurses and offer a broad range of health screening and diagnostic services for their employees. Some of the health centers in larger businesses and industries offer fitness centers, counseling, and other health services.

Community mental health centers are generally organized as outpatient facilities for the diagnosis and treatment of mental and emotional disorders. These centers provide counseling services for patients who can continue to live in society but are in need of specialized treatment.

Health Care Service

Health care service is a term used to describe the actual delivery of health care by health care workers. Health care service includes the prevention, diagnosis, and treatment of illnesses. It also includes providing care during an illness. Health care service can take many forms: a surgeon who performs an appendectomy, a nurse who provides home care, a dietitian who plans the week's menu for a nursing home, a hospital administrator who orders equipment for the physical therapy department, a public health nurse presenting information to a community group on cancer prevention, a volunteer in a hospice facility, and an LP/VN bathing a patient. All are delivering health care services.

✔ *In 2012, there were about 2,824,641 RNs and more than 750,000 LP/VNs in the United States.*

You will be a member of a team delivering health care services. Your contributions as a member of that team are vitally important to the success of the health care service. The health care team is the topic of Chapter 8.

Health Care Regulation, Approval, Accreditation, and Standards of Excellence

Health care regulation is a term used to describe methods designed to control not only the quality of health care but also the cost. The need to regulate the quality and cost of health care can be attributed, in part, to increasingly complex technology, social and ethical issues, consumer demand for more services, and the high cost of providing medical services. Regulations that affect the health care industry are usually developed by governmental bodies, which have the legal authority to close down those who don't comply.

✔ *Each state has laws and regulations that a health care facility must follow to retain a license to operate.*

Health care approval is a term used to describe minimum regulatory standards that a facility must meet to admit or treat patients or residents. Facilities that offer health care services must be approved to operate by the state in which they are located. For example, a hospital operating in the state of Pennsylvania must be approved to operate by the Pennsylvania Department of Health. Every state has a similar office whose purpose is to evaluate health care facilities and approve or allow them to operate.

Health care accreditation is a term used to describe a process in which an accrediting agency uses their written standards of excellence to examine the operation of a health care facility or organization. Accreditation lets the public know that the accredited organization exceeds the minimum state regulatory standards for operation. In some cases, accreditation is voluntary. Accreditation of providers and facilities that receive Medicare and Medicaid funds from patient care or other federal or state government money for education and research is mandatory.

Standards of Excellence certificates are awarded for performance that exceeds the requirements for both approval and accreditation. The American Nurses Credentialing Center awards Magnet designation to health care organizations that demonstrate quality patient care, nursing excellence, and innovations in professional nursing practice. The Baldrige Performance Excellence Program is an award that gives recognition for quality and productivity in US organizations, including health care. The Standards for Excellence Institute awards a Seal of Excellence to nonprofit organizations, including health care organizations and facilities, that meet their rigorous criteria in ethics, effectiveness, and accountability.

As a health care worker, it is likely that you will be working for a health care facility that is seeking approval and accreditation or even applying for a Standards of Excellence certificate. Understanding the purposes of each of these processes will help you make appropriate and valuable contributions to this process.

✔ *Approval is mandatory; accreditation is usually voluntary.*

Regulation and Primary Health Care Providers

You will recall that primary health care providers are usually those who are first to see the patient, such as a physician, a nurse practitioner, a dentist, or any one of a number of other health care providers. Primary health care providers must be licensed by the state in which they practice their profession.

Licensure is mandatory. This means that someone can't say that he or she is a physician and use the initials MD (doctor of medicine) or DO (doctor of osteopathy) or DDS (doctor of dental surgery) unless licensed to do so. A license is usually obtained after the candidate for licensure has met educational and practice requirements and has passed a licensing examination in that particular profession.

Agencies that directly regulate the practice of primary health care providers are the licensing boards of individual states. It is the responsibility of each state's board to protect the citizens of that state. Therefore, the board examines applicants for licensure and issues, renews, and revokes licenses. Although licensing boards have many other responsibilities, regulating the practice of licensees is one of their major ones. Primary health care providers are also regulated by the ethical codes of their professions. Codes of ethics are discussed in more detail in Chapter 10.

✔ *A license lets the public know that the person has met the minimum education and practice requirements for that occupation.*

Approval and Accreditation of Hospitals

Each state evaluates and approves the activities of hospitals. To accept patients and offer medical care, hospitals must be approved by the state department of health or a similar organization. Standards specific to hospitals are applied during the evaluation process. A hospital that meets these standards is then approved to operate in that state.

About 90% of accredited hospitals and other health care facilities are accredited by the Joint Commission (JC). The American Osteopathic Association (AOA) as well as several other organizations also provide accreditation services for general and specialized hospitals. Accreditation is a voluntary process and indicates that the hospital has met the accrediting agency's specific standards and criteria for operating a health care facility. Accreditation of a hospital is mandatory if the hospital wants to sponsor medical educational programs and receive payment from Medicare and several other public and private health insurance plans.

Approval and Accreditation of Long-Term Care Facilities

As is the case with hospitals, long-term care facilities must be approved to operate in the state in which the facility is located. State approval guidelines and standards for accreditation are designed to evaluate the unique health care activities that occur in long-term care.

Facilities that accept Medicare or Medicaid funds for their services must be accredited by an appropriate accrediting agency such as the JC.

Approval and Accreditation of Home and Community Health Care Organizations

Home health and community health organizations are also required to be approved to operate by the state. Those that comply with state regulations are issued a license to operate within the state in which the organization is located.

Several organizations accredit home and community health care organizations. In 1992, the Community Health Accreditation Program (CHAP) became the first organization to receive government approval as a home health accrediting agency. CHAP began providing accrediting services for hospice and community and public health organizations in 1999. The JC also accredits home health and community agencies.

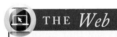 THE *Web*

> The Community Health Accreditation Program provides details on their accrediting programs on their Web site.

Approval of Other Health Care Facilities

Among the organizations and facilities that must be approved to operate by the state are boarding homes and residential treatment facilities, group homes, clinics, adult and child day care centers, hospice centers, pathology and clinical laboratories, behavioral health care organizations, ambulatory care providers, health care networks, home care agencies, assisted living facilities, and community mental health centers.

The JC, AOA, and CHAP are just three of the several organizations that are approved to provide accreditation services for these other health care facilities. Just about every organization or facility that offers health care must meet the guidelines for approval and often accreditation to operate.

Regulation of Agencies That Receive Medicare and Medicaid Payments

The federal government pays, through Medicare, Medicaid, and the State Children's Health Insurance Program, the health care costs of a large number of citizens. To ensure that adequate services are provided at a reasonable cost, the government has established regulations affecting those hospitals, nursing homes, physicians, and other providers of health care that receive reimbursement for services directly from one of these insurance plans. Many of the regulations originally established by the federal government are now being adapted for use by private insurance companies, such as Blue Cross and Blue Shield, as well as HMOs, PPOs, and other managed care organizations. Although many of the regulations developed by the government are complex, they are intended to help control the cost of health care in the United States.

✔ More than 62 million people are enrolled in Medicare with benefits costing more than $512 billion in 2014.

Quality Assurance, Peer Review, and Risk Management Programs

One aspect of approval and accreditation of health care providers who are paid for their services through Medicare, Medicaid, or other government funds is the requirement for developing a mechanism to ensure that patients receive quality care in a safe environment. Safety and quality patient care is a goal shared by all members of the health care team, but providing safety and quality in a complex health care system with many recent technologic advances is not as easy as it may seem. The purpose of quality assurance (QA) programs in health care facilities is to evaluate and improve the level of service to patients to ensure that at least minimally accepted levels of service are provided at the lowest cost possible.

✔ Committees can describe quality of care, but only you can provide it.

Continuous quality improvement (CQI) through QA and quality improvement (QI) programs is part of a continual evaluation process and is required by some accrediting agencies such as the JC. Although there are similar programs designed to improve the quality of care, the CQI program is the most common.

Continuous quality improvement is a term used to describe the overall plan for improving the quality of care. It includes activities such as QA and QI. The CQI group or committee reviews reports from the QA and QI committees and reviews patient charts, incident reports, patient surveys, and costs of care. They look for and implement ways to improve the quality of care provided in their facility.

Quality assurance sets minimal standards of care. This is usually done by a committee of people who are experts in a particular area. For example, nurses who have an extensive educational background in maternity nursing and several years of experience working with women in a maternity department meet together and define, in writing, standards of nursing care that would ensure safe care.

Quality improvement is intended to help an organization move beyond minimal standards to higher standards of care. This is often done through patient surveys, staff questionnaires, and patient chart reviews. The result of this evaluation process leads to changes in procedures, which lead to greater patient satisfaction and lower costs.

Peer review can be described as the examination of someone's work by other people of equal standing. As a result of peer review, many expensive diagnostic and laboratory tests are no longer done, and many surgeries are now performed on an outpatient basis. This has eased the financial burden for both the patient and the health care system.

Risk management programs are intended to prevent financial loss to the organization or facility. This is done by identifying situations that result in longer lengths of stay in the facility; injury to patients, visitors, or staff; and incidents of patient care errors. Based on the findings of the risk manager, changes in policies and procedures are made to reduce the financial risk to the organization.

Because CQI, peer review, and risk management programs in health care facilities are the rule rather than the exception, you will most likely be employed in an agency that has these programs. Your employer will expect you to provide a certain standard of care, to keep accurate written records, probably to serve on special committees, and perhaps to participate in a peer review program. Your contributions will go a long way toward making yourself an important part of the health care team.

HEALTH CARE FINANCING

Health care financing is a term used to discuss how the costs for health care are paid. The cost of health care during the 1980s grew at a rate of about 11% a year. Rapidly escalating costs placed a heavy burden on the health care system as well as on consumers, and because of these rapid increases, a number of new cost-containing measures were put in place. As you can see in Table 7-1, costs more than doubled between 1980 and 1990 and almost doubled between 1990 and 2000. Spending for health care in 2010 was $2.6 trillion. The cost of health care is expected to increase to be about $4.6 trillion by 2020. Figure 7-3 shows the high cost of medical services for a partial day of inpatient treatment in a hospital intensive care unit.

Two major ways that people pay for health care are private health insurance and government health insurance. Although health insurance pays much of the cost of health care, in 2012, about 48 million Americans did not have any health insurance coverage.

✔ *In 2012, about 48 million people had no health care insurance.*

The findings presented in Table 7-2 show that in the years between 1987 and 2014, the percent of people with private health insurance decreased. The percent of people with government health insurance increased during that same time period. The percent of people without health insurance steadily increased from 1987 to 2009 and then dropped by about 3% by 2014.

One of the reasons for the recent decrease in the percent of people without health insurance is the result of recent legislation called the Patient Protection and Affordable Care Act (also known as the Affordable Care Act or ObamaCare). The Affordable Care Act (ACA) requires everyone, with certain exceptions, to have health insurance by 2014. The ACA will be discussed later in this chapter.

✔ *The ACA was signed into law by President Obama on March 23, 2010.*

Private Insurance

Private medical insurance is the type a person buys as an individual or as a member of a group. This type of insurance is sold by commercial insurance companies and others in the same way that life, homeowner's, and automobile insurance are sold. The two basic types of private medical insurance plans are indemnity insurance and prepaid insurance. In 2014, there were more than 2,000 companies offering private health and disability insurance.

Fee-for-service plans (also called indemnity plans) pay their policyholders or assignees (someone authorized to receive payment, such as a health care provider) the amount stated on the policy when an approved claim is made. This amount may pay for all or part of the claim, depending on the amount of

TABLE 7-1 Rising Cost of Health Care From 1960 and Projected to 2020	
Year	Annual Health Care Cost per Person
1960	$147
1970	$356
1980	$1,110
1990	$2,855
2000	$4,878
2010	$8,411
2020	$13,708[a]

[a]*Projected.*

Data from Centers for Medicare and Medicaid Services, National Health Expenditure Data, 1960–2020.

DESCRIPTION OF SERVICE	AMOUNT BILLED
MEDICAL CENTER CLAIM WAS RECV'D ON 07/27/15	
06/16/15 INTENSIVE CARE	58,932.00
06/16/15 MEDICAL - INPATIENT	1,932.00
06/16/15 MEDICAL - INPATIENT	375.00
06/16/15 MEDICAL - INPATIENT	1,500.00
06/16/15 SUPPLIES	412.75
06/16/15 DURABLE MEDICAL EQUIPMENT	3,200.00
06/16/15 LABORATORY	12,200.00
06/16/15 LABORATORY	64.00
06/16/15 LABORATORY	1,823.00
06/16/15 LABORATORY	3,214.00
06/16/15 LABORATORY	460.00
06/16/15 MEDICATIONS	1,720.00

FIGURE 7-3. ● This sample patient bill illustrates the high costs of health care.

coverage purchased. Cost of the policy will vary with the amount of coverage desired, deductible amount, the insured person's age and health, and other factors. Blue Cross and Blue Shield is an example of one company that offers fee-for-service insurance. Most indemnity insurance plans pay only for purchased services that result from a claim specifically covered in the policy. Usually, the insured person may choose the care provider, as long as that provider or the services provided aren't specifically excluded.

The second type of private insurance, prepaid insurance, often stresses the importance of disease prevention. These plans are generally referred to as managed care plans and they provide a range of prepaid services to their policyholders. HMOs, point of service (POS) groups, PPOs, and high-deductible health plan (HDHP) groups are examples of plans that offer prepaid insurance.

Beginning in 2003, people who had HDHP health insurance could put money into a Health Savings Account (HSA). This money was not subject to federal tax and could be used to pay for doctor's fees, obstetrical expenses, dental braces, drugs, psychiatric care, and hundreds or other health-related expenses. It is estimated that nearly 17.4 million people are enrolled in an HSA.

✔ Blue Cross health insurance was first offered in 1929.

✔ In 2013, more than 262 million people belonged to an HMO, PPO, POS, or HDHP insurance plan.

TABLE 7-2	Percentage of US Population Insured From 1987 to 2014[a]		
Year	Private Insurance (Including Managed Care)	Government Insurance (Including Medicare)	Uninsured
1987	75.5%	23.3%	12.9%
1990	73.2%	24.5%	13.9%
2000	72.6%	24.7%	13.7%
2005	68.5%	27.3%	15.3%
2009	63.9%	30.6%	16.7%
2014	63.9%	32.6%	13.9%

[a]Total exceeds 100% due to individuals having more than one type of health insurance.
Source: U.S. Census Bureau; Income, Poverty, and Health Insurance Coverage in the United States: 2014.

In managed care, the policyholder pays a set monthly (or other period) charge. This payment entitles the policyholder to use the plan's services for routine health care and hospitalization as needed. Some plans include long-term care and other services. Cost of the plan varies according to services offered. Some plans limit the amount of money they will pay, either annually or over a lifetime, for certain services. The term used to describe limiting the amount a policy will pay is *capitation*. The policyholder usually doesn't get to choose a primary health care provider. Primary health care providers (e.g., physicians, nurse practitioners) are usually salaried employees of the managed care group or work under contract. The managed care employee salary may or may not be directly related to the profits (or losses) of the organization.

Each type of insurance has advantages and disadvantages. With indemnity insurance, the insured person can choose a provider and health service facilities. The managed care member must receive treatment by member providers. On the other hand, indemnity insurance doesn't generally pay for preventive care as managed care groups do. This distinction is diminishing and will probably continue to do so as studies show that preventive measures actually reduce hospitalization and the accompanying costs.

Government Insurance

In 1965, the US government passed legislation that made it a major health care insurance provider. The Social Security Act of 1965 included Titles XVIII and XIX, better known as Medicare and Medicaid. Medicare is a federally funded health insurance program, whereas Medicaid is a jointly funded federal–state health insurance program. Title XXI, titled State Children's Health Insurance Program (SCHIP), was passed in 1997 to provide low- or no-cost health insurance for children of low-income families. All three of these insurance programs are administered by the government's Centers for Medicare and Medicaid.

Medicare is a hospital and health care insurance plan for persons 65 years of age and older. Money for this program comes from Social Security taxes paid by workers and their employers to the federal government. Services provided under Medicare are the same nationwide.

Medicaid, a state-administered program, pays for health care services for the disabled or poor of any age with funds that come from both the state and the federal governments. Because Medicaid is administered by the state, services that are provided can vary from state to state.

✔ *In 2014, 35% of the cost of personal health care was paid for by federal and state governments through Medicare, Medicaid, and SCHIP.*

SCHIP is jointly financed by the federal and state governments and administered by the states. Within broad federal guidelines, each state determines the design of its program, eligibility groups, benefit packages, payment levels for coverage, and administrative and operating procedures.

Individuals participating in Medicare, Medicaid, and SCHIP programs may choose their health care services and facilities from participating health care providers. Although not all health care providers accept these insurances as payment for services, the majority do.

A major portion of the Affordable Care Act (ACA) is related to health care insurance and regulation of health care insurance companies. The ACA created the Health Insurance Marketplace, which allows individuals to compare health plans and find out if they are eligible for tax credits for private insurance or if they are eligible for insurance through programs like SCHIP. The Marketplace also provides information so consumers can compare the cost of insurance premiums from one company to another. Health care insurance companies can no longer drop people who require expensive medical care, nor can they deny coverage because of pre-existing conditions.

CONTROLLING HEALTH CARE COSTS

Consumers, politicians, and health care providers have been attempting to find ways to control the continuing increase in health care costs for many years. As you saw in Table 7-1 on page 144, the annual cost of health care for each person in the United States in 2020 is expected to be $13,708 or 12 times more than in 1980. The health care system is complex and the task is monumental. Some of the ways to try to control the cost of health care have been around for some time, and newer ways to control costs are emerging.

One of the newer ways to control the cost of health care is the ACA. Many provisions in the ACA aim to curb the rising cost of health care through greater competition among health plans, taxes on high-priced insurance coverage, measures to cut waste, abuse and fraud, prevention and wellness promotion, and provider incentives. Whether the ACA will slow down the escalating cost of health care remains to be seen. History indicates that health care spending dropped from 6.3% in 2007 to 3.8% in 2009 and stayed at that rate through 2012. Proponents of the ACA attribute the steady lower rates to this law and an improving economy; those opposed to ACA believe that this is a temporary lull and that costs will skyrocket as time goes by.

Diagnosis-Related Groups

One of the older ways of controlling costs is the diagnosis-related groups (DRGs) method of payment that was developed by the federal government. From 1965 to 1983, the federal Medicare program paid health care providers (e.g., physicians, hospitals, nursing homes) for services provided to people who were eligible for health care under the Medicare program. This system, called retrospective payment, meant that the health care provider ordered any and all medical care he or she believed was necessary or desirable without consideration of the cost. The providers were reimbursed by Medicare for their costs. As a consequence of rising health care costs, the DRG payment system was instituted in 1983. This system, called the prospective payment system (PPS), was developed by the federal government in an attempt to control health care costs associated with the Medicare program. The principle of prospective payment is to set rates for health care services in advance, rather than after the service has been delivered.

✔ *The DRG system of payment takes age, complications, and multiple health problems into consideration.*

For example, under a PPS, the cost for an appendectomy would be calculated and fixed ahead of time. The calculated cost would allow for appropriate patient care and for an ordinary profit for the treating facility. If treatment was provided below the fixed rate, the agency or physician would keep the difference, but if actual costs exceeded the allowable rate, the agency or physician would have to bear the extra expenses themselves. CMS uses separate PPSs for reimbursement to acute inpatient hospitals, home health agencies, hospice, hospital outpatient, inpatient psychiatric facilities, inpatient rehabilitation facilities, long-term care hospitals, and NFs.

The government's payment system for acute hospitalized patients is made up of 25 major diagnostic categories (MDCs) and over 900 DRGs. For example, the MDC for an appendectomy is 06 (Digestive System) and the related DRG

MS-DRG[a]	MDC[b]	Type	MS-DRG TITLE
338	06	SURG	APPENDECTOMY W COMPLICATED PRINCIPAL DIAG W MCC
339	06	SURG	APPENDECTOMY W COMPLICATED PRINCIPAL DIAG W CC
340	06	SURG	APPENDECTOMY W COMPLICATED PRINCIPAL DIAG W/O CC/MCC
341	06	SURG	APPENDECTOMY W/O COMPLICATED PRINCIPAL DIAG W MCC
342	06	SURG	APPENDECTOMY W/O COMPLICATED PRINCIPAL DIAG W CC
343	06	SURG	APPENDECTOMY W/O COMPLICATED PRINCIPAL DIAG W/O CC/MCC
344	06	SURG	MINOR SMALL & LARGE BOWEL PROCEDURES W MCC
345	06	SURG	MINOR SMALL & LARGE BOWEL PROCEDURES W CC
346	06	SURG	MINOR SMALL & LARGE BOWEL PROCEDURES W/O CC/MCC
347	06	SURG	ANAL & STOMAL PROCEDURES W MCC
348	06	SURG	ANAL & STOMAL PROCEDURES W CC
349	06	SURG	ANAL & STOMAL PROCEDURES W/O CC/MCC
350	06	SURG	INGUINAL & FEMORAL HERNIA PROCEDURES W MCC
351	06	SURG	INGUINAL & FEMORAL HERNIA PROCEDURES W CC
352	06	SURG	INGUINAL & FEMORAL HERNIA PROCEDURES W/O CC/MCC
353	06	SURG	HERNIA PROCEDURES EXCEPT INGUINAL & FEMORAL W MCC
354	06	SURG	HERNIA PROCEDURES EXCEPT INGUINAL & FEMORAL W CC
355	06	SURG	HERNIA PROCEDURES EXCEPT INGUINAL & FEMORAL W/O CC/MCC

TABLE 7-3   List of Medicare Diagnosis-Related Groups (DRGs)—FY 2010

[a]*Medicare Severity Diagnosis-Related Group.*
[b]*Major Diagnostic Category.*
Adapted from: List of Diagnosis-Related Groups (DRGs)—FY DRG MDC Type. http://www.cms.hhs.gov

are 338, 339, 340, 341, 342, or 343 depending on complications, age, and other factors. See a partial list of selected DRGs in Table 7-3.

By knowing the amount of reimbursement that will be received for services to patients, health care facilities and health care providers can control how much they spend and thus ensure a profit while still providing necessary health care.

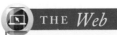 THE *Web*

The Centers for Medicare and Medicaid Services provides a complete list of the 999 MS-DRGs (Medicare Severity Diagnoses-Related Groups).

Other Cost-Controlling Programs

Utilization review, quality management, critical pathways, care maps, pay for performance, improvements in managed care programs, governmental legislation such as the ACA, and yet to be proposed programs will try to control the costs of health care. You will be learning more about each of these as you continue your nursing education and as you participate in providing patient care. In general, each of these programs is designed to outline the most efficient and best care for an individual at the least cost to the insurer and to the patient. The goals are to maximize quality of care, to better use resources, and to minimize costly delays in treatment.

✔ *When you become a nurse, you will be expected to participate in cost-controlling practices.*

U.S. DEPARTMENT OF HEALTH AND HUMAN SERVICES

The federal government became active in health care for citizens of the United States when medical care was authorized for American merchant seamen in 1798. Since then, the federal government has been involved with many health-related issues in areas of regulation, prevention, and control.

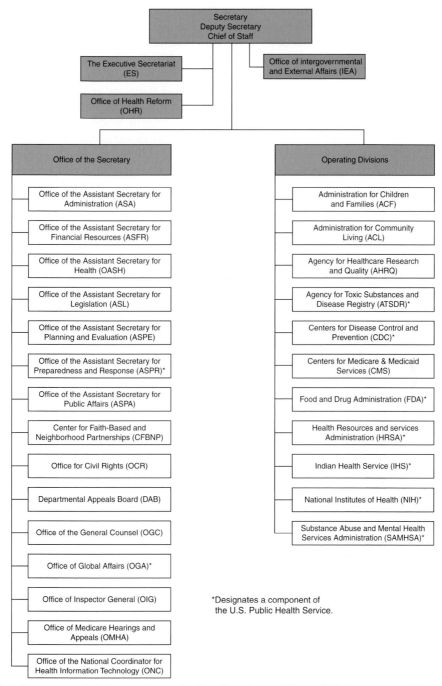

FIGURE 7-4. ● Department of Health and Human Services Organizational Chart. (U.S. Department of Health and Human Services. Available at http://www.hhs.gov, keywords DHHS Organizational Chart.)

✔ There are 10 CDC facilities in the United States with more than 15,000 employees and contractors and a budget in excess of $11.2 billion annually.

✔ The FDA has nearly 15,000 employees who inspect more than 100,000 FDA-regulated businesses.

✔ The HRSA is working with other organizations to resolve the shortage of health care workers.
✔ Founded in 1887, the NIH awards over 50,000 research grants each year.

✔ The IHS provides health care services for approximately 1.9 million American Indians and Alaskan Natives who belong to 566 federally recognized tribes.

✔ CMS provides health insurance for over 100 million people through Medicare, Medicaid, SCHIP, and the Health Insurance Marketplace programs.

The U.S. Department of Health, Education, and Welfare was created in 1953 to address the health, education, and social concerns of Americans. This department was divided into the Department of Health and Human Services (DHHS) and the Department of Education in 1980. The DHHS has 11 agencies and a number of offices and departments that support the work of these agencies. Figure 7-4 shows the organizational chart of the DHHS.

Several of the 11 operating divisions in the DHHS are of interest to nurses. **The Centers for Disease Control and Prevention (CDC),** headquartered in Atlanta, Georgia, is the agency to which communicable diseases are reported. The mission of the CDC is to promote health and quality of life by preventing and controlling disease, injury, and disability. This agency collects data and maintains statistics on diseases and their spread and supports research for controlling communicable diseases in the United States and around the world.

The Food and Drug Administration (FDA), through its various bureaus, protects the public from impure and unsafe foods, medications, and cosmetics, regulates the use and labeling of medicines and devices for preventing and treating diseases, sets standards for food additives and labeling, conducts research, develops policy, fosters the development of medical products to counteract public health threats, and provides information to the public. The FDA regulates over $1 trillion worth of products in the United States.

The Health Resources and Services Administration (HRSA) is the primary federal agency for improving access to health care by strengthening the health care workforce, building healthy communities, and achieving health equity.

The National Institutes of Health (NIH) is composed of 27 separate institutes and centers. The National Cancer Institute, the National Center for Complementary and Alternative Medicine, the National Institute on Aging, and the National Institute of Nursing Research are examples. Each agency is engaged in research to uncover new knowledge that will lead to better health for everyone.

The Indian Health Service (IHS) is primarily concerned with the health of Native American Indians and Alaskan Natives. This branch of the government provides a variety of health care services on many reservations throughout the United States.

The Health Care Financing Administration was renamed the **Centers for Medicare and Medicaid Services (CMS)** on June 14, 2001. This is the federal agency that administers Medicare, Medicaid, the State Children's Health Insurance Program (SCHIP), a major portion of the ACA, and the quality improvement and accreditation operations. The CMS is the largest agency in the DHHS and it provides services that affect millions of Americans every day.

The other six agencies of the DHHS are focused on children and families, aging, health care research and quality of care, community living, registration of diseases and toxic substances, and substance abuse and mental health. Through these agencies and the other offices of the DHHS, the health of all Americans, especially those who are least able to help themselves, is tended to.

THE *Web*

Visit the Web site of the individual agencies within the DHHS to learn more about the services they offer.

STATE AND LOCAL HEALTH DEPARTMENTS

State governments are also involved in the delivery of health care services. A commissioner of health, a secretary of health, or someone with a similar title is assigned the responsibility of overseeing state health programs. This office also administers the state Medicaid and the SCHIP for residents with low incomes or disabilities.

State health department functions may also include the licensing of health care workers, hospitals, nursing homes, pharmaceutical manufacturers and distributors, and other health care agencies. State health departments also disseminate information and educational material, such as films, books, and pamphlets, on health matters to both the general public and health care agencies.

✔ *Local and state health departments report communicable disease data to the CDC.*

Divisions of the state health department may include public health, communicable diseases, vital statistics, maternal and child health, mental health, and other programs. State health departments in some areas have a direct relationship with local health departments.

Local health departments place their emphasis on health care needs of people living in specific geographic areas. Their jurisdiction may include a town, a city, a parish, a county, a borough, or some other clearly defined area. Functions of the local health department include reporting communicable diseases, keeping vital statistics, managing sanitation, providing a safe water supply, providing child and school health services, and managing other matters of local public health.

PRIVATE ORGANIZATIONS THAT SUPPORT THE HEALTH CARE SYSTEM

Many additional types of health care are provided through a variety of private organizations. Although these services are not the typical ones that come to mind when we think of the health care system, they do contribute to the health of our society. Some of them include adult and child day care centers, Meals on Wheels, suicide prevention hotlines, child abuse hotlines, family planning services, homemaker services, and specialized transportation services for ill and disabled persons.

Private groups organized to provide emotional and psychological support for individuals and families with health-related problems include Alcoholics Anonymous, Women Organized Against Rape, Women Against Abuse, Reach to Recovery (for patients recovering from mastectomies), Sudden Infant Death Syndrome Foundation, the Susan G. Komen Breast Cancer Awareness Organization, the Zipper Club (for patients recovering from heart surgery), and Mothers Against Drunk Driving.

✔ *Private organizations and volunteer groups make enormous contributions to the health of the people of the United States.*

A large assortment of private organizations dedicated to meeting specific health care needs of the population include the American Heart Association, the American Cancer Society, the March of Dimes Birth Defects Foundation, the United Way, and many more. Financial support for these organizations comes from fund drives, individual contributions, business and corporate gifts, and donations raised through radio and television marathons. Although these organizations don't generally provide health care, they do contribute millions of dollars to support research and treatment of specific diseases.

Private funding for health care services also includes community drives that raise money to help an identified individual or family cope with a catastrophic and expensive illness. You've probably been approached by a friend or neighbor and asked to contribute to a health care fund for a needy individual in your community. These people-to-people programs do a great deal to improve the health of this society.

In 2014, individuals contributed over $300 billion for charitable purposes, which include funding to conduct medical research, improve technologies, and treat diseases. These contributions to the health care system must be recognized, supported, and appreciated by everyone.

ISSUES AND CONCERNS

The ACA legislation is a step toward health care for all Americans, but this alone will not address all of the issues and concerns about health care that confront the people of the United States. Some of those issues and concerns are discussed in the remainder of this chapter.

Health Care System

The capitalistic system in the United States encourages private ownership, free enterprise, and private profit. An advantage of this system is that it creates many choices and options. While we enjoy having all of these choices, in health care choices can be confusing. Multiple organizations, a diversity of private providers, a wide variety of facilities, cumbersome regulations, and complex procedures and policies confuse the public and make it difficult for people to navigate their way through the maze of available choices and options.

To address these concerns and confusions, a case or coordinated care manager, most often a registered nurse or social worker, can help patients and their families meet their health needs by explaining options and services, identifying medical and financial resources, and identifying providers and facilities. The case manager works to coordinate care that utilizes the best options for the individual patient. Many case managers take an examination to be a Certified Case Manager.

You will most likely have patients and families who are struggling to understand all of their health care options. Keeping up with current events in health care and knowing who and what resources are available, both in your workplace and in your community, will help you deliver care that goes beyond meeting basic physical needs.

Health Care Providers

A persistent concern has been the geographic concentration of primary care providers and an overabundance of doctors specializing in anesthesiology, radiology, and emergency medicine. In many areas of this country, no doctor is available for hundreds of miles, whereas large cities and major medical centers have a high physician/person ratio. While nurse practitioners and nurse-midwives have done much to alleviate the shortage of primary care doctors, the shortage remains significant. There are new incentives in the ACA to expand the number of primary care doctors, advanced practice nurses, and certified nurse-midwives, including funding for scholarships and loan repayments. It will be several years before this incentive will have an impact on underserved areas, but it is a step toward reducing the shortage of primary health care providers.

The future role of other health care providers such as the multipurpose worker and the cross-training of current health care workers are also a concern. Multipurpose workers are those who are taught to perform the skills usually performed by workers in other job classifications. Cross-training means that workers are trained to perform several different jobs. Issues related to these workers include concerns about their educational preparation for the skills they perform and how their practice is regulated. It is important for practicing nurses to vigorously oppose the delivery of nursing care by nonnursing personnel. The American Nurses Association Online Journal of Issues in Nursing article titled "Overview and Summary: Delegation Dilemmas: Standards and Skills for Practice" describes many of the issues and concerns related to delegating nursing duties to others.

✔ As of 2015, 14–18 million Americans gained health insurance coverage under the ACA.

✔ Quality health care for all citizens is a national goal.

✔ In 2014, more than 12 million people were employed in health care.

✔ Delegation of nursing duties to nonnursing personnel is a concern for all nurses.

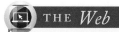 THE *Web*

Overview and Summary: Delegation Dilemmas: Standards and Skills for
Practice is available on the American Nurses Association Web site using the
search term "Delegation Dilemmas."

Health Care Facilities

A few of the major issues confronting hospitals include financial challenges,
implications related to implementing the ACA, care for the uninsured and charity care, personnel shortages, quality of services, and patient safety. A few of the
issues confronting long-term care facilities include lack of staff, lack of training
for staff, and lack of supervision of staff in nearly every nursing home in the
country. Rehabilitation facilities, ambulatory surgical centers, dialysis centers,
and group medical practices are just a few of the many facilities that continue to
wrestle with issues related to prospective payment systems, insurance regulations, government regulations, costs of accreditation, and malpractice claims.

✔ Between 2007 and 2013, more than 600 acute care hospitals either merged or were acquired by another group.

Health Care Services

Another major concern has to do with equal access to health care services for all
citizens. The ACA is designed to provide reasonably priced high-quality health care
to all Americans. Figure 7-5 provides a list of the significant highlights of the ACA.

✔ The ACA includes provisions to improve access to quality health care for all Americans.

It is likely that we will see more services offered in community health centers
and other outpatient facilities. Health care services in school-based health clinics
will become the rule rather than the exception. Incentives to primary care providers, including nurse practitioners, to practice in underserved geographic areas
may help improve the public's access to health care.

Health Care Approval, Accreditation, and Standards of Excellence

As patients continue to express dissatisfaction with the cost and quality of the
health care they receive, more regulations will appear. These regulations will most
likely be aimed at improving the quality of care through CQI programs, containing
the cost of care through extensive peer review, and generally raising the standards
of care through approval, accreditation, and standards of excellence programs.

- Prohibits health insurance companies from dropping people except for fraud.
- Eliminates lifetime limits on insurance coverage.
- Eliminates charging more for health insurance because of a pre-existing condition.
- Covers preventive services and immunizations if your insurance plan is subject to these requirements.
- Extends dependent health insurance coverage up to age 26.
- Requires individuals to maintain Minimum Essential Coverage or pay a penalty at tax time.
- Establishes the Health Insurance Marketplace.
- Promotes prevention, wellness, and public health.
- Funds scholarships and loan repayment programs to support and expand education of the health care workforce.
- Prevents providers who have been penalized in one state from setting up in another.
- Ends anti-competitive behavior by drug companies that keep effective and affordable generic drugs off the market.

FIGURE 7-5. ● Selected Highlights of the Affordable Care Act. Adapted from HealthCare.gov available at www.healthcare.gov

Approval of health care programs is generally granted by the state department of health or another similar department within the state in which the health care facility is located. Efforts to improve the quality of health care are ongoing; therefore, approval and accreditation standards are frequently updated. To learn about current approval requirements, go to the specific state Web site for further information. To learn more about current accreditation requirements, use the term "CMS-approved accreditation organizations," select the accreditation agency you would like to know more about, and then proceed to that Web site.

Although accreditation is important to maintaining quality and eligibility for reimbursement from private and government insurance plans, it is also costly. Most accrediting organizations charge an organizational membership fee, an application fee, and a base fee plus an additional amount per member or per agency. They also charge per person for the on-site reviewers and their expenses, and some require extensive reports for the years between the on-site reviews. For example, the Joint Commission charges an ambulatory surgery center with approximately 6,000 visits per year nearly $16,000 in annual fees. This does not include the cost of salaries for time spent in implementing compliance programs, completing the accreditation application, and documenting progress in meeting accreditation standards.

✔ *Organizations that offer superior care and service might not seek national accreditation or might not apply for a Standards of Excellence certificate because of the cost.*

Health care administrators are in a difficult position when it comes to national accreditation. In many cases, accreditation is a requirement for reimbursement from insurance companies, especially Medicare, Medicaid, and SCHIP. Lack of accreditation may mean that the number and types of patients that can be served are restricted. If an agency does seek accreditation, the costs of this process are passed on to the patient in the form of higher costs for medical or nursing services.

The costs associated with achieving Standards of Excellence certificates can also be quite expensive. While the actual application and evaluation process are costly, the cost of maintaining the standards between evaluations can also be expensive.

Costs for accreditation and Standards of Excellence certificates are going to have to be controlled to help contain the escalating cost of health care.

Health Care Financing

Spending for health care reached $2.9 trillion in 2013. There are several reasons why it is difficult to control or reduce spending. One of the most significant is the increased number of elderly people in America. In 2000, 4.2 million people were age 85 or older. By the year 2030, the number of Americans age 85 and older is expected to be about 8.7 million. Increasing age doesn't necessarily mean illness, but many older people do have extensive and expensive health care needs. Because the primary source of health insurance for older Americans is Medicare, many are concerned that Medicare funds will be depleted in the near future.

✔ *About $8,411 was spent on health care for each person in the United States in 2010.*

Other factors that are increasing the cost of health care are related to the various treatments that are prescribed for expensive illnesses. The 2012 cost of prescription drugs was nearly $326 billion or about $898 per person. Organ transplants are extremely expensive procedures, and the annual cost of drugs a patient must take to prevent rejection is enormous. The lifetime cost to treat an HIV-positive person is about $650,000.

✔ *Financing the cost of health care will remain a serious national issue over the next years.*

The cost of finding cures for diseases such as cancer and heart disease is becoming more expensive, and the cures, when found, will no doubt be very costly. The increase in the number and settlement costs of medical malpractice lawsuits places a heavy burden on the health care system. New drugs that are very effective in treating diseases are also very expensive.

Advances in technology require large investments in equipment, which also increases the cost of health care. For example, an x-ray machine costs about $190,000, whereas a computed tomography/positron emission tomography scanner costs about $3,000,000 plus an additional $100,000 a year in maintenance costs. Simple open surgery costs about $14,000, while robotic surgical devices cost more than $1.5 million each with a $100,000 yearly maintenance fee.

Electronic Health Records

The health care industry is far behind the finance, retail, manufacturing, and transportation industries in using computer-based records. Some of the advantages of using electronic health records (EHRs) include having all of the information about a patient in one place, being able to quickly find and read the record, being able to search for specific activities, being able to conduct medical research more efficiently, and having up-to-date information immediately available. One cannot argue with the benefits of an EHR; however, there are a number of reasons why creating these records is so difficult. Probably, the biggest barrier to creating an EHR is cost. The computer equipment, scanners, software programs, maintenance, and training are very costly and many health care facilities do not have all of the money that is needed to implement such a system. For this reason, the ACA contains financial incentives for those health care providers who implement an approved EHR system by 2015. The incentive for a Medicare-eligible hospital is based on a number of factors beginning with a $2 million base payment.

There are also concerns about confidentiality, security, and incompatibility between systems.

The ACA includes a provision that will institute a series of changes to standardize billing and requires health plans to begin adopting and implementing rules for the secure and confidential electronic exchange of health information. In 2009, only 11.9% of hospitals were using EHRs, and of those, only 2% would meet the federal government's standards for EHRs. By the end of 2013, 80% of eligible hospitals were using approved EHR systems.

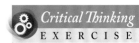

Critical Thinking
E X E R C I S E

You have learned a lot about the health care system in this chapter. What challenges and opportunities does this provide for you in the next 5 years? The next 10 years? How can you use what you have learned as you plan for your career in nursing? Use appropriate Characteristics of Critical Thinking in Box 1-2 on pages 18–19 to develop your response to these questions.

SUMMARY

The health care system in the United States is complex and sometimes difficult to understand. It is important that nurses and other health care providers be able to help their patients and clients find the right care at the right price and at the right time. To do this requires a continuing effort to learn all you can about the issues and concerns surrounding the health care system.

The Affordable Care Act contains many provisions some of which are intended to provide health care to people who could otherwise not afford it and to correct some of the worst abuses by the health insurance industry. No matter what direction health care reform takes, the goals of the health care system in the future will be to provide safe, efficient, and effective care at the least cost and to restore health in the shortest possible time. You will be in a position both to affect and to be affected by changes in the health care system. You will affect it by the efficiency with which you provide care; you will be affected by what health care services you can afford for yourself and your family.

APPLY
Critical Thinking Skills

1. In the opening story at the beginning of this chapter, Mary found a lump in her breast. If Mary asked you what she should do, what would you suggest and why?

2. List as many different local facilities as you can where health care services are provided. (You might use GPS or the Internet or walk around your neighborhood for additional information.)

3. How is the practice of primary health care providers (physicians, nurse practitioners, and hospitals) regulated in your state?

4. Try a short peer review after your next clinical day. Ask one of your classmates to evaluate your performance during the day. How does your classmate's assessment of your performance compare with facility standards and with your standards?

5. Ask some of your family, friends, or relatives to describe their health care insurance. Do they know what services are excluded? How much does their insurance cost, and does their employer pay any part of the cost?

6. Discuss the DRG method of payment for health care with your classmates. What are the advantages and disadvantages of this system to both the patient and the health care provider?

7. List some of the ways you can directly contribute to controlling health care costs, both as a nurse and as a consumer of health care.

8. List 10 reasons for supporting (or not supporting) the Affordable Care Act.

Read More
ABOUT IT

Ellis JR, Hartley CL: Nursing in Today's World: Trends, Issues, and Management, 10th ed. Philadelphia, PA: Lippincott Williams & Wilkins, 2011.

Estes CL, Chapman SA: Health Policy: Crisis and Reform, 6th ed. Boston, MA: Jones & Bartlett, 2012.

Goldsteen R, Goldsteen K: Jonas' Introduction to the US Health Care System, 7th ed. New York, NY: Springer Publishing, 2012.

Nickitas D, Middaugh DJ, Aries N: Policy and Politics for Nurses and Other Health Professionals, 2nd ed. Boston, MA: Jones & Bartlett, 2014.

Shi L, Singh D: Essentials of the U.S. Health Care System, 3rd ed. Boston, MA: Jones & Bartlett, 2013.

Sultz HA, Young KM: Health Care USA: Understanding Its Organization and Delivery, 8th ed. Boston, MA: Jones & Bartlett, 2013.

Zephyros Press: Obamacare Simplified: A Clear Guide to Making Obamacare Work for You. Berkeley, CA: Callisto Media, 2013.

The Health Care Team

LEARNING OBJECTIVES

When you complete this chapter, you will be able to:

1. Describe the function of several health care team members.

2. Define the term health care team and describe the educational preparation of several of its members.

3. List the members of the nursing team and describe their major responsibilities related to patient care.

4. Explain and describe differences in case, functional, team, and primary nursing care delivery models.

Alice parked her car in the lot behind Riverview, the nursing home where her grandmother lived, and hurried inside.

As she approached her grandmother's room, she saw her sister, Jeanne, in the doorway. "They're taking Grandma to the hospital," Jeanne said in a worried voice. "She's having trouble breathing." The two women accompanied the stretcher to the waiting ambulance. The elderly woman's breathing was labored. Alice spoke to the emergency medical technician (EMT) as the stretcher was put into the ambulance. "I'm a licensed practical nurse," she said. "May I go along?" "Sure, get in," the EMT said.

The ambulance delivered Alice's grandmother directly to the emergency department of the hospital. Alice was soon joined by her sister, who had followed in her car. "What's going to happen?" Jeanne asked. She was clearly worried.

"Don't worry," Alice said reassuringly, as she patted Jeanne's shoulder. "Grandma will get the best of care here." The two women went to the admitting office, where a clerk took the necessary information about their grandmother. Then they returned to the emergency department.

"How is my grandmother?" Alice asked one of the nurses on duty.

The nurse smiled. "They took her up to the Coronary Care Unit. It's her heart. The doctor wants to change her medications and monitor her heart rate for a few days."

Alice and Jeanne went upstairs. One of the staff nurses was speaking with their grandmother's physician. A lab technician stopped at the nurse's station. He spoke briefly with the unit secretary, who gave him a tray of freshly drawn blood samples. As they spoke, a nursing assistant appeared. He handed a package from the hospital pharmacy to the clerk, who read its label and made a notation on a chart. The doctor left the unit.

An LPN emerged from a room down the hall carrying a tray of medications. A maintenance worker, who was pushing a repair cart, hurried by. Others moved through the halls, each with a task to do.

Jeanne watched all the activity in amazement. "Is it like this every day?" she asked.

Alice shook her head. "No," she said. "Some days it gets busy!"

A week later, the sisters met again. This time they were taking their grandmother home. Not to Riverview, but to Alice's home. A home care plan had been arranged through the hospital's social service department.

"Is this something special they did because you're a licensed practical nurse?" Jeanne asked, as Alice poured tea for her sister and their grandmother.

Alice smiled. "No. It's all a part of a team effort that works inside the health care system," she said. She winked at her grandmother, who lay propped up on a rose-colored pillow in bed, and said, "And I'm proud to be a member of the health care team."

THE HEALTH CARE TEAM

The term *health care team* refers to all of the personnel in all of the departments of any type of health care facility. When we think of people who provide health care services, we immediately think of doctors, nurses, x-ray technicians, and lab technicians.

But it takes more than doctors and nurses and technicians to provide health care services. There are people who work in administration, medical records, social services, food services, purchasing, research, education, risk management, management information systems, finance, pharmaceuticals, and building maintenance. You will find these job titles and more in the more than 540,000 health care facilities in the United States.

All health care facilities, regardless of type, size, sophistication, or service, depend on the people who staff them to deliver health care services. The biggest, best-equipped health care facility is no better than the team that runs it and delivers care there because health care comes from people, not from the tools and technology used to provide it.

The primary function of a health care facility is to deliver health care services to its patients, clients, or residents. The patient, client, or resident has to be the center of attention of everyone who works in that facility. Health care workers are individuals who have personal problems and concerns just like everyone else, but when they are at work, the focus has to be on the patients and their needs.

✔ The *Dictionary of Occupational Titles lists more than 240 different job titles in health care.*

PERSONAL QUALITIES OF HEALTH CARE WORKERS

In addition to special skills, people who provide health care services must have special personal qualities. They must arrive for work on time and keep personal problems and concerns to themselves. They must like to work with people and be able to get along with others. They must be willing to work on holidays, weekends, evenings, and nights. Additional qualities are listed in Box 8-1. A constant assessment of your personal qualities will help you make changes that will enhance your ability to provide the best nursing care possible.

Health care workers also must be able to function as a member of a team that includes nurses, physicians, assistants, and others. Take the self-assessment test "Are You Ready To Be a Team Member?" on page 160 to determine your team member skills.

✔ *When at work, health care workers must be able to put the needs of their patients before their own.*

ORGANIZATIONAL ARRANGEMENTS

Every business, including health care, has its own specific organizational arrangement. Depending on the size of the organization and on the types of services provided, the organizational arrangement may be simple or it may be very complex. An organizational chart is a tool used to present a visual picture of the administrative structure of a business. Examples of organizational charts are shown in Figures 8-1, 8-2, 8-3, and 8-5.

BOX 8-1	Personal Qualities of the Health Care Worker

Dependable	Uses good judgment
Empathetic	Concern for others
Effective communicator	Patience
Practices good personal hygiene	Good listening skills
Reasonable moral standards	Flexible
Keeps information confidential	Kind
Respects coworkers and patients	Considerate
Organized	Role model
Problem solver	Ethical
Uses critical thinking skills	Creative
Abides by rules and regulations	Energetic

Critical Thinking EXERCISE

One of your classmates is always talking about himself and his problems. You feel as though you should be given an honorary degree in counseling because he talks to you so much. You have noticed that he does the same thing on the clinical unit to his patients. Is this situation none of your business or do you have a responsibility to do something about it? Describe at least three actions you could take in this situation. Include the possible outcome of each action. Use appropriate Characteristics of Critical Thinking in Box 1-2 on pages 18–19 to develop your responses to these questions.

| ASSESS YOURSELF | Are You Ready To Be a Team Member? |

Mark each of the following statements "True" or "False."

Question. It is easy for me to ask others for help.
  a. True
  b. False

Question. I enjoy helping others with their work.
  a. True
  b. False

Question. I think other people work as hard as I do.
  a. True
  b. False

Question. I like to assist with scheduling, organizing, and prioritizing work.
  a. True
  b. False

Question. When I have a choice, I prefer to do things with others rather than alone.
  a. True
  b. False

Question. I like to teach things I know to other people.
  a. True
  b. False

Question. Most people can work cooperatively.
  a. True
  b. False

Question. I enjoy working with people from other cultures.
  a. True
  b. False

Question. Everyone on the team is responsible for the work of others.
  a. True
  b. False

Question. I find it easy to trust other people to do a good job.
  a. True
  b. False

SCORING

Each "True" answer is worth 1 point; each "False" answer is worth 0 point.

0–5 points: You are missing some of the qualities needed to be a member of a team. You should work on those areas in which you scored 0 point.

6–8 points: You have many of the qualities needed to be a team member. Look at the areas in which you scored 0 and think about what you could do to improve your score.

9–10 points: You are the type of person who can really help a team work well together. Continue to develop your team-building skills.

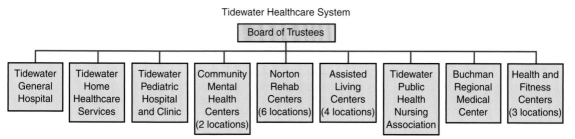

FIGURE 8-1. ● Organizational chart of a typical health care system.

Health Care Networks and Systems

A health care network or system is made up of a few to many facilities or organizations that provide a variety of health services. There are currently more than 400 integrated health care systems and networks nationwide. Mergers and acquisitions cause the number of networks to vary from month to month. These networks may operate in a confined geographic area, or they may own national or international health care facilities.

A board of trustees generally heads health care networks or systems. The members of the board make major business decisions regarding such issues as purchasing new facilities, selling facilities they already own, finding operating funds, and identifying places where their facilities can prosper. The networks may be nonprofit or for-profit businesses. Figure 8-1 is an organizational chart of a typical health care network.

Each facility within a network has its own administrator. This administrator may have the title of administrator, chief executive officer, chief operating officer, director, or president; this person is responsible for the day-to-day operation of the facility. To find out if a network owns any of the health care facilities that you use, you will probably have to read the fine print on the informational publications written by the facility.

THE *Web*

Using a search engine or the Web address of a local health care network or system, determine the number of facilities and/or centers owned by the company and the number of employees who work for that network.

Hospitals

Hospital administrators are responsible for the overall daily operation of the hospital. Departments within the hospital provide specific services or functions for the facility. Each department has a manager or department head who is responsible for the operation of his or her department.

Figure 8-2 is an example of how a typical hospital might be organized. To determine who reports to whom, start at the bottom of the organizational chart and work toward the top. This is known as the chain of command, and it outlines lines of authority and accountability.

Most health care administrators get their authority from a board of directors or a board of trustees. Hospitals that are a part of a larger network or system get their authority from the network board of directors. The board members are a group of responsible individuals who may or may not have day-to-day

✔ *Organizational charts identify the chain of command within an organization.*

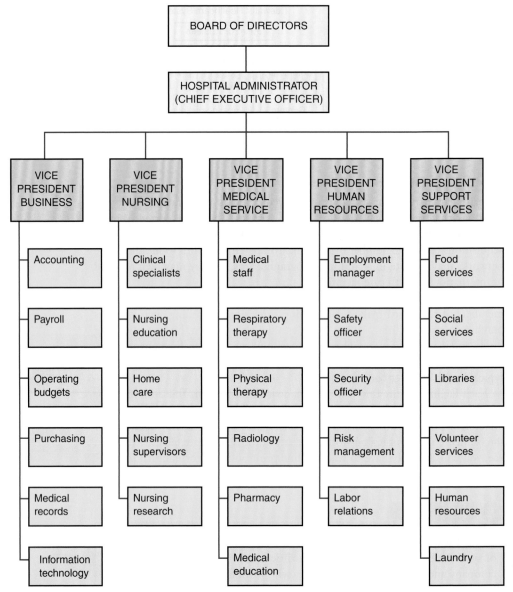

FIGURE 8-2. ● Organizational chart of a typical large hospital.

involvement with the facility's operation. They set the overall objectives and see that they are carried out. A board of directors has ultimate control of a facility. In some situations, the board of directors may be a group of local people, whereas in the case of an integrated health care system, the board of directors may be hundreds or even thousands of miles away and they may live in different parts of the country.

The activities that occur in a health care facility are usually divided into several major areas of service. These areas of service include, but are not limited to, business, nursing, medical services, human resources, and support services. These departments are often headed by vice presidents.

In this organizational chart, business matters are under the direction of a vice president for business. This person oversees offices that manage payroll,

✔ *The person at the top of the organizational chart is ultimately responsible for the operation of the organization.*

purchasing, medical records, accounting, budgets, and information technology. Educational preparation for this position includes advanced degrees in business and accounting.

The nursing department is under the direction of a professional nurse who has advanced degrees in nursing, business, and management. Those who report to the vice president (or director) of nursing may include clinical nurse specialists, nursing supervisors, and nurse educators. Figure 8-3 outlines a simple organizational chart for a typical nursing service department.

The medical services department is under the direction of a physician (or a group of staff physicians). The vice president for medical services oversees all

✔ Knowing the organizational chart where you work will help you know who to go to with work-related issues.

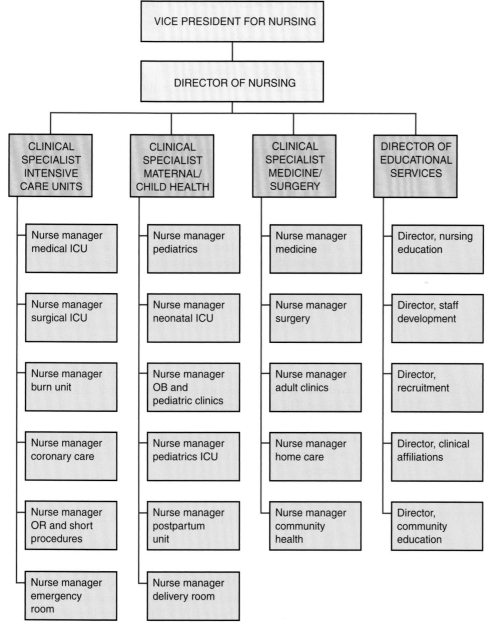

FIGURE 8-3. ● Organizational chart of a typical large hospital nursing service department.

departments that provide medical care in the facility. The heads of each medical specialty department are accountable to the medical director. Educational preparation for the position of medical director is completion of medical school and business school plus several years of experience in practicing medicine.

Other services include human resources and support services. Although this organization is typical, it may not be identical to the organizational chart of the facility to which you are assigned for clinical experience or where you will work.

It is important to understand the organizational chart of the facility in which you work. As a worker, you are expected to follow the chain of command and discuss any work-related problems or concerns with the person to whom you report.

MEMBERS OF THE HEALTH CARE TEAM

A health care team at a typical facility will include some or all of the following. Keep in mind that advances in technology and health care management continually generate the need for skilled personnel with new job titles.

- Administrator—A physician, nurse, or college graduate with a degree in business or hospital administration. This person is often the manager or director of one of the several departments in a health care facility.
- Aides/Assistants—Nearly every health care occupation has an aide or assistant. Educational preparation for being an aide or assistant varies from on-the-job training to formal classroom instruction. For example, physical therapy assistants must have at least an associate degree, whereas medical laboratory aides usually learn the required skills on the job.
- Case Manager—Most often an experienced professional nurse with additional education related to financing of health care. The case manager's job is to monitor a patient's health care in an effort to provide safe and effective care and at the same time contain costs. Case managers may specialize in fields such as geriatrics, pediatrics, obstetrics, or adult health.
- Dentist (DDS)—A state-licensed practitioner of dentistry with a 4-year undergraduate degree plus 4 years of dental school. Dentistry is the treatment and prevention of disorders and diseases of the teeth and related structures of the mouth, including repair, replacement, and restoration of teeth.
- Dietitian—A 4-year college graduate specializing in dietetics. Dietetics involves food, nutrition, and diet planning and preparation according to sound nutritional principles, especially as they relate to health and disease. A registered dietitian is a person who has passed a certification exam that has been approved by the American Dietetic Association.
- Electrocardiograph (ECG) Technician—One who is trained in the use of an ECG, a device used to record heart muscle activity to detect cardiac (heart) problems or to monitor the heart activity of patients known to have cardiac problems.
- Health Unit Coordinator—Sometimes called unit secretary; manages the clerical work at a nursing station.
- Hospitalist—A physician who works only in a hospital and treats hospitalized patients.
- Laboratory Assistant—One trained to perform simple laboratory tests and procedures; usually a high school graduate.
- Laboratory Technicians and Technologists—May be required to have a college degree and, in some states, certification and licensure.
- Licensed Practical/Vocational Nurse (LP/VN)—A state-licensed graduate of an approved LP/VN program, which is approximately 1 year in length.

- Medical Assistant (MA)—A person who performs administrative, clerical, and/or clinical tasks to support the work of physicians and other health professionals.
- Medical Doctor (MD)—A state-licensed graduate of 4 years of college and 4 years of medical school. After a medical residency lasting 3–6 years, the physician can enter practice. A general practitioner or primary care physician is a nonspecialist who provides general health care. A specialist has additional education in a special area and limits practice to that specialty.
- Medical Technologist-American Medical Technologist (MT-AMT)—A person trained and certified to work in a medical laboratory under a pathologist's supervision. A medical technologist has a minimum of 4 years of college education plus 1 year of approved laboratory experience and has passed the American Medical Technologist certification examination.
- Nurse Aide/Nurse Assistant—A person whose primary function is to assist the nursing team with patient care; receives instruction on the job and in the classroom. Nurse aides/assistants who work in Medicare-funded health care organizations must complete a training program and pass a competency examination developed by the state in which they will be working.
- Nurse Practitioner (NP)—A registered nurse who has advanced education in a specialty such as geriatrics, obstetrics, pediatrics, oncology, school health, or adult health. NPs may be primary care providers who work independently or with a physician. In all 50 states, NPs are permitted to write prescriptions for certain medications and diagnostic tests.
- Nurse, Clinical Specialist (RN-BC)—Nurses who pass certification tests such as those offered by the American Nurses Credentialing Center are permitted to use the title Registered Nurse, Board Certified (RN, BC) in their documentation.
- Occupational Therapist—One who has a minimum of 4 years of college education and helps patients readapt to daily life after illness or injury.
- Optometrist (OD)—A licensed specialist in eye examination and prescribing and fitting eyeglasses.
- Osteopathic Physician, Osteopathic Surgeon (DO)—A physician trained and licensed in osteopathy, a practice of medicine that emphasizes the role of the body's organs, muscles, and skeletal system in treating disease.
- Patient Care Technician (PCT)—A multidisciplinary technical worker trained to provide basic nursing assistant care as well as other skilled functions usually performed by staff from several different departments such as nursing, phlebotomy, EKG, and respiratory.
- Pathologist—A licensed physician who specializes in the nature and causes of disease.
- Pharmacist—One who has a bachelor of science (BS) degree with several additional years of college, and who is a licensed and registered specialist in compounding and dispensing medications.
- Physical Therapist—One who has a minimum of 4 years of college education and works with patients to regain full physical function through exercise, massage, and other techniques, after illness or injury.
- Physician's Assistant (PA)—One who is specially trained in approximately 26 months to provide assistance to a physician under the physician's direction and supervision; also called physician's associate, medex, or medic. Most PAs practice primary health care.

- Podiatrist (DSC, PODD)—A college graduate who completed four additional years of education in a college of podiatric medicine and is licensed to specialize in the treatment of foot disorders.
- Psychologist—A graduate (master's or doctoral degree) who specializes in diagnosis, treatment, and counseling of patients with mental, emotional, or emotionally caused physical problems.
- Radiologic Technologist (RT)—One trained in the use of x-ray equipment, fluoroscopy, and radiation therapy and the administration of radioisotopes.
- Registered Nurse (RN)—A graduate of a diploma, associate degree, or baccalaureate program with a major in nursing. Graduates are qualified to apply for the licensing exam to become an RN. RNs are also known as professional nurses.
- Respiratory Care Practitioner (RCP)—A graduate of a 2-, 3-, or 4-year approved program that provides training in the use of gases, drugs, and equipment under medical supervision to restore normal pulmonary function in patients recovering from illness or injury. More than 45 states require licensure of RCPs.
- Risk Manager—Often an experienced professional nurse who has specialized training in how to identify and correct situations that may make the health care facility at risk for unnecessary or avoidable costs such as lawsuits from personal injury or malpractice.
- Social Worker—One who has a minimum of 6 years of college education and helps patients and their families adjust to personal problems.
- Unit Manager—A person in charge of the clerical management of several units who works under the supervision of a hospital administrator.

Accountants, attorneys, human resources managers, building engineers, librarians, pastors, information management specialists, and a variety of others fill out the staff of a large health care facility.

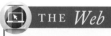 THE *Web*

Both CareerOneStop and the O*Net Online Center provide information on tasks and the educational preparation for careers in the United States.

THE NURSING TEAM

A nursing team may have many or few members and varies from institution to institution (Fig. 8-4). Regardless of the number of people on the team, each person is responsible for his or her own performance. It is each member's personal obligation to do the assigned work at or above accepted standards of practice for health care workers at his or her level of education and competence. Education should not be confused with competence. A job title or assignment to perform a specific task does not necessarily qualify that person to do it.

On the other hand, someone with the required skill to do a procedure does not automatically have the right to do it. Because you are personally and legally responsible for what you do at all times, for your own protection and the protection of your patient and employer, never perform nursing acts beyond your competencies.

✔ *Always work within your level of nursing competence.*

How the nursing team is organized will vary from facility to facility. It will be your responsibility to learn the organization of the nursing department where

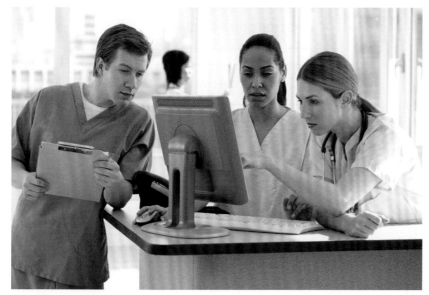

FIGURE 8-4. ● Nursing teams plan patient care.

you are employed and to conform to the lines of authority and responsibility it sets. An example of the organization of a typical nursing team is shown in Figure 8-5.

Clinical Nurse Specialist

Many larger health care facilities hire clinical nurse specialists, who are specially trained and certified RNs, to work with nurse managers to plan care and solve clinical problems related to their patients. The American Nurses Credentialing Center accredits over 360 organizations that offer certification in specialty areas for nurses. To be certified, a nurse must meet the certifying agency requirements for education, experience, and continuing education and must pass a competency examination.

Nurse Managers

Nurse managers (also known as head nurses or charge nurses) are RNs who are appointed to their job by the director of nursing and are responsible for directing those working under their authority.

✔ *A nurse manager is responsible for the total operation of his or her unit.*

   Nurse managers generally have the responsibility for planning, supervising, and evaluating nursing care in a single patient care unit, such as the emergency department, obstetrics, or the surgical unit. They are also responsible for managing their own budget, hiring staff, and coordinating work schedules. In large nursing units, assistant nurse managers or charge nurses may assume some of the responsibilities of the nurse manager.

Team Leaders

Patient care units that have more than 10 or 12 beds are often divided into two or more parts. Nursing teams (as outlined in Fig. 8-5) are assigned to care for the patients who reside in one of the divisions of the nursing unit. Team leaders in hospitals are most often RNs; experienced LP/VNs frequently work as team leaders in long-term care facilities.

✔ *The team leader is directly involved in providing patient care.*

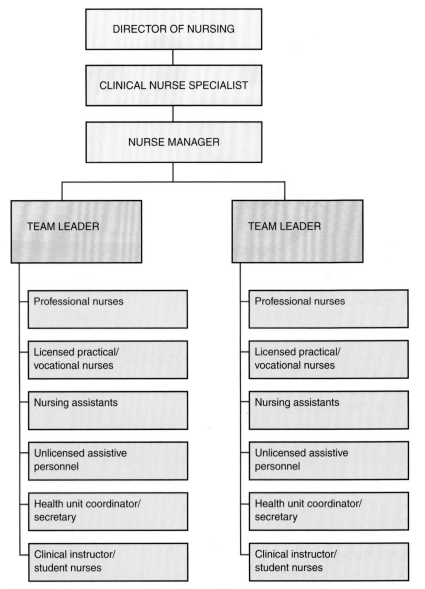

FIGURE 8-5. ● Organizational chart of a typical patient care unit in a hospital.

The team leader is responsible for being certain that appropriate care is provided for the patients on his or her team. The team leader supervises staff, evaluates care, teaches patients as well as staff, and conducts patient care conferences. The team leader is also responsible for ensuring that all supplies and equipment needed to provide patient care are readily available.

Professional Staff Nurses

Staff nurses, or professional nurses, are RNs who usually have direct responsibility for patient care. Typical functions of a staff nurse include assessing a patient's physical and psychological condition, administering medications, monitoring vital signs, providing personal hygiene, documenting progress, teaching patients and families, and carrying out treatment regimens. In addition, staff nurses develop nursing care plans based on nursing diagnoses and collaborate with physicians to resolve medical problems. Staff nurses collaborate with their nurse manager and clinical specialists to solve nursing problems.

The staff nurse is a patient advocate and, as such, communicates with other hospital departments to meet the many needs of a person receiving services in the health care system.

✔ *A staff nurse is one who provides nursing service to patients.*

Licensed Practical/Vocational Nurses

Under the supervision of other licensed personnel, LP/VNs provide nursing services for which they are licensed and qualified. The source of supervision is clearly defined in the nurse practice acts of the state in which each LP/VN works. Many state nurse practice acts require that LP/VNs work under the direct supervision of a licensed physician, professional nurse, or dentist.

The LP/VNs working as members of the nursing team are expected to be contributing members of their teams. Providing direct patient care and assisting the professional nurse in meeting the needs of the patients in a particular health care facility require excellent communication and observation skills. The beginning skills of the LP/VN are discussed in Chapter 4.

✔ *The National Association for Practical Nurse Education and Service offers certification exams for practical nurses in pharmacology, long-term care, rehabilitation, and intravenous therapy.*

Nursing Assistants

Nursing assistants, as members of the nursing team, help RNs and LP/VNs by providing basic nursing care to patients. Nursing assistants may also be called aides, orderlies, or attendants. Their functions generally include making beds; measuring temperatures, pulses, respirations, and blood pressures; filling water carafes; distributing and collecting meal trays; and feeding some patients.

Nursing assistants who are employed in long-term care facilities that receive Medicare funds must complete a state-approved course of classroom and clinical instruction and must pass a written and performance examination. Those who pass the examination are listed on the nurse aide registry of the state in which they passed the examination.

✔ *Nursing assistants who work in Medicare-funded long-term care facilities must complete a state-approved training program.*

Unlicensed Assistive Personnel

Unlicensed assistive personnel (UAP) are those who are taught to perform specific tasks associated with patient care. Some of their duties include making beds, taking vital signs, feeding patients who need assistance, and bathing patients. Unlike the nursing aide/assistant, the UAP receives little training, does not take a state-administered certification test, and is not listed on a state registry. Licensed nurses are legally responsible for making sure that the UAP is capable of safely performing the tasks they are assigned. The delegation of duties to UAPs is discussed in Chapter 13.

✔ *The National Association for Practical Nurse Education and Service offers a certification exam titled Allied Health Professional—Certificate in Long-Term Care (AHP-CLTC) for unlicensed assistive personnel.*

Health Unit Coordinators

Health unit coordinators, or unit secretaries, provide secretarial services for a particular nursing unit. Their duties include answering the telephone, preparing patient charts, accessing information through the computer network, ordering equipment and supplies, and serving as a receptionist. In some health care facilities, unit clerks transcribe doctor's orders.

✔ *The unit secretary manages the clerical aspect of the nursing unit.*

Student Nurses

Student nurses, whether in a professional or a practical/vocational nursing education program, learn clinical skills under the instruction of a clinical instructor.

✔ *Student nurses can, in certain situations, be held personally liable for their actions.*

The clinical instructor, in turn, works closely with the nurse manager and other members of the nursing team. Clinical instructors are legally responsible for the actions of their students and, for this reason, are careful to observe and evaluate student performance.

Student nurses do not replace staff nurses and LP/VNs on the nursing team, but they are a part of that team. As such, student nurses are expected to provide safe and competent patient care. Student nurses are expected to seek the assistance of their clinical instructor when questions regarding patient care arise.

Multiskilled Workers

A multiskilled worker, sometimes called a medical assistant or a PCT, is a person who has completed the educational and, if required, licensing requirements for a specific job. Through cross-training, this person is given additional training in skills that are not a part of his or her basic job. For example, a unit secretary may be taught to perform electrocardiograms, draw blood samples, and take and record vital signs. This concept is controversial, but some health care administrators believe these workers could help reduce the cost of health care by decreasing the need to retain staff whose skills are limited.

✔ *Multiskilled workers must work within the rules and regulations of the state in which they are employed.*

The effect multiskilled workers will have on health care remains to be seen. Issues related to these workers involve certification, state licensing laws, definitions of scope of practice, and regulation of the length and content of cross-training educational programs. For these reasons, most nursing organizations are opposed to the use of multiskilled workers in health care facilities.

THE MULTIDISCIPLINARY TEAM

A multidisciplinary team includes a number of health care workers who work together to solve problems, increase efficiency, decrease lengths of stay, and enhance the quality of care. This team provides a single point of contact for the patient. The team provides information to the patient on all of the treatment options for a particular illness, as well as on rehabilitation and aftercare.

✔ *A good team can help a patient efficiently access appropriate health care.*

Which health care providers are included on this team depends on the patient's diagnosis, as well as on the individual's other health care needs. In addition to the patient's primary nurses, the multidisciplinary team may include physicians, clinical nurse specialists, social workers, physical therapists, dietitians, home health nurses, and hospice nurses.

You may hear the terms multidisciplinary team, interdisciplinary team, or transdisciplinary team being used in the hospital where you have your clinical experience. All of these teams are made up of health care workers with different areas of expertise all working together to benefit the patient (Fig. 8-6). The differences in these three types of teams are very minimal and are generally related to the different roles and working relationships among team members.

NURSING CARE DELIVERY MODELS

✔ *Care is often delivered through a combination of case, functional, total patient care, and team nursing.*

Models or methods of providing nursing care can be divided into a number of different types or categories to ensure the highest level of care performed in the most efficient and economical manner. The method used by one facility may differ from that of another. Which method of nursing care an institution uses is based on type and degree of illness of the patients, the availability of staff and equipment, size and nature of the physical plant, and administrative and nursing philosophies.

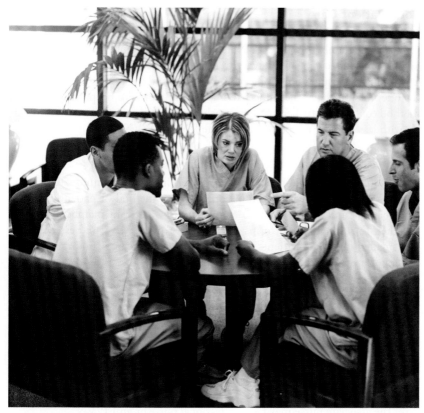

FIGURE 8-6. ● The multidisciplinary team meets to coordinate the preadmission through the postdischarge plan of care.

As a student, and later when you enter practice, you will most likely be assigned to a unit where one of the following general nursing care delivery methods is followed: (1) case method, (2) functional nursing, (3) total patient care, (4) team nursing, or (5) primary nursing.

Case Method

The case method is the oldest approach to nursing care delivery. In this method, the nurse is responsible for the entire care of one or more patients for one shift in a 24-hour period. This method is frequently used in intensive care units and home care nursing and is always used in private duty nursing. It is often the method used with student nurses during their clinical experience.

✔ *Case management and primary nursing are often practiced together.*

Functional Nursing

Functional nursing is a system in which each nursing team member is assigned a specific function or task. For example, one team member takes the vital signs of all the patients on the unit, other team members make all the beds, and so forth. Functional nursing is sometimes efficient, but it is a fragmented approach to patient care. Patients often have a difficult time establishing a relationship with the nursing staff because so many members of the staff provide for their care.

Total Patient Care

In this pattern of care, an RN or LP/VN is assigned to provide all of the care for a specific number of patients. Nurses enjoy this structure because they get to know their four to six patients very well. The disadvantage is that most patients are not in the hospital for a long period of time, and with time off, it is difficult for one nurse to have the same patients during an entire hospitalization. This method could be costly because many tasks that could be performed by individuals with less training are performed by the RN or LP/VN.

Team Nursing

Team nursing, instituted in the mid-1950s, was intended to minimize the fragmentation associated with the functional nursing method of patient care. The large patient unit is divided into smaller units with team members working together. Each member performs the duties for which they are best prepared. The smaller number of patients, team conferences, and team planning make this system of providing care different from functional nursing.

Primary Nursing

✔ *Nurses conduct research to identify nursing care delivery models that will provide the kind of nursing care the public expects to receive.*

The most recently developed nursing care delivery method is called primary nursing. In primary nursing, a professional nurse has total responsibility for a particular patient or group of patients, 24 hours a day, 7 days a week, for the entire time the patient is in the hospital through discharge. This model's purpose is to provide continuity and coordination of care. When the primary nurse is not physically present in the health care facility, an associate nurse provides patient care. The associate nurse may be a professional nurse or an LP/VN.

Functions of a primary nurse include performing an admission assessment; developing, planning, implementing, evaluating, and revising the nursing care plan; providing directions for care in his or her absence; collaborating with physicians and families; making referrals; teaching health concepts; and making discharge plans.

THE CHANGING ROLES OF NURSES IN HEALTH CARE

At those times in our history when the supply of nurses was low and patient care was suffering, new types of health care workers were introduced. An increase in the number of LP/VN schools during World War II, the opening of associate degree programs during the nursing shortage in the 1950s, and the introduction of UAPs, multiskilled workers, patient care assistants, and cross-training of nurses in the 1990s were all attempts to make up for a shortage of professional nurses. The addition of these workers eliminated some of the nurse's duties but added new concerns about the quality of patient care and safety.

The cost of nursing salaries has increased significantly over the past 20 years. Those looking to cut health care costs often take the position that RNs are too expensive and that many of their duties can be performed by less costly staff members. By assigning some of the RN's duties to others, the number and therefore the cost, of registered nurse staff assigned to provide patient care are lower. Professional nurses continue to object to reducing nursing staff because all studies show that patient care declines when the nurse-to-patient ratio is reduced.

As the health care system continues to evolve, the nursing profession is responding. Titles such as nurse practitioner, clinical nurse specialist, and primary nurse are terms used to describe the modern nurse. Nursing research has led to the development of career ladders, nursing diagnoses, critical pathways, care maps, nursing care plans, specialty nursing journals, nurse licensure compacts, and laws regulating workload, lifting, staffing ratios, and overtime. Nursing educators and nursing administrators are continuing to work to develop even more innovative nursing approaches that will not only change the role of the nurse but also positively influence the quality of patient care and the health care system.

SUMMARY

Roles and responsibilities have changed and will continue to change over the years. As new roles are created and additional responsibilities are added to existing roles, the public is becoming more and more confused about who is providing care and just what qualifications and education they have for these roles. Your understanding of the roles and functions of various members of the health care team will help you answer your patients' questions.

Through all of this transition and turmoil in health care, it is your responsibility to be as knowledgeable and competent as you can be as you perform your duties, however much they may change, during your career in nursing.

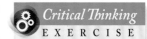
APPLY
Critical Thinking Skills

1. In the opening story at the beginning of this chapter, Alice commented on the number of people who seemed to be in and around the nurse's station. With two of your classmates, station yourselves near a medical or surgical nurse's station. (It is recommended that you conduct this activity during the middle of a typical weekday.) Two of you should ask those who walk by to give you their position and reason for being on the unit while the third records the information. After 15 minutes, what conclusions could your team draw from this activity?

2. Using the hospital in which you will receive the primary portion of your medical and surgical clinical experience, find out how many different job titles there are.

3. Complete the same information requested in question 2 for a local nursing home.

4. In addition to those members of the health care team discussed in this chapter, how many additional members can you list? Also list their educational preparation and their major function.

5. Obtain an organizational chart for the nursing service department in one of the health care facilities to which you are assigned. How do the job titles of the various members of the nursing department differ from those in Figure 8-3?

6. What nursing care delivery method is used in your clinical affiliation? Is this the same method used in all patient care units in the facility?

Critical Thinking
EXERCISE

You have a patient who was admitted yesterday with multiple fractures he received in a car accident. He is in pain and worried about something. As he starts to confide in you, you are interrupted every few minutes by a different member of the health care team. First, it is the respiratory therapist; next, the UAP to do an electrocardiogram and draw blood; and then the dietitian to review the menu. After that, the doctor examines him; then the professional nurse checks his pain medication. The building engineer comes to repair a faulty wall vacuum fitting. A volunteer brings him a fruit basket, and someone from the business office stops by to confirm his insurance information. Finally, the patient says he cannot take it anymore and does not want all of these strangers parading through his room all day. What do you say to him and why? Use appropriate Characteristics of Critical Thinking in Box 1-2 on pages 18–19 to develop you responses to this situation.

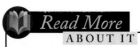
Read More
ABOUT IT

American Hospital Association: AHA Guide 2014 (American Hospital Association Guide to the Health Care Field). Chicago, IL: American Hospital Association, 2014.

American Medical Association: Health Care Careers Directory 2012–2013, 40th ed. Chicago, IL: American Medical Association, 2012.

Cherry B, Jacob SR: Contemporary Nursing: Issues, Trends & Management, 6th ed. St. Louis, MO: Mosby, 2013.

Robbins A: The Nurses: A Year of Secrets, Drama, and Miracles with the Heros of the Hospital. New York, NY: Workman Publishing, 2015.

Sultz HA, Young KM: Health Care USA: Understanding its Organization and Delivery, 8th ed. Boston, MA: Jones, Bartlett Learning, 2103.

Tankt K, Usher S: Nurse: Past/Present/Future: The Making of Modern Nursing. London, UK: Black Dog Publishing, 2010.

Theory, Culture, and Diversity in Nursing Care

LEARNING OBJECTIVES

When you complete this chapter, you will be able to:

1. Describe nursing behaviors that demonstrate caring.

2. Outline the position of at least two nursing theories on person, environment, health, and the profession of nursing.

3. Apply your understanding of nursing theory, nursing process, and the concepts of transcultural nursing in your practice of nursing.

4. Conduct research to find examples of how a specific cultural or social diversity influences a patient's response to illness.

Luca was aware of the butterflies in her stomach as soon as she opened her eyes that morning. It was her first day on her new job as a licensed vocational nurse, and she had a case of the jitters at the thought of putting into practice all she'd been learning this past year. What if she forgot something? "Maybe if I walk to work it will help calm me down," thought Luca. "Central Memorial Hospital is only 20 minutes away, and it's a lovely day."

Steve Jamison, known as "Old Steve" to his friends, was at his usual spot, watching the neighborhood activity. His wheelchair was drawn up next to his first-floor window so that he could see clearly up and down the street. The disabled man waved to Luca as she passed. "On your way to school?" he asked.

Luca smiled. "I graduated last week," she said proudly. "Today's my first day on the job." "Good luck," Steve called after her.

Luca heard the shouts of children playing as she approached the playground. She stopped for a minute to watch the lively ball game before she continued on. "Children are such a precious gift," she thought. "How could anyone ever harm a child?"

A dirty, disheveled woman in a ragged coat and floppy sneakers several sizes too large for her was pawing through a trash can on the corner. "That poor woman could certainly use a bath and some tender loving care," thought Luca. It seemed she saw more and more such people every day, pushing their shopping carts filled with the castoffs of the city, shouting and mumbling in turn to exorcise their particular demons.

Luca spotted a small crowd outside the Hill Street Clinic, a small neighborhood health facility. A man was handing out flyers to anyone who would accept them. A young woman attempted to enter the building. "Abortion is wrong," said the pro-life demonstrator, trying to block the clinic door. The woman shook her head and quickly slipped past the man into the building.

Farther down the street, a volunteer sat at a table collecting signatures of passersby. "Please sign the petition to the governor asking for additional funds for addiction research. We need more money to help find a cure." The man's words sent a chill down Luca's spine. Drugs and alcohol were ruining the lives of so many people.

"Excuse me," a wistful voice said. "I'm late for school and I can't find the day care center." It was a young girl with her small child. Luca put her hand on the girl's shoulder. "It's across the street," the young nurse said, pointing to a storefront with a simple sign in the window. The girl thanked Luca and hurried across the street with the child in tow.

In the next block, softly ringing church bells sounded a counterpoint to the traffic noise. Two elderly women reverently entered St. Mary's Church. On the next corner, a bearded young man wearing a yarmulke was sweeping the walk in front of the synagogue. He paused to exchange greetings in Hebrew with another man.

As she reached the entrance to Central Memorial Hospital, Luca thought, "I wonder who my first patients will be?" She recalled each of the people she had seen as she walked to work. "Everyone is so different and has such different needs. I just hope that I will always remember to try to understand where my patients are coming from and know that what is best for me may not be best for them."

NURSE–PATIENT INTERACTIONS

Medicine is primarily concerned with the diagnosis and treatment of disease or, in other words, with curing disease. Although nurses are involved with curing disease, nursing's unique duty is caring for patients. The curing part of nursing includes tasks such as performing treatments and procedures, giving medications, assisting with activities of daily living, meeting nutrition and elimination needs, and teaching about self-care. The caring part of nursing goes beyond these technical skills.

✔ *Medicine cures; nursing cares.*

Caring, in the context of nursing, means protecting and looking after the well-being of another person. Caring requires creating an interpersonal relationship with another person. Caring means that the caregiver respects and accepts the other person's freedom to make decisions. Caring means that the caregiver has the knowledge and skills needed to carry out the duties of his or her position in a legal and ethical manner.

Being able to let your patients know that you care about them and how events are affecting them and their families requires energy, self-understanding, and self-confidence. Without confidence in your abilities and a good understanding of yourself, you may be reluctant to use the technical skills you have learned.

Your confidence in and understanding of yourself will be what cements your relationships with your patients. You will be able to draw on your own feelings of caring and understanding as you relate to your patient as another human being. The nurse who is shy, insecure, self-serving, or more concerned with meeting personal needs than patient needs will not be able to provide the caring part of nursing. Your obligations as a student nurse are to get the best education you can and to develop a self-awareness that will allow you to interact with your patients as a skilled, empathic, sensitive, and caring human being.

✔ *Caring involves developing a relationship with another person.*

The interpersonal relationships you establish between yourself and your patients can provide great rewards to you in your career as a nurse. Almost anyone can be taught to perform the technical skills your patients will need. But not everyone, and unfortunately not every nurse, will be skilled in providing caring and compassionate nursing care. Work on your caring skills and try to remember that you may be the only person in the health care system that is in a position to provide both physical and emotional care.

NURSING THEORY

Although caring nurses have been providing for the physical and emotional needs of people for centuries, it was only recently that nurses began to study and describe exactly what nursing is.

✔ *A theory attempts to explain the nature of something.*

Research into what nursing is and what nurses do began with Florence Nightingale in the mid-1850s and then remained dormant until the mid-1950s when a number of nurses became interested in describing what nursing is. These researchers knew that nurses did something unique and special for people, and they attempted, in their nursing theories, to describe what they thought and observed.

A *theory* is an explanation of the nature of something. A nursing theory attempts to describe or explain the nature of nursing. Nursing theory guides the practice of nursing by providing the foundation on which the principles and practice of nursing as a profession are developed.

✔ *Learning some of the major points of a few nursing theories will be the foundation for more detailed learning later in your nursing career.*

You may hear the term *conceptual model* used interchangeably with the term *nursing theory*. Although there are some differences between theories and models, both attempt to describe or explain the nature of nursing. Therefore, in this book, nursing theory and nursing model are used to mean the same thing.

A specific nursing theory or combination of nursing theories has been used as the basis for the design of your educational program. Nursing theories also provide the foundation on which nursing services in health care facilities are designed.

By studying different nursing theories, you will develop an understanding of why your nursing education is organized in a certain way and why your clinical facilities use a particular system for delivering nursing services.

Major Theorists

The first theory of nursing was developed by Florence Nightingale in 1859, and her views on nursing prevailed for almost 100 years. It was not until the 1950s that an interest in nursing theory development reappeared. Since then, a number of theories of nursing have been proposed, studied, and refined.

Five well-known nursing theories are briefly summarized in Table 9-1. Currently, more than 40 nursing theories and conceptual models are being studied and used by nurses in a variety of clinical settings around the world.

Nightingale

Nursing care in England and in the United States was based for many years on Florence Nightingale's nursing theory. Her theory was based on her observations and experiences as a nurse in the Crimean War. Her best-known work describing her theories, *Notes on Nursing: What It Is and What It Is Not*, was originally published in 1859.

✔ *Nightingale developed the first theory of nursing.*

Nightingale believed that if a patient was put in the right environment, he or she would get better through natural health processes. A nurse's duty was to provide the right environment.

Her theory of nursing was based on environment because at the time during the Crimean War, and also during peace, people lived in crowded, unsanitary conditions, epidemics of disease were common, social conditions were strained, and medicine as a science was still in its infancy. When she and her nurses provided a clean and sunlit environment, their patients seemed to recover.

Henderson

Virginia Henderson described her theory of nursing in a book titled *The Nature of Nursing: A Definition and Its Implications, Practice, Research, and Education*,

TABLE 9-1	Selected Nursing Theories and Models				
Theorist	Theme	Person	Environment	Health	Nursing
Nightingale, Florence 1859	Environment affects health	Has physical, intellectual, and spiritual attributes	Those aspects outside the person that affect health	Being free of disease	Putting the person in the best condition for nature to act on him or her
Henderson, Virginia 1955	Fourteen principles or components of nursing care	Mind and body are inseparable	Can be either a negative or positive influence on the person	Ability to function independently in the physiologic, environmental, and social aspects of life	Deliberate plan to meet the 14 components of nursing care
Orem, Dorothea 1958	Basic human needs are met through self-care activities	An integrated whole, with physiological, psychological, and sociological components	Created by society; includes values and expectations	Ability to meet self-care needs	Nursing education gives nurses the legitimate right to assist patients to meet self-care needs
Roy, Sister Callista 1964	Stressors affect how a person adapts	Biopsychosocial being in a changing environment	All internal and external influences that affect the human being	Health and illness are relative terms and exist at different times in differing degrees	Nurses' role to help the person adjust to changes in stimuli
Neuman, Betty 1972	Systems approach to meeting human needs	An integrated whole in a constant state of change because of dynamic interrelationship of many variables	An external and an internal environment, both of which constantly affect the development of the person	Health seen as relative, depending on physiological, psychological, sociocultural, and developmental state of the person	Concerned with total person and attempts to either reduce or minimize effects of external or internal stress on the person

which was first published in 1955. In her second edition, published in 1966, she defined nursing as follows:

The unique function of the nurse is to assist the individual, sick or well, in performance of those activities contributing to health or its recovery (or to a peaceful death) that he/she would perform unaided if he/she had the necessary strength, will, or knowledge. And to do this in such a way as to help him/her gain independence as rapidly as possible.

✔ *Henderson's theory identifies 14 components of basic nursing care.*

Henderson believed that health is basic to human functioning, and an individual's ability to function independently depends on health. She listed 14 components of basic nursing care that are intended to contribute to a patient's independence, as follows:

1. Breathe normally.
2. Eat and drink adequately.
3. Eliminate body waste.
4. Move and maintain a desirable position.
5. Sleep and rest.
6. Dress, undress, and select suitable clothing.
7. Maintain body temperature by adjusting clothing and environment.
8. Keep the body clean and well groomed, and protect the skin.
9. Avoid changes in the environment and personal safety.
10. Communicate to express emotions, needs, fears, or opinions.
11. Worship.
12. Work to acquire a sense of accomplishment.
13. Play or participate in various forms of recreation.
14. Learn, discover, satisfy curiosity for normal development and health, and use health care facilities.

Each of these components, according to Henderson, should be individualized to accommodate the uniqueness of each patient. The goal of nursing care is to assist the patient until he or she is able to perform these components independently.

Orem

Self-care—the things people do "on their own behalf in maintaining life, health, and well-being"—is the main theme of Orem's nursing theory, first published in 1958. Orem saw humans as functioning biologically, symbolically, and socially, with specific needs in each of these areas. To her, health meant being able to meet these needs for oneself. Orem's universal self-care requisites or needs are somewhat similar to the 14 components identified by Henderson. When a person's ability to perform self-care is impaired, in whole or in part, nursing care is indicated to compensate for this deficiency and to increase the person's potential to live in his or her environment. How much nursing is required is determined by the person's specific needs.

✔ *Orem's theory says that the nurse helps patients meet self-care deficits.*

Orem divides nursing intervention into three categories:

1. In wholly compensatory nursing, the nurse provides virtually all of the patient's self-care needs, as in intensive care and total care situations.
2. In partly compensatory nursing, the patient and the nurse work together to make up for the patient's limitation. As an example, the patient may be able to bathe unassisted but needs a nurse to change a dressing.
3. In supportive–educative nursing, the patient can provide self-care or could learn how to do so but needs help to learn or to adjust. Teaching a patient how to live normally within the limits of a diabetic diet is an example of this type of nursing.

In Orem's theory, nurses, by virtue of their education and training, have a legitimate role in helping patients meet their self-care needs.

Roy

Sister Callista Roy proposed that a person's ability to adapt to the environment is the basis of an effective nursing model. Her adaptation model, which she introduced in 1964, says that people face a constantly changing environment and must adapt to it. Conflict between the changing environment and the need to adapt to it produces stress. A person's response to stress is observable behavior combining physiologic, intellectual, and behavioral reactions. How well or how poorly the person copes with the stress determines how much stress is reduced or eliminated which, in turn, affects health.

✔ *Roy's theory says that people's ability to adapt to their environment determines health.*

Health, for Roy, can be represented by a continuous line from very ill to very healthy. Successful coping with stress produces better health; unsuccessful coping produces worse health. The nurse's goal is to help the individual cope so that better health can be gained. The nurse does so by first assessing the patient's needs and then intervening to see that those needs are fulfilled, which is done with the person's active participation.

Neuman

In Betty Neuman's health care systems model, first published in 1972, the person is viewed as a whole being of many parts in an environment consisting of internal, external, and interpersonal elements. The combination is a system in which all its parts are constantly interacting. This health care model implies that to understand one thing about a person, you must consider everything about that person.

✔ Neuman's theory states that stressors upset an individual's stability.

Forces, or stressors, as Neuman calls them, act on people from both inside and outside. They may benefit or harm the individual they act on, and they can be either strong or weak. They tend to upset the individual's stability, which is the ideal condition to be in.

To remain stable, the person reacts to stress by using energy. A person's health is defined by the amount of energy available to respond to stress. It is determined by comparing normal conditions with present conditions. High energy is good health; low energy is illness; no energy is death. A person maintains good health, called stability or harmony, by using energy to balance the effects of stress.

In this model, nursing's aim is to identify a patient's stressors being produced by any part of the system and then to intervene to reduce or eliminate them. Interventions should (1) prevent stressors from reaching the person, (2) treat stressors after they reach the individual, or (3) return the patient to good health after treatment.

Relationship to Nursing Practice

Trends in nursing theory development can be identified and are evident in today's nursing practice. Nightingale was more concerned with environment than with person, health, or nursing. The Henderson and Orem models emphasize the concept of nursing as having a duty to the person within the context of his or her environment. Roy and Neuman focus on the person in a fluctuating state of health, with the nurse being the one who helps the person adjust to these fluctuations.

Because of the work of these and other nurse theorists, nurses began recognizing that there was more to nursing than performing treatments and procedures. These theories provide the basis for continuing research on how nurses can be more effective in helping people maintain their health or recover from an illness.

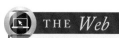 THE *Web*

> The Clayton State University School of Nursing and the Hahn School of Nursing maintain Web sites that provide links to information on more than 40 nursing theories and models.

NURSING PROCESS

One of the ways that nursing theories and models are translated into practice is through the nursing process. The nursing process is a systematic, organized method of providing nursing. The nursing process consists of five steps:

1. Assess the patient.
2. Formulate the nursing diagnosis.
3. Plan nursing care.
4. Implement the plan.
5. Evaluate the effectiveness of nursing care.

✔ The nursing process provides the framework for nursing care.

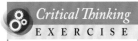

Critical Thinking
E X E R C I S E

Your good friend from high school knows you are in nursing school. When you run in to him in the pizza shop, he says to you, "By the way, I've been meaning to ask you a question." "And just what question might that be?" you ask. "Well," he says, "I was wondering if you could tell me what it is that makes a nurse a nurse. I mean, is there something special that nurses do that no one else does?" How would you answer your friend?

Use appropriate Characteristics of Critical Thinking in Box 1-2 on pages 18–19 to develop your response to these questions.

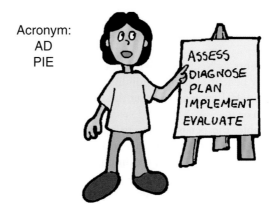

Acronym:
AD
PIE

ASSESS
DIAGNOSE
PLAN
IMPLEMENT
EVALUATE

The first step, assessment, is done by observing patients and asking questions of them, their families, or their significant others. Things you can see are called objective observations; things that a patient says are called subjective reports. Objective observations include vital signs, skin condition, body language, and physical characteristics, such as height and weight. Subjective reports include a patient's description of pain, symptoms, or discomfort.

The second step in the nursing process is formulating a *nursing diagnosis*, a statement describing an existing or potential health problem that nurses can treat separately from a physician's order. A nursing diagnosis is made on the basis of information collected during the assessment phase.

The National Conference Group developed the first written nursing diagnoses in 1973. To more accurately describe their work, the name of the organization was changed to the North American Nursing Diagnosis Association International (NANDA-I) in 1982. Members of this organization discuss, review, and study research reports on proposed nursing diagnoses before including them in the NANDA-I-approved list of accepted nursing diagnoses. The 2012–2014 edition of Nursing Diagnosis Definitions and Classifications contains 217 distinct nursing diagnoses.

 THE *Web*

NANDA-I maintains a comprehensive Web site that describes their efforts to create standard language related to nursing diagnosis throughout the world.

Planning, the third step in the nursing process, includes setting priorities and writing the *nursing care plan*. Each health care facility chooses or creates its own forms for the written nursing care plans. Some use paper forms, whereas others use computerized forms. Some have standard care plans that are specific to one nursing diagnosis with additional information individualized to each patient; others develop individualized plans for each patient. Some health care facilities use different types of care plans in different departments within the same facility.

✔ *Review sample nursing care plans in your nursing textbooks.*

Nursing care plans can be created in a few ways. One of the ways is for the professional nurse responsible for admitting patients to a particular unit or service to create the nursing care plan. Another way is for the primary nurse responsible for planning a particular patient's comprehensive care to write the nursing care plan. The nursing care plan may also be created through a formal patient care conference, which may consist of only nursing team members or may incorporate multidisciplinary members. A multidisciplinary conference includes nurses, social workers, physicians, pharmacists, dietitians, physical and occupational therapists, and others who are involved in providing care for a particular patient. Often, the family of the patient is involved as well. In either case, a meeting is held to develop a plan of care based on the patient's total needs.

Regardless of how the nursing care plan was initially created, everyone providing care and service to a patient is expected to contribute to the continual revision of the initial plan. The nursing care plan communicates to all members of the patient care team any changes in the patient's condition and needs and must be continually updated. Your clinical instructor will help you learn to understand and contribute to the nursing care plans in the clinical facilities to which you are assigned.

The fourth step, *implementation*, is the step in which the care plan is put into practice. Nursing team members should implement (put into practice) the recommendations made in the nursing care plan. Problems in implementing the care plan should be reported to the professional nurse responsible for the patient unit or department.

The fifth and last step in the nursing process is the *evaluation* of the effectiveness of the care. At this point, the nurse is able to evaluate how well nursing interventions have worked in assisting the patient to achieve health goals. Evaluation of the care plan and how it is implemented is a constant process based on continual reassessment of the patient, revision of some or all nursing diagnoses, and changes in the nursing care plan.

✔ As a patient's condition changes, the nursing care plan changes.

Planning patient care by using the nursing process helps you organize your approach to the patient. It requires you to integrate your knowledge of person, environment, health, nursing, and medicine to best serve the needs of the patient. It helps you communicate with other members of the nursing team and helps them communicate with you. Above all, the patient benefits from the quality of care that the nursing process encourages.

TRANSCULTURAL NURSING

Culture refers to values, beliefs, customs, rituals, attitudes, roles, and behaviors that are shared by a large group of people and are passed from generation to generation. Another way that nursing theories and models are translated into practice is through the continuing investigation of culture as it relates to the individualization of care to meet the needs of every patient. A leader in research in this area is Madeleine M. Leininger, a nurse and an anthropologist.

In looking for an answer to how nurses could be more effective in meeting the individual needs of patients, she found that how people respond to health and illness is strongly influenced by their culture.

Leininger coined the phrase *transcultural nursing* to describe nursing care that incorporates all aspects of a person's culture in planning and providing care. The Transcultural Nurse's Prayer, which was written by Dr. Leininger, concisely describes the meaning of transcultural nursing.

Transcultural Nurse's Prayer

Divine spiritual master, help us to make transcultural nursing care meaningful and relevant to those served worldwide. Help nurses to facilitate transcultural understanding, peace, healing, and love among people of diverse and similar cultures in the world. Where there is hatred, fear, prejudice, racism, or violence, help nurses to lessen or remove these barriers through the use of transcultural caring knowledge and skills. In all of our endeavors, let nurses be guided by knowledge reflecting transcultural sensitivities, compassion, understanding, and other differential caring skills to promote holistic healing of cultural wounds, pain, or human suffering. We are, indeed, grateful that you fashioned the universe with diversities so that we could come to your creative design in nature, and in different environmental contexts. For these gifts we are most grateful, but we need your continued help so that the full meaning, goals, and practices of transcultural nursing will be realized for your glory and for the benefit of all beings worldwide.

Transcultural nursing encourages an appreciation of all cultures and discourages imposing your own cultural practices on others. It means respecting other cultures and adapting nursing care to meet the needs of people from cultures other than yours. Transcultural nursing is indeed the application of those nursing theories that stress understanding the whole person in the context of total environment. Nurses who consider their patients' values, beliefs, spiritual practices, and customs before planning nursing care are practicing transcultural nursing.

Attention to transcultural awareness is needed because of the growing diversity of the population in the United States. Diversity among people in this country can be attributed in part to immigration, changes in social values, changes in technology, and changes in the economic system.

Immigration from different parts of the world has kept the racial and ethnic composition of the United States in flux. In the early 1700s, people emigrated primarily from England and Germany; in the early 1800s, most immigrants were from Ireland and Germany; and in the late 1900s, a large number of people came to the United States from Italy, Russia, and central European countries. Since 2000, nearly 54% of immigrants have come to the United States from Mexico, China, the Philippines, India, Vietnam, Cuba, El Salvador, Dominican Republic, Canada, and Korea. If immigration laws are not changed and immigration and birth rates continue to increase at the current rate, the population of the United States is expected to increase from 321 million today to 400 million persons in 2050.

The United States Census Bureau also predicts that by 2060, minority groups will make up just over 50% of the population of the United States. Just over 43% of the population is projected to be white; about 31% of the population will be of Hispanic origin; nearly 15% will be African American; about 8.5% will be from Asia or the Pacific Islands; and just over 6% will be categorized as other.

✔ *The United States is made up of people from diverse cultural heritages.*

It is quite likely that you will be working in an environment where you will be expected to provide nursing care for people who speak a variety of languages and who have social customs and values that are different from yours. Giving care that respects and incorporates an individual's uniqueness will require that you continue to learn all you can about how you can effectively provide culturally competent nursing care.

According to Leininger, the goal of transcultural nursing care is to preserve, accommodate, or repattern the culture of the patient. When cultural beliefs and values do not have a negative effect on care, nurses must make every effort to help the patient preserve his or her culture. For example, a Jewish patient who follows a kosher diet must have that aspect of his culture preserved.

In some situations, it may be necessary to make accommodations to preserve the culture of the patient and the family. For example, in a culture in which the man has no role in homemaking or child care and the woman is unable to carry out her duties in the home, a housekeeper may provide an accommodation that permits the male and female roles of the culture to be preserved.

Repatterning the culture of the patient requires the patient to essentially change his or her way of life. For example, in a culture where foods high in cholesterol and fat are routinely eaten, the nurse must provide detailed information on how continuing this diet will affect the cardiovascular system. Working with the patient who needs to make such drastic changes requires patience and understanding on the part of the nurse. Changing a part of one's culture is not an easy thing to do.

Whether you are preserving, accommodating, or repatterning the culture of a patient, it is essential that the patient be involved in making decisions about his or her health care. Nurses who respect cultural differences are more likely to succeed in getting their patients to practice healthier lifestyles.

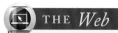 THE *Web*

The Transcultural Nursing Society provides a comprehensive resource for information related to transcultural nursing activities around the world.

Working with culturally diverse people provides you with great opportunities to grow, not only as a person but also as a nurse. Learning about the values, traditions, and beliefs of others; finding ways to communicate with people who may not fully understand the language you speak; and helping people retain their culture and at the same time benefit from all of the technology and treatment available in the US health care system can be as challenging as they are rewarding. Complete the self-assessment test "How Do You Relate to Various Groups of People in the Society" on pages 186–188 to determine how you might feel about working with different types of people.

Cultural Characteristics

From the moment of birth, children begin to learn the culture of their family and, as they grow older, the culture of their society. They learn what kinds of behaviors are right and what kinds of behaviors are wrong; which attitudes are acceptable and which are not; what is expected of them in their roles as child, adult, parent, spouse, and worker; and what are acceptable social behaviors.

Unlike opinions, preferences, and attitudes, which change, cultural characteristics are deeply rooted and are difficult or impossible to alter. They are tightly woven into an individual's personality and character. Your patients reflect their cultural heritage each time they interact with the world around them. In a situation that is alien to them (e.g., a health care setting), their differences may seem magnified because, in stressful situations, most people cling more tightly to what they are familiar with to protect themselves against the unknown.

People's reactions to circumstances vary according to culturally learned behaviors. Customs and values reflect behavior that is correct within a culture. Therefore, behaviors that are correct or expected in one culture may be very different from those of another culture. This is particularly true in the American health care system. Many health care providers direct their treatment plans

ASSESS YOURSELF	How Do You Relate to Various Groups of People in the Society?

The purpose of the following list of individuals is to help you determine how you might respond at different levels to different persons. The levels of response are defined below. Try to respond as you honestly feel, not as you think might be considered socially or professionally desirable. Your answers are only for your own personal use in clarifying your initial reactions toward different people. You can substitute other categories of people "types" according to your work experience, community setting, or the like. For example, Haitian American could be substituted for Islamic fundamentalist (28) or Prostitute for Homeless person (12).

DIRECTIONS

Take one level of response at a time and follow it through the complete list of individuals in the left column. Place a check mark (✓) in the proper column only if you would answer NO or *if you hesitate before answering YES.* Quickly go through the complete list of individuals using response level 1, then repeat with level 2, and so on through level 5.

LEVELS OF RESPONSE

1. I feel I can *greet* this person warmly and welcome him or her sincerely. If **NO**, place a check mark in column 1 of LEVEL OF RESPONSE columns.
2. I feel I can honestly *accept* this person as she or he is and be *comfortable* enough to listen to her or his problems. If **NO**, place a check mark in column 2 of LEVEL OF RESPONSE columns.
3. I feel I would genuinely try to *help* the person with his or her problems as they might relate to or arise from the label–stereotype given to him or her here. If **NO**, place a check mark in column 3 of LEVEL OF RESPONSE columns.
4. I feel I have the *background* of knowledge and/or experience to be able to help this person. If **NO**, place a check mark in column 4 of LEVEL OF RESPONSE columns.
5. I feel I could honestly be an advocate for this person. If **NO**, place a check mark in column 5 of LEVEL OF RESPONSE columns.

Check Mark for No Answers Only	Level of Response				
Individual	1 Greet	2 Accept	3 Help	4 Background	5 Advocate
1. Italian American					
2. Child abuser					
3. Jew					
4. Amputee					
5. Neo-Nazi					
6. Mexican American					
7. Divorced person					
8. Catholic					
9. Senile elderly person					
10. Teamster Union member					
11. Native American					
12. Homeless person					
13. Jehovah's Witness					
14. Cerebral palsied person					
15. Abortion rights activist					
16. Vietnamese American					
17. Gay/lesbian					

ASSESS YOURSELF

How Do You Relate to Various Groups of People in the Society? *continued*

Check Mark for No Answers Only	Level of Response				
	1 Greet	2 Accept	3 Help	4 Background	5 Advocate
Individual					
18. Atheist					
19. Blind person					
20. Political correctness extremist					
21. African American					
22. Unmarried pregnant teenager					
23. Protestant					
24. Person with AIDS					
25. Skinhead					
26. White Anglo-Saxon American					
27. Alcoholic					
28. Islamic fundamentalist					
29. Person with facial disfiguration					
30. Pro-life proponent					

You have completed the previous chart to see if you have difficulty in working with specific clients at various levels. The 30 types of individuals described above can be grouped into five categories: ethnic/racial, social issues/problems, religious, physical/mental disability, and political/social. TRANSFER your check marks to the following forms. If you have a concentration of checks within a specific category of individuals or at specific levels, this may indicate a conflict or lack of knowledge that could hinder you from rendering effective professional help.

Check Mark for No Answers Only	Level of Response				
	1 Greet	2 Accept	3 Help	4 Background	5 Advocate
Individual					
Ethnic/Racial					
1. Italian American					
6. Mexican American					
11. Native American					
16. Vietnamese American					
21. African American					
26. White Anglo-Saxon American					
Social Issues/Problems					
2. Child abuser					
7. Divorced person					
12. Homeless person					
17. Gay/lesbian					
22. Unmarried pregnant teenager					
27. Alcoholic					

continued on page 188

ASSESS YOURSELF	How Do You Relate to Various Groups of People in the Society? *continued*

Check Mark for No Answers Only	Level of Response				
	1	2	3	4	5
Individual	Greet	Accept	Help	Background	Advocate
Religious					
3. Jew					
8. Catholic					
13. Jehovah's Witness					
18. Atheist					
23. Protestant					
28. Islamic fundamentalist					
Physical/Mental Disability					
4. Amputee					
9. Senile elderly person					
14. Cerebral palsied person					
19. Blind person					
24. Person with AIDS					
29. Person with facial disfiguration					
Political/Social					
5. Neo-Nazi					
10. Teamsters Union member					
15. Abortion rights activist					
20. Political correctness extremist					
25. Skinhead					
30. Pro-life proponent					

QUESTIONS FOR YOUR CONSIDERATION

1. Is there a particular category of people or level of response that may present a conflict/difficulty for you? Identify.
2. What could you do to reduce such difficulty, that is, how could you improve your level of rendering effective professional help?
3. If you have a single group or category of groups that you *do not* believe you could work with:
   a. Clarify your reasons.
   b. How would you refer a person from this group for help? To whom/where?
4. If you have strong perceptions (thoughts and/or feelings) about a particular grouping, you might consider what sources within your own culture and/or the society reinforce those perceptions. How and by what means does such reinforcement occur? How easy or difficult do you think it would be to change one's opinion in the face of such influence? What might be the potential risk of such a change in perception?
5. Would it be likely for you to find work in an agency in which you would be assigned the kind of client you don't like (or can't) work with? What would you do?

From Accessing Awareness and Developing Knowledge, Foundations for Skill in a Multicultural Society, 3rd edition by AXELSON and McGrath. 1999. Reprinted with permission of Brooks/Cole, a division of Cengage Learning.

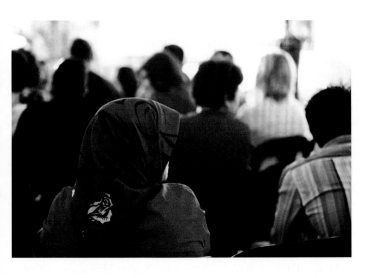

FIGURE 9-1. ● The US population includes people from diverse cultural and ethnic backgrounds.

toward middle-class white Americans. They tend to ignore the cultural diversity of their patients and then wonder why treatment regimens are not followed. Finding ways to incorporate cultural differences in health care will result in better health care for everyone (Fig. 9-1).

Ethnic Characteristics

Ethnic is an adjective applied to cultural subgroups. These subgroups, although part of the larger culture, have certain distinguishing characteristics.

An ethnic group shares, for example, food preferences, racial similarities, religious practices, a common ancestry, clothing preferences, language and linguistic styles, and mannerisms. Although cultural characteristics vary little, there are wide variations in ethnic characteristics. These variations depend in part on the education of the group, their geographic location, and the number of members in the group. An example is the differences seen between an ethnic group found in the southern part of the United States and one found in the northern part of the United States. Both groups may share similar religious practices, racial characteristics, and mannerisms, but they may have different language patterns and accents.

✔ *Nurses must avoid imposing their culture on their patients.*

Although cultural and ethnic distinctions can be made, they are often both studied under the topic of culture. In the context of this book, the term *culture* includes both cultural and ethnic behaviors.

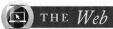 THE *Web*

The "Related Links" section of the Transcultural Nursing Society Web site provides links to information about some of the health care practices of various cultural and ethnic groups.

Language

Language is common to everyone, but not everyone shares the same language. Differences in language and how words are used can lead to misunderstanding. When a patient speaks a different language or English is not the native language,

✔ *Dr. Mehrabian estimates that 7% of communication is verbal, 38% is vocal, and 55% is nonverbal.*

or the patient uses a different dialect of English, it does not mean the patient's needs are different, only that the language is different.

When a patient's language difference is enough to seriously limit communication and understanding, take the time to ensure that you understand what the patient is trying to communicate. In addition, give the patient an opportunity to let you know that you are being understood. If necessary, obtain an interpreter or family member to assist in communicating with the patient, because not being understood and not understanding what is being done to you and why can be a very frightening experience.

Because much of our communication is nonverbal, you can provide reassurance and comfort without speaking. A smile will go a long way toward comforting those who do not understand your spoken language.

Race

✔ *Race is important in physical assessments but not in providing nursing care.*

The U.S. Census Bureau defines five major racial groups: American Indian or Alaska Native, Asian, Black or African American, Native Hawaiian or Other Pacific Islander, and White. Distinctions among races are physical, such as skin color, eye shape, hair color and texture, nose and lip shape, and stature. The United Nations dropped the term "race" in 1950 and since then has referred to "ethnic groups" of which there are more than 5,000 in the world.

Although race may predispose people to certain illnesses, nurses must recognize that race is only a physical distinction. Knowing the race of a person will not assist you to better understand that person's cultural or ethnic background.

Views on Aging

The U.S. Census Bureau projects that approximately 2.5% of the population will be age 85 or older in 2030. That percent is expected to increase to 3.7% in 2040 and 4.5% in 2050. As people grow older, they tend to have a more frequent need to seek health care. Whether the ill elderly seek health care or not is often based on cultural values. In some cultures, people believe that to get old is to get sick and that nothing can be done for them. Other cultures stress the value of health care, and their members make every effort to maintain their health.

In some cultures, the elderly are respected for their age and wisdom. In others, the elderly are often treated with disrespect, ignored, and even abused. In some cultures, it is the absolute responsibility of the family to care for the ill elderly at home; however, members of other cultures do not feel the same sense of responsibility.

If the culture of an older family member requires that younger female family members care for him or her and the younger family members have their own families and job responsibilities, the potential for a conflict in cultural values is a real issue.

Recognizing the vast array of cultural variations in the role of the elderly person in the family will help you as you learn to work with families to solve these problems.

Views on Childbearing

Many cultural variations are related to pregnancy and childbirth. To avoid deformities and even the death of a fetus, some cultures believe that certain foods should not be eaten during pregnancy; others believe that photographs should not be taken of the mother. Some believe that the mother should not witness any emotionally upsetting event; others believe that sexual intercourse should be avoided during pregnancy. The list of do's and don'ts for the pregnant woman goes on and on and is as varied as the cultures in which the mothers live.

In many cultures, the anatomic position for delivery is squatting or sitting. In the Anglo American culture, until very recently, the position for delivery was supine. In some cultures, the father is not expected or even wanted during the delivery process; in others, the father is a part of that process. In many cultures, laywomen or midwives deliver the baby at home; in others, the delivery occurs in a hospital or a birthing center.

How the infant is treated immediately after birth also depends on the cultural background of the parents. In some cultures, the infant is immediately given to the mother, and in others, the baby is placed in a bassinet and cared for by someone else. How the cord is cared for, how the episiotomy is managed, whether the baby is breast- or bottle-fed, and when the baby begins to eat solid foods all depend on the culture into which the child is born.

Behaviors surrounding pregnancy, birth, and childrearing are culturally learned and personal to the parents. If, in your practice as a nurse, you encounter people from cultural groups other than your own, you must learn as much as you can about their childbearing practices so that the family's culture will be included in your plan of care.

✔ How a baby is delivered varies from culture to culture.

Religion

Religion is an area of individual preference and a part of a person's culture that must be accommodated in any health care setting. It can be an especially sensitive issue because religious beliefs are among the most fundamental beliefs people have. People facing immediate questions of health, life, and death will frequently turn to their religion for answers. Circumstances in a hospital, nursing home, or other health care setting can make it difficult for patients to continue to practice their religion. No one should stand between the patient and his or her beliefs. Patients should be given every opportunity possible to practice or express their religious beliefs and rituals. This includes extending an open mind and every courtesy to the patient's priest, minister, rabbi, or other religious representative.

There are more than 4,300 different faith groups covering all parts of the world. Although the three largest organized religions by population in the United States are Catholicism, Protestantism, and Judaism, there are many other faiths that are not as large in numbers, but are just as significant to those who practice them. It is important to remember that to each of your patients, his or her religion is "the" religion. Remember, too, that many people do not belong to organized religious groups and may not practice or acknowledge any established religion. This does not mean they are antireligion or not spiritual.

✔ Religious beliefs may influence a patient's choice of treatment.

Although you cannot be expected to know all the differences among the more than 1,200 religious organizations in the United States, it will be helpful to you to become acquainted with basic religious convictions of a few. Religious practices of some groups are described below. To facilitate the practice of lesser known religions, your patients will probably be the best sources of information.

In all religions, the patient's religious representative should always be informed that the patient has entered your health care facility when requested by the patient and when circumstances suggest that spiritual counseling is required. The best way to ensure that this important need is not overlooked is to ask the patient what his or her wishes are. It is perfectly appropriate to ask, and it also shows your concern for the whole person beyond his or her immediate physical and medical needs.

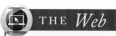

Most organized religions maintain Web sites that describe their beliefs and practices. Use a search engine to access information directly from the religious organization.

Catholicism

The basic tenet of the Catholic religion is that God, as Jesus Christ, lived, died, and was resurrected so that all of humankind could attain eternal salvation. Various rites known as sacraments (sacred) are performed at appropriate times by Catholic priests. Among the sacraments you may encounter in a health care setting are Baptism, Eucharist, Reconciliation, and Anointing of the Sick.

✔ *Approximately 24% of Americans belong to the Catholic Church.*

Baptism is administered only once in a Catholic's life. The parents of a hospitalized infant who has not been baptized may request that a priest perform this sacrament in the hospital.

The Eucharist is also called the Holy Eucharist or Holy Communion. A patient preparing to take this sacrament is required to abstain from food or drink for an hour before the rite, although water and medications are allowed at any time. If a patient is unable to attend church or chapel, the Eucharist may be brought to him or her. Also, if a patient requests the Eucharist preceding surgery, inform your supervisor, the hospital chaplain, or the patient's priest.

Reconciliation is a rite for the forgiveness of sins. The patient's confession is heard by a priest, who then pronounces absolution. It is a private matter and should be respected as such.

The Anointing of the Sick, in which the patient is anointed with holy oil, is frequently misinterpreted as the "last rites" given to someone facing imminent death. This is not the case, and most Catholic families understand this. However, assurances to the patient's family and others that the sacrament is intended for restoration of physical and spiritual health and is not a preparation for death will help dispel fear and misunderstanding.

Protestantism

Hundreds of separate denominations and sects constitute the faith known as Protestantism. Some of these denominations include Baptist, Episcopalian, Lutheran, Methodist, Presbyterian, United Church of Christ, Mennonite, and Seventh Day Adventist. A number of their practices differ, although they have many others in common.

Baptists do not practice infant baptism. For them, baptism is a rite to be given only after a believer confesses his or her faith. They believe that this can be done only by someone who is old enough to understand the significance of baptism. Baptism is performed by full immersion in water rather than by sprinkling.

Episcopalians share a number of similarities with Catholics, including Reconciliation, Anointing the Sick, Holy Communion, and Baptism, although each differs somewhat. Anointing the Sick, for example, is more often given as a healing sacrament, although it is also administered to those facing death.

✔ *Approximately 51% of Americans belong to a Protestant church.*

Episcopalians believe that a dying infant should be baptized, following a ritual similar to that described for Catholics. The usual administration of these sacraments is by Episcopal priests.

Lutherans practice baptism of children and adults by sprinkling. They also celebrate Communion, at which they believe Christ is present in spirit. Personal faith plays an essential role in their religion, which holds that Christ is both God and man.

Methodists acknowledge the baptismal rites of other religions and practice both infant and adult baptism by sprinkling and by immersion in water. For them, religion is a matter of personal belief; they use conscience as a guide for living.

Presbyterians also practice Communion (at which Christ is believed to be present in spirit) and baptism (generally by sprinkling). Salvation is believed to be a gift from God.

Members of the United Church of Christ practice infant baptism and Communion.

Seventh Day Adventists do not believe in infant baptism. They practice public and private worship, as well as private and group Bible reading. They are generally vegetarians, although some may eat meats that are specified in the Bible. This preference should be respected in the health care setting and notification should be given to your supervisor or to the dietary department.

✔ *Beliefs of Protestants vary widely from one sect to another.*

Judaism

Judaism, which is the religion and the ethnic way of life for Jewish people, is based on the five books of Moses called the Torah. Culture and religion are deeply intertwined in the Jewish faith. As a result, ritual, tradition, ceremony, religious and social laws, and the observance of holy days (holidays) are often major influences in Jewish daily life.

There are three groups in Judaism: Orthodox, Conservative, and Reform. Although all share the fundamental teachings of Judaism, they vary in how strictly they follow the traditions. Orthodox Jews are the strictest in following Jewish tradition. The Conservative group is less strict, and the Reform group even less rigid. The rabbi is the spiritual head of a Jewish congregation and is the representative to inform when a patient of the Jewish faith requests it.

✔ *Approximately 1.7% of Americans belong to a Jewish synagogue.*

Because there are wide differences among Jews in the observance of customs, rituals, and laws of Judaism, ask your Jewish patients what their preferences are. When you show a genuine interest and willingness to personally care for the physical, emotional, and spiritual needs of any patient regardless of his or her religion, beliefs, or background, most patients will respond.

The Jewish Sabbath, a day devoted to prayer, study, and rest, begins at sunset on each Friday and lasts until sunset Saturday. The Sabbath meal is an important occasion.

Circumcision, a religious custom in Judaism, is performed on male infants 8 days after birth by a pediatrician or a rabbi. In some instances, the procedure is done by Jewish religious representatives specially trained for the ritual. Jewish boys receive their name at this ceremony. Jewish girls receive theirs at their parents' synagogue (house of worship).

Dietary practices vary among the three Jewish groups. These practices are derived from traditional observances dating from early Jewish history. Kosher (meaning clean or fit to be eaten) restrictions apply to meats, fish, and dairy products and to the utensils with which they are prepared and served. The dietary department in health care facilities will observe these restrictions for your patients when they are informed to do so.

✔ *In the Jewish religion, to visit the sick is a "mitzvah" of service.*

Various procedures regarding death are observed in Judaism, although not all by each of the three groups. Generally, all believe that a dying person should not be left alone. Autopsies and embalming are not allowed by Orthodox and

Conservative Jews. Funerals are held on the day after the person dies, before sundown, but burial on the Sabbath and some holidays is not permitted.

Islam

The religion of Muslims (also known as Moslems) is Islam. Islam holds that Allah is the supreme deity and that Mohammed, the founder of Islam, is the chief prophet. Moslems follow strict dietary rules and seek edible and nonedible consumer products that carry the symbol H-MCG to identify the Halah (lawful) status of the product.

✔ *Approximately 0.6% of Americans belong to a mosque.*

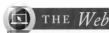

THE *Web*

The Muslim Consumers Group Web site provides detailed information on Halah certified food and drug products.

Buddhism

✔ *Approximately 0.7% of Americans practice the teaching of Buddha.*

Buddhists believe in Buddha, or the "Enlightened One." There are a number of Buddhist sects in the United States, each having some differences from the others. The primary emphasis of Buddhism is for each individual to find what is right and, through that discovery, to achieve Nirvana, or supreme tranquility.

Other Religions

Members of other religious groups that you may provide care for include Mormons (Church of Jesus Christ of Latter Day Saints), Jehovah's Witnesses, and Christian Scientists.

Mormons do not believe in baptizing infants or in the use of caffeine (e.g., tea, coffee, cola drinks), alcohol, or tobacco. Baptism occurs at age 8 years, when it is believed the child has reached the age of reasoning. Mormons who are worthy to enter the temple wear a special type of underclothing called a garment. Mormons are permitted to remove this garment when necessary health care procedures require it.

✔ *Approximately 1.7% of Americans belong to the Mormon Church.*

The Mormon blessing of the sick is performed by two elders. One anoints the person with oil, while the other offers a prayer for healing. During this blessing, both elders place their hands on the head of the patient.

Members of the Mormon Church usually have a number of visitors who represent the church. These visitors are important, and you should provide as much privacy for their visits as possible.

Jehovah's Witnesses are prohibited from receiving any blood or blood products and from coming into contact with any equipment that has been in contact with the blood of someone else. They also believe that Jesus Christ is King. For that reason, they do not participate in any political activities such as voting, pledging allegiance, or serving in the military.

✔ *A Christian Science family is unlikely to agree to treatments that would prolong life indefinitely.*

Christian Scientists belong to the Church of Christ, Scientist. There are no ordained or appointed leaders of the church. Many larger cities have Christian Science reading rooms where literature is available to the public.

The basic premise of the Church of Christ, Scientist is that healing, both spiritual and physical, is a result of drawing closer to God in how one lives and thinks. Christian Science practitioners are available to pray with those who are ill for their healing. Christian Science nurses provide the physical care that may be needed for people who are unable to meet their own needs. Most Christian

Scientists do not use medications and do not accept blood or blood products. In general, any measures that interfere with the natural progression of life are avoided.

Secular and Nonreligious Groups

There is a large number of Americans who do not believe in a supernatural power and do not belong to any organized or formal religious groups. As with those who have firm religious beliefs, it is important to provide nursing care that includes accommodating, to the extent possible, a patient's personal beliefs.

Views on Pain

From your experience as a nursing student or as a nurse, you know that people express pain in different ways. There are those who say nothing and refuse medication and those who moan and groan loudly and beg for medication. How one responds to pain is often as much a result of one's culture as it is of one's personality and emotional state at the time.

You will no doubt care for many patients who are in pain. As a nurse, you must be careful to avoid expecting your patients to express their pain in the same way you do. In some cultures, it is considered a weakness to cry when in pain; in others, crying is permitted and even encouraged for even mild pain.

For these reasons, it is important for nurses to consider more than physical expressions to assess pain. A patient may physically appear to be in excruciating pain; however, a careful assessment may indicate that a change of position reduces the pain to the point where medication is not needed. On the other hand, a patient whom you believe should have some complaints of pain may be lying quietly in the bed. A careful assessment of this patient may reveal rather intense pain.

A good rule of thumb is to ask the patient if he or she is in pain. If the answer is yes, make an assessment and recommend an action. If the patient is not comfortable with your recommendation, it is appropriate to ask what measures he or she would prefer to use to relieve the pain. Narcotics, barbiturates, biofeedback, acupuncture, herbs, guided imagery, religious rituals, and therapeutic touch are just a few of the measures that can be used to alleviate pain.

Views on Nutrition

Guidelines published by the U.S. Department of Agriculture identify the number of servings that should be eaten from each group of food each day. Although these guidelines may work well for Anglo Americans, they are not guidelines that are incorporated by many other cultures.

People in some cultures use various foods to cure illnesses or ward off evil spirits. In some cultures, men and women eat separately, and in others, it is unheard of to eat alone. People in some cultures eat diets high in rice or beans. Some make no distinction between breakfast and dinner foods. Some eat five or six times a day, and others eat every other day.

To assess a patient's diet, it is more appropriate for the nurse to ask what the patient ate and when rather than what he or she ate for breakfast, lunch, and dinner.

Adequate nutrition is important to the healing process. If your patient is not eating, it is necessary to find the reasons. If it is a dislike of the types of foods being served, you might suggest that a dietitian work with the patient and family to find a more agreeable diet.

✔ *Approximately 16% of Americans report being atheist, agnostic, or secular or as having no religious belief.*

✔ *Nurses should be aware that their own culture may influence their attitudes toward a patient's pain.*

⚙ Critical Thinking
E X E R C I S E

You have been caring for a thin, 60-year-old Asian man who immigrated with his wife and children to the United States 1 year ago. Since being admitted to the hospital, he has not been eating and has lost 4 lb. When you ask him why he doesn't eat, he smiles politely and tells you he is not hungry. Describe exactly where you could find resources that would help you understand how his cultural heritage might be contributing to his smiling and saying he is not hungry. What could you say to him to encourage him to talk about his food preferences?

What will you do if he tells you what foods he would eat but you know that they are not normally available in your facility? Use appropriate Characteristics of Critical Thinking in Box 1-2 on pages 18–19 to develop your response to this situation.

Views on Death and Mourning

Death is viewed in different ways by different cultures. For some cultures, death is a natural extension of life; for others, it is a time of great loss. Regardless of how death is perceived, all cultures prefer that people who are dying do so with dignity.

Nurses are in a unique position to provide dignity in the last moments of a person's life. Respecting the wishes of the patient and family for privacy, permitting the family to carry out religious or cultural rituals, limiting interruptions, and providing gentle and compassionate care are just a few things nurses can do to help the patient die with dignity.

But not all deaths can be anticipated. In those situations where death is a result of an accident or violence and family members have not had time to prepare, not having a chance to say goodbye to their loved ones is particularly difficult, regardless of the cultural background. The nurse can give support to the family in this situation by providing a private area and offering to contact people who would be able to support the family during a time of crisis.

Care of the body after death is deeply rooted in cultural and religious traditions. In some cultures, there is a ritualistic washing of the body; in others, certain clothing is required for burial; and in others, the body is quickly buried. If you are uncertain of how to handle the body after death, ask a family member or a religious representative before doing anything.

Mourning is the cultural expression of grief, and all cultures have rituals associated with mourning. The nurse must recognize that his or her own personal ways of mourning are not the only ways people mourn the loss of a loved one. Understanding that there are wide variations in how different cultures cope with death and that mourning rituals also vary widely within cultures and ethnic groups will help the nurse provide support for the relatives and friends of the deceased.

✔ *Kübler-Ross's book, Questions and Answers on Death and Dying, should be required reading for all nurses.*

✔ *Mourning is a cultural behavior that varies widely from one group to another.*

Cultural Assessment

Many health care facilities have printed forms (tools) to use to complete a cultural assessment. Find out if your clinical affiliation has a cultural assessment tool, and if so, begin using it to develop a better understanding of cultures other than your own.

When collecting information for a cultural assessment, it is important to use common sense and good interviewing skills. Much of the information about a person's values and beliefs related to health care and religion can be obtained informally through conversation. Some information, such as folk remedies that have been tried, can be obtained only through a formal interview. Other information about a person's culture may be irrelevant to the situation and should not be requested.

It is impossible to completely know every cultural variation of the people for whom you will provide care. The best way to provide culturally appropriate health care is to use an assessment tool and to involve your patient and the family in determining the plan of care. If a treatment, medication, diet, or procedure is unacceptable, it will be necessary to work with that patient to find an alternative that will be acceptable.

SOCIAL DIVERSITY

Nurses who work with socially diverse people need to learn about the needs of these groups and apply many of the same skills they use when caring for people from culturally diverse groups.

Some socially diverse groups have had the benefit of extensive research and investigation of their situation, but others have not. The nursing needs of a few of what might be called socially diverse groups are discussed on the following pages.

The Child

Children may experience a lot of fear in their lives because so much of what they do is new to them. Not all fear is registered as open-eyed trembling. In a hospital or other health care setting, children may appear to be perfectly normal—sitting quietly or doing just what they've been told to do. Or they may scream and fight any efforts to hold them, especially when facing a procedure that might hurt, such as having blood drawn. Whether quiet or screaming, chances are good that children in health care settings are generally afraid.

Talking to a child to determine whether he or she is afraid may not work because a young child, or one who is very frightened, may not be able to communicate effectively. A nod or a shake of the head from the child will not provide enough information if you have to make a clinical judgment about the child's physical and mental condition.

✔ *Most children who need health care are frightened.*

It is better to assume that a child is afraid and treat the child accordingly than to neglect the possibility. If it turns out that the child is not afraid, no harm has been done. If the child is afraid, your actions will help him or her deal with the fear.

To help children deal with fear, you must try to make them feel secure by being warm, open, friendly, and honest. Although you are not a relative or even a family friend, you may be in an excellent position to help a child ward off or calm fears. Holding, touching, praising a child, and attempting to reduce fear by quiet reassurance are the kinds of behaviors a child should get from a parent. When a parent is not present, those needs remain. You may be able to meet at least some of them to a certain extent (see Fig. 9-2).

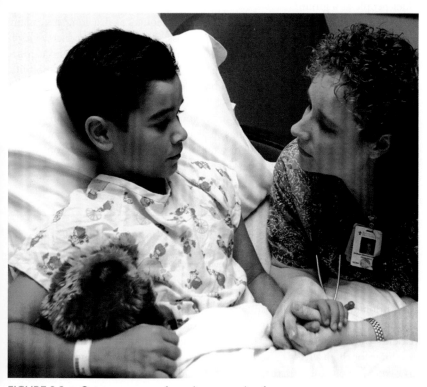

FIGURE 9-2. ● Quiet reassurance from the nurse calms fears.

You can be equally important to the child's well-being by establishing good relationships with parents and other family members. A smile, an answered question, reassurance, and a willingness to listen to parents' concerns can help the child learn to trust you.

The Child Who Is Abused

At some time, you may find yourself caring for a child who has been abused. Abused children who are hospitalized need more love and attention than do others. They may have an induced fear of adults that could be overwhelming when combined with the normal fear some children have of hospitals and other health care facilities. Most states have laws mandating that physicians, nurses, teachers, and others report suspected child abuse. Consult with your instructor or supervisor when you suspect that a child has been abused. Also learn whether you, when you become licensed, will be obligated to report child abuse.

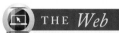

THE *Web*

The *Safe Kids* Web site provides a lot of suggestions about how to keep kids safe.

The Patient Who Is Elderly

An older person is not an old child. It is inaccurate to use words such as hopeless, obstinate, demanding, confused, irrational, slow, or stubborn to describe older people. Although older people are as different from one another as are younger people, there are some physical and social changes that generally tend to affect older people as a group.

It is important to understand that as a consequence of a long life, many changes, including losses, occur. A partial loss of hearing or reduced vision affects many older people. The incidence of arthritis, osteoporosis, and cardio-pulmonary diseases increases with advancing age and can lead to loss of mobility. Other losses may include the loss of a home or driver's license and the loss of a spouse through death. In general, most elderly people have suffered some losses. Therefore, it is important for you to treat your older patients in a manner that will reduce further loss. Simple things such as the loss of privacy may not affect a younger patient, but an older patient who loses privacy may be losing one of the few important things he or she has left.

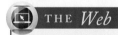

THE *Web*

The American Association of Retired Persons Web site provides information about the concerns and activities of the elderly.

Independence is a strong characteristic of people in a free society. Institutionalization (being hospitalized or confined to a health care facility such as a nursing home), by its nature, reduces one's independence. To limit elderly patients' independence further by treating them as though they're unable to do anything for themselves is a serious blow. An older patient may need assistance, and your responsibility is to provide it. But don't make the assumption that a

patient who has gray hair or who walks more slowly than you do is totally dependent. Learn by observing and by asking your older patients what you can do to
help them.

For many reasons, the elderly people you meet in a health care facility may
show more than average loneliness, depression, confusion, and a sense of being
rejected. In many cases, these symptoms have medical causes that can be allevi-
ated. For example, it is not uncommon for elderly people to neglect their diet.
Certain dietary deficiencies can produce depression. Careful assessment may
provide clues to the causes of depression.

Elderly persons constitute a highly visible population in health care settings
and especially in long-term and extended care facilities. The elderly population is
growing very rapidly, and the likelihood is that you will encounter more elderly
than young patients in your nursing practice. It will be to your benefit to closely
study aging and its associated factors.

Greater understanding and knowledge will help improve your relationships
with older patients, assist you in making clinical decisions in helping older
patients, and increase your career opportunities.

The Patient Who Is Having an Elective Abortion

Abortions are a combination of a physical event (the abortion itself) and the
postabortion period that follows. They are often emotionally charged events in
a woman's life and can be very upsetting. A nurse caring for a woman having
an abortion should provide extraordinary understanding along with the routine
nursing care required.

Many factors are associated with abortion, including legal, medical, religious, social, emotional, family, and other concerns. You are not expected to be
a specialist in these areas, but compassionate understanding in all of them is
important.

Regardless of your personal feelings about elective abortion, it is legal in the
United States. Although as a nurse you are required to provide nursing care,
you may be exempt from assisting with this procedure. There are differences in
state abortion laws. You can learn what they are in your state by asking your
instructor or the legal representative of your health care facility after you are
employed.

The Patient Who Is a Single Parent

The increasing number of single parents has significant implications for nurses.
The number of single mothers increased from 3 million in 1975 to a little over
12 million in 2014; over the same time period, the number of single fathers
increased from 393,000 nearly 2.5 million.

Single parents have multiple concerns but being able to financially afford to
care for their children is their biggest concern. A low-income, single parent will
pay approximately $157,410 to raise a child to the age of 17. Although federal
programs provide some financial assistance for single parents, many work more
than one job just to afford the bare essentials.

When a single parent is ill and needs health care, you will need to be sensitive
to his or her concerns about his or her children. Some single parents will forego
their own health to attend to their children. Be certain that your instructor is
informed of any behavior changes you see in your patient, and if the situation
develops beyond your experience or capacity to manage it, be sure that a qualified
professional is notified.

The Patient Who Is Homosexual

For many years, homosexuality was so carefully hidden that virtually no one could say with certainty who was homosexual and who was not. With the openness that is now common, male and female homosexuals are less likely to hide their sexual preference, although many still do.

A patient may tell you he or she is homosexual, or you may learn it through other sources. The important thing to keep in mind when you are caring for a homosexual patient is that your obligation is to the patient as a person who requires health care.

If you have a patient who tells you that he or she is homosexual, acknowledge it and discuss it freely. Let the patient be the guide as to how much discussion is permissible because privacy is a right of all patients. It is particularly important to protect the patient's right to privacy by keeping this information confidential if so requested.

To the homosexual patient, the partner is the significant person in his or her life. You should recognize this relationship and handle it as you would for all of your patients and their families.

The issue of homosexuality has taken on new dimensions as a result of acquired immunodeficiency syndrome (AIDS). Many AIDS patients are homosexuals. However, it must be underscored that having this disease does not mean the patient is homosexual. Heterosexuals, children, hemophilia patients, and intravenous drug users are also AIDS victims. There are no medical or legal distinctions to categorize homosexuals, and you owe it to your patient not to make any of your own.

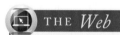
THE *Web*

The *Straight for Equality in Healthcare* Web site offers suggestions for creating an atmosphere of inclusion in health care.

The Patient Who Chooses Complementary and Alternative Forms of Treatment

Increasing numbers of Americans are using nontraditional approaches to maintain or improve health or to treat illness. Complementary forms of treatment include treatments that are used along with traditional Western medicine. An example would be using behavior modification with blood pressure medications. Alternative forms of treatment are those treatments used in place of traditional Western medical treatments. An example would be using acupuncture in place of surgery for lower back pain.

Using herbs, diets, vitamins, stress reduction techniques, acupuncture, behavior modification, meditation, and consulting with faith healers, chiropractors, nutritionists, naturopaths, masseurs, and exercise physiologists can be complementary, alternative, or both. Although many traditional health care providers may dismiss some or all of these as a waste of time, the federal government is providing money to investigate the value of nontraditional approaches to health care.

The National Center for Complementary and Alternative Medicine was formed in October 1998. The name was changed in December 2014 to the National Center for Complementary and Integrative Health (NCCIH). This change in name reflects the Center's commitment to studying promising health approaches already in use by physicians and the American public.

NCCIH is 1 of 27 institutes and centers that make up the National Institutes of Health within the U.S. Department of Health and Human Services In 2015, the federal government appropriated almost $125 million to NCCIH for research and to study the effectiveness of complementary and alternative methods of treatment.

Appendix D is a dictionary of terms related to complementary and alternative medicine. A review of these pages will increase your awareness of the many alternative and complementary forms of health care treatment. Hundreds of books, journals, and Web sites provide information about each of these complementary and alternative methods of treatment. Just as with traditional medical advice, patients must learn as much as they can about the proposed treatment, so they can make their own decision about what is best for them.

When you have patients who are using complementary or alternative methods of treatment, you must stress to them the importance of sharing all of the information about what they take or do with their physician. Herbs and certain diets and biologic products can cause lethal interactions with some treatments and medications.

 THE *Web*

The National Center for Complementary and Integrative Health, a division of the National Institutes of Health, provides information on current research projects and accurate information about the effectiveness of complementary and alternative treatments.

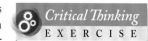
Critical Thinking
E X E R C I S E

You are assigned to care for a 24-year-old patient who was admitted for the surgical repair of a broken arm that she sustained in a motorcycle accident. Her surgery was yesterday, and she should be discharged tomorrow. As you enter her room, you see her inhaling something from a small vial. You aren't sure what it is, so you decide to ask her. She says she is inhaling peppermint oil to help with postoperative nausea and the pain from her surgery. What will you do and why? Use appropriate Characteristics of Critical Thinking in Box 1-2 on pages 18–19 to develop your response to this situation.

The Patient Who Is Mentally Ill

Everyone has an emotional side and a physical side. When both are in relative balance, a person is considered well. When either one or both are not balanced, a person is ill. Emotional or mental illness is a disease and must be treated as such. There is no place in a health care setting for words such as crazy, loony, or nuts when one is describing behavior.

Many health care facilities in the United States are devoted exclusively to the care and treatment of mentally ill patients. In addition, many hospitals have psychiatric units especially designed to care for those who have mental illnesses.

Even if you don't work in a psychiatric setting, as a nurse, you will surely encounter emotionally disturbed patients. A health care facility often has an effect on people's emotional states. For example, someone who is facing a life-threatening situation but who is otherwise emotionally stable may become depressed. A patient who is anticipating major surgery may become extremely anxious. While waiting for test results with lifelong implications, a patient may become withdrawn and uncommunicative. And patients with known psychiatric conditions may get worse; for example, a person with depression may develop thoughts of suicide.

✔ *There are many forms of treatments to improve the lives of people who are mentally ill.*

Not all expressions of extreme emotion are clinical (i.e., having psychiatrically verifiable causes). An elderly patient with no relatives, who has no visitors, and who spends the day wistfully in her room may say, "I might as well be dead." Such statements may not always represent feelings of suicide, but they should always be reported to your instructor. Often, they are cries for attention. You should not be the one to judge whether a patient's expressions of wanting to die are suicidal or are statements of loneliness.

Sometimes, quietly listening to someone who is emotionally distraught is sufficient. Sometimes, a gentle touch on the shoulder lets the patient know that someone cares. Sometimes, providing the privacy to cry alone is what the patient needs. Sometimes, the suggestion of a visit by a religious advisor is helpful to the patient. If these usual nursing measures do not help the patient who is dealing with intense emotions, a psychiatric evaluation may be needed. Again, your instructor or team leader must be informed of your observations and assessments so that appropriate measures can be taken to benefit the patient.

The Patient Who Is Withdrawn

✔ *Never assume that the patient who does not ask for anything does not need anything.*

Some patients in a health care facility may ask for little or nothing from the nursing staff. However, it is a disservice to overlook any patient who is not clamoring for attention or mentioning a need. For example, an elderly patient who is lying on a painful pressure sore may suffer in silence rather than impose on you, or a patient who has soiled the bed may be too embarrassed to ask for help.

To avoid these and other situations in which nursing care is needed but may not be requested by the patient, you must make your patients understand that you want to help them meet their needs. Let them know that it is okay to tell you what is going on with them, what they need, and what they want. If you are open and direct with your patients, those who might otherwise go unnoticed will get the full benefit of your care.

The Patient Who Is Hostile

There is another group of patients in health care facilities who are anything but unnoticed. They are the opposite of the shy, undemanding patient, and they may be disruptive as well. The disruption may be merely vocal, or it may also be physical. The solution is not to ignore the demanding shouts, grumbling complaints, or overt physical acts that are meant to get your attention, but to deal with the patient calmly. Avoid either encouraging the behavior by yielding to the demands or fanning the flames by becoming angry yourself.

✔ *Attend training programs to learn how to deal with violent behavior in the workplace.*

Disruptive, complaining behavior is often a cry for attention. If you and your instructor can determine the underlying cause and satisfy the need, the patient will probably calm down. Seriously disruptive behavior should be reported because it may indicate deeper problems than just a lack of attention.

When behavior becomes truly abusive or hostile, and you, other patients or staff, or the patient himself is threatened with harm, the matter should be reported immediately to your supervisor. If the behavior is violent, as in the case of someone who is mentally disturbed or who is reacting to alcohol or drug abuse, protect yourself and other patients and call for help at once. Don't attempt to restrain a patient who is violent or threatening violence without qualified assistance.

The Patient Who Abuses Alcohol or Drugs

The substance-abusing patient may have psychological, medical, and legal problems all at the same time. People do not become addicted to drugs for pleasure or because they are thrilled with how their lives are going. They have underlying needs that are being inappropriately met through chemical interventions that eventually become addictive.

Your duty as a nurse is to provide care for any patient regardless of what caused him or her to need your care. Most people have strong feelings about substance abuse. Yours may be even greater because you know the dangers of substance abuse and you see the end result of years of abuse. You must not let those feelings come between you and your patient, as difficult as this may be.

Substance abuse is a disease and must be treated as such. Sometimes, the consequences of a substance abuser's acts may cause outrage; for example, a drunk driver may run over and injure or kill a child. It will take an exceptionally strong commitment on your part, but you cannot turn your back on the abuser, any more than you could turn your back on the injured child.

Any person with a diagnosis of substance abuse needs more care than you alone can give. If your patient is not already under special care for substance abuse, see that such care is given by informing your instructor of the need and by providing information to the patient or the patient's family about where such care can be obtained.

The Patient Who Is Dying

Saving lives is one of the goals of health care, but dying and death are facts that cannot be overlooked by health care personnel. The number of dying patients that you will care for will depend on the type of work you do after you enter practice. In some fields, death is remote, whereas in others it is a regular occurrence. You may never get used to working with dying patients, but there are ways to make the situation more comfortable for your patients, their families, and yourself.

When you are caring for someone who is dying, the most important thing you can do is to be secure with your own feelings. You must confront your own feelings about death before you can be of much help to others. As difficult as it may be for some of us to accept, death is inevitable. Whenever it occurs, it is usually an emotionally wrenching experience.

Death in a health care setting comes in two general types: expected, as in the case of terminally ill patients, and unexpected, as in the case of accident victims, heart attack victims, and others who, except for the immediate cause, would not have died. The latter group includes patients who die suddenly during an otherwise positive recovery.

Little can be done to prepare for unexpected deaths except to know that they may happen and, when they do, to get past your own shock and disbelief so that you can continue to care for your other patients and also provide solace for the deceased's family and friends.

✔ *Learn to accept the behaviors associated with the five stages of dying.*

A patient who is known to be dying—as in the case of someone with a long-term illness—will pass through a series of stages that, if completed, will prepare him or her for death. Dr. Elizabeth Kübler-Ross distinguished five stages of dying in her book *Questions and Answers on Death and Dying*. These stages are as follows:

1. Denial
2. Anger
3. Bargaining
4. Depression
5. Acceptance

The first stage, denial, may last a short or a long time. It expresses the patient's unwillingness to accept a serious illness and its likely consequences.

When the reality of what is happening can no longer be denied, the patient will become angry. This anger may be expressed by demanding, difficult, critical, and unpleasant behavior. This second stage may be difficult for you to deal with because one common reaction to someone who is being objectionable is to respond in the same way. You must not. It is in this situation that your objectivity will get you through. The patient's behavior toward you is not personal, although it may sound that way. Realize that the patient must express this anger to progress toward full acceptance of events he or she cannot control.

As the patient understands more fully that death is inevitable, bargaining for time is a common behavior. This can take the form of making promises to society, to God, to a church, or to someone on the health care facility staff. These promises can take any form, but the offer is usually to exchange something (e.g., a donation to a cause, a promise to be good) for more life.

When it is even clearer that nothing can be done to change what is happening, the patient may become depressed. This may be expressed through crying, through silence, or by mourning past life events—things that the patient feels should have been done differently or losses already experienced. This kind of depression is similar to that which everyone experiences from time to time. As time passes, the nature of the patient's depression changes as the patient begins to mourn his or her own death. It is a grief that cannot be shared because the dying patient is grieving over the impending loss of everyone and everything she knows, and only someone who is dying can know what that must be like. However, the patient must be allowed to express this grief. You can encourage this expression by making it okay to cry or to talk about this grief if the patient desires.

If the preceding stages are allowed to be completed by the patient, and when denial, anger, bargaining, and grief are finished, the patient may reach the stage of acceptance. Acceptance of death does not mean willingness to die, but it does mean that the patient is in some way ready.

Dr. Kübler-Ross believes that all patients sense they are terminally ill, even if they have not been told. It is not your responsibility to inform a patient that he or she is dying. However, knowing what the patient has been told about his or her condition will improve your ability to help the patient through the process of dying. Ask your instructor or supervisor whether your patient has been told if he or she is dying. If so, you can deal with the situation openly.

In the course of a terminally ill patient's care, you will also get to know family, friends, and other regular visitors. They may rely on you for information, for trust, and as someone to whom they can express their feelings. Your best preparation is to have a thorough understanding of your own feelings and the knowledge that you can interact with compassion and empathy while maintaining the required objectivity that allows you to function efficiently.

✔ If appropriate, include family members and significant others in the care of the dying person.

SUMMARY

✔ Begin including what you have learned in this chapter in the care of your patients.

This chapter provides the foundation on which you can individualize patient care. Understanding the needs of diverse groups helps you focus on general needs, but you must never overlook the individuality of each patient. Not all substance abusers want help, and not all withdrawn patients will ask for assistance just because you encourage them to do so.

You will be more effective and feel better about the nursing care you provide when you take the time to approach each person under your care as a unique human being with his or her own special needs.

APPLY
Critical Thinking Skills

1. In the opening story at the beginning of this chapter, Luca sees a lot of different people on her way to work. Think about two or three ideas about which you have very strong opinions. What do you do/say/think when classmates or friends or neighbors disagree with your ideas on these subjects? How are you going to handle situations in which patients have ideas that are very different from yours?

2. Identify the nursing theory that was used as the basis for your nursing education curriculum. How are the concepts of this theory evident in your curriculum?

3. Ask a nurse who graduated from nursing school 40 or more years ago to describe changes in how nurses plan care for their patients.

4. Read several actual nursing care plans for patients in your clinical facility. Can you provide the rationale (reasons) for the nursing orders?

5. Think about the following situation: A 35-year-old man who immigrated to the United States from Mexico 6 months ago is admitted to the emergency room of a short-term (acute) care hospital after an automobile accident. He was alone in the car, his family and home are in a city 100 miles away, and he has never been in a hospital before. His most serious injury appears to be a broken leg; however, the doctors are considering the possibility of internal injuries. What do you think some of his thoughts and feelings might be while he is waiting for their diagnosis? How might you as a student nurse help this patient during this crisis?

6. Several special groups of patients were discussed in this chapter. Think of a group not discussed, and outline some of the more significant characteristics of that group. What are some of the special nursing considerations for this group?

7. Ethnic differences exist in almost every culture. What are some of the ethnic differences in wedding ceremonies of students in your class?

8. How many different religious organizations are there in your community?

9. Make a list of your beliefs about the things a pregnant woman should and should not do during pregnancy. Then ask someone from a different cultural background to do the same. What are the similarities and what are the differences? Are any of the practices considered unhealthy or dangerous to the baby?

10. Attend a social event being held by a social group different from yours. What were you able to learn from the experience?

11. Develop a plan to teach a diabetic diet to a person who is not a member of your cultural group. Where can you find resources to help you and the patient select foods that are culturally acceptable and at the same time meet the requirements of the prescribed diet?

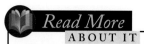

Read More ABOUT IT

Allgood MR: Nursing Theorists and Their Work, 8th ed. St. Louis, MO: Elsevier, 2014.

Andrews MM, Boyle JS: Transcultural Concepts in Nursing Care, 7th ed. Philadelphia, PA: Lippincott Williams & Wilkins, 2015.

Arnold E, Boggs KV: Interpersonal Relationships: Professional Communication Skills for Nurses, 7th ed. St. Louis, MO: Elsevier, 2015.

Balzer-Riley J: Communication in Nursing, 7th ed. St. Louis, MO: Elsevier, 2011.

Benner P: From Novice to Expert: Excellence and Power in Clinical Nursing Practice, Commemorative Edition. Upper Saddle River, NJ: Prentice Hall, 2001.

Carpenito JY: Handbook of Nursing Diagnosis: Application to Clinical Practice, 14th ed. Philadelphia, PA: Lippincott Williams & Wilkins, 2012.

Giger JN, Davidhizar RE: Transcultural Nursing: Assessment and Intervention, 6th ed. St. Louis, MO: Elsevier, 2012.

Henderson V: Principles and Practices of Nursing. New York, NY: Macmillan, 1978.

Kübler-Ross E: Living with Death and Dying. New York, NY: Simon & Schuster, 1997.

Kübler-Ross E: Questions and Answers on Death and Dying. New York, NY: Simon & Schuster, 1997.

McFarland MR, Wehbe-Alamah HB: Leininger's Culture, Care, Diversity, and Universality: A Worldwide Nursing Theory, 3rd ed. New York, NY: Jones and Bartlett, 2014.

Milliken ME, Honeycutt A: Understanding Human Behavior: A Guide for Health Care Providers, 8th ed. Clifton Park, NY: Delmar, 2012.

NANDA: Nursing Diagnoses 2015–17: Definitions and Classifications. Indianapolis, IN: Wiley Blackwell, 2014.

Neuman B, Fawcett J: Neuman Systems Model, 5th ed. Upper Saddle River, NJ: Prentice-Hall, 2011.

Nightingale F: Notes on Nursing: What It Is and What It Is Not, Commemorative Edition. Philadelphia, PA: Lippincott Williams & Wilkins, 1992.

O'Brien ME: Spirituality in Nursing: Standing on Holy Ground, 5th ed. New York, NY: Jones & Bartlett, 2013.

Orem DE: Nursing: Concepts of Practice, 6th ed. St. Louis, MO: Mosby-Year Book, 2001.

Purnell LD: Transcultural Health Care: A Culturally Competent Approach, 4th ed. Philadelphia, PA: F A Davis, 2012.

Purtilo R, Haddad A, Doherty R: Health Professional and Patient Interaction, 8th ed. St. Louis, MO: Elsevier, 2014.

Roy C, Andrews HA: The Roy Adaptation Model, 3rd ed. Upper Saddle River, NJ: Prentice-Hall, 2009.

Sheldon LK: Communication for Nurses: Talking With Patients, 3rd ed. Boston, MA: Jones & Bartlett Learning, 2013.

Spector RE: Cultural Diversity in Health and Illness, 8th ed. Upper Saddle River, NJ: Prentice-Hall, 2012.

PREPARING FOR
Successful Practice

Ethical Issues in Health Care

LEARNING OBJECTIVES

When you complete this chapter, you will be able to:

1. Define the word ethical.

2. Describe what is meant by individual, societal, and situational ethics.

3. Explain why a study of ethics and ethical behavior is important in nursing.

4. State the purposes of a code of ethics.

5. Paraphrase the National Federation for Licensed Practical Nurses (NFLPN) and the National Association for Practical Nurse Education and Service (NAPNES) statements regarding ethical behavior of practical/vocational nurses.

6. Explain personal responsibility and accountability as they relate to ethical behavior.

7. Outline the process for making decisions related to ethical dilemmas.

8. Apply guidelines for ethical decision making in your practice of nursing.

9. Participate in discussions regarding ethical issues in the work environment.

Jim and Jeannie started practical nursing school 2 months ago. They were already good friends, and they often studied together. Jim was doing very well. His lowest grade was a 92. Jeannie's was a different story. Her grades were generally poor. In fact, if she did not pass the upcoming exams, she would be dismissed from the program.

Jim was concerned for his friend. "The exam is next week," he said. "I'll help you study this weekend, if you like." "Oh, that's very nice of you, Jim," Jeannie said as they chatted over coffee after their last class on Friday. "I just don't think I'll have time. I have some shopping to do tomorrow. And I've got a date tomorrow night." She thought for a moment. "But Sunday would be fine. Can you call me then to set up a time?" "I sure will," Jim said. "One day of study is better than none. Especially for you, Jeannie. It could mean your whole nursing career." Jeannie nodded. "I know," she said. She was very serious.

On Sunday morning, Jim called Jeannie. "What time do you want to meet me?" he asked.

There was silence for a moment. Then, Jeannie spoke. "For what?" she said.

"We were going to study for the exam today," Jim said.

"Oh, I can't," Jeannie said. "I didn't get in until early this morning. I'm so tired I can't even think of studying." "Do you want me to come by later this afternoon?" Jim asked, unwilling to let his friend miss her last opportunity to prepare for the exam.

"Sure," Jeannie said. "That's a good idea."

When Jim went to Jeannie's that afternoon, there was a note on the door. It said: "Jim. I forgot I had to go to my mother's for dinner. See you in class tomorrow. J." The next day, Jim met Jeannie in the hall. "I left a set of my notes under your door," he said. "Did you get a chance to read them?" Jeannie smiled. "That was so sweet, Jim. But, I just couldn't find the time. It was late and to be perfectly honest, I'm not really worried about this exam." "Well, I am," Jim said. "And I'm only trying to keep my average up. Not keep from getting put out of the program." Jeannie squeezed his hand. "You worry too much," she said.

Later, when the class was assembled for the exam, Jim nodded to Jeannie. "Good luck," he said.

"Thanks," she whispered back.

The instructor distributed the exam papers. Jim glanced through it to familiarize himself with its content and to estimate how much time he would need to complete it. Other students did the same, although some started writing their answers immediately.

About halfway through the exam, Jim glanced across the aisle at Jeannie. He was astonished by what he saw. In her hand was a 3 × 5 index card. She looked at it and then slipped it out of sight before answering a test question. She did this a number of times during the exam. She was still writing when Jim turned in his paper and left the room.

Jeannie joined him a few minutes later. "That wasn't so hard after all, was it?" she said.

"You didn't think so?" Jim asked in surprise. "Maybe it wasn't the hardest exam we've had, but it sure wasn't the easiest. I know I couldn't have winged it." Jeannie said nothing.

"Did you get a chance to go over the notes I left?" Jim asked. Jeannie's hand shot up. "Oh, there's Diana," she said, waving her arm. "I have to talk to her about something. Diana! Wait up!" She turned to Jim. "See you tomorrow." The hall emptied as the last of the students left the exam room.

Soon it was very quiet. Jim was deeply concerned. A flurry of questions raced through his mind. Did Jeannie cheat on the exam? What should I do? Should I tell her what I saw? Should I ask her if she used notes? Should I report her? Is it my business to snitch on someone if I think she cheated? Is it my business to report someone if I know she cheated? What if we were on duty and I saw Jeannie do something dishonest that would harm a patient, like writing on a chart that she did something but really didn't? Would I be responsible? Jim shook his head sharply. I'll have to make Jeannie talk to me about this, he said to himself.

Jim's decision was guided by what he and his class were discussing at great length: the ethics of people who accept the responsibility of caring for others.

ETHICS

For many years now, you have been developing personal standards of conduct and making decisions based on your personal beliefs and values. Before you entered nursing school, your personal standards of conduct, your beliefs, your values, and your prejudices probably had little influence on others. Perhaps those who did not agree with your opinions were not your friends; those who did not approve of the way you conducted yourself did not associate with you.

But now that you have decided to become a nurse, you must closely examine yourself—your heart and your soul. By becoming a nurse, you agree to provide certain services to other human beings, and human beings have certain rights that are absolute. That means that these rights apply equally to every human being. Human rights are absolute privileges that people have and that they have the right to expect because they are human. There are many human rights. Some are specific to individuals; others are specific to groups.

People are neither more nor less human because of their income, their occupation, their sex, their race, or any of an infinite number of factors that make people different. Although people are different in what they think, how they behave, the language they speak, and the clothes they wear, certain characteristics are common to all. All humans bleed when they are cut and all need air, food, and water. All are born and all die. All have hearts and lungs and livers.

✔ *Ethics is the study of what is right and wrong related to human conduct.*

The fundamental characteristics common to all humans raise certain philosophical questions that have been debated for centuries. What rights does a human being have just by being human, and what responsibilities are associated with these rights? Ethical questions are directly related to these philosophical questions. The word *ethical* comes from the Greek word *amethikos* and means knowledge of right and wrong related to human conduct. Decisions based on this knowledge of right and wrong may be related to the individual, the society, or the situation.

Individuals make many decisions on the basis of what they personally believe is right or wrong. These beliefs begin developing early in life and generally evolve from what a child is taught by parents, friends, culture, religion, school, and society in general. This is a personal value system. Healthy individuals change their value system over a lifetime. What individuals believe about relationships with, and responsibilities to, other people changes as they learn and live in society.

Decisions regarding what is right and what is wrong are also made by society. These decisions may be carried out through changes in customs and behaviors, or they may be written as laws. There are many examples of how society continually redefines the rights of its people. Abolition of slavery, the right to vote, women's rights, the rights of the disabled, and the right to die with dignity are just a few examples of how our society has redefined human rights over time.

✔ *What is right and what is wrong vary depending on the individual, the society, and the situation.*

Decisions about what is right and what is wrong can also be situational. That is, what is right in one situation may be wrong in another. As you become more involved in providing nursing care, you will be confronted with many situations in which there is no clear right or wrong action. Incredible advances in technology, complex social issues, and complicated work environments force us to ask questions about what is right and wrong more often than we might realize.

This is by no means an exhaustive discussion of ethics or ethical decisions. You should realize that human beings have fundamental rights and that society gives nurses a responsibility for protecting those rights. Many of your nursing responsibilities to society will involve ethical decisions.

THE *Web*

For general information on ethics in health care, visit the Hastings Center Web site. For information on the position of various religious groups on ethical issues in health care, visit the National Catholic Bioethics Center, Islamic Medicine Online, the Jewish Virtual Library, and other Web sites maintained by specific religious organizations.

NURSING AND ETHICS

Society has, through nurse licensing laws, given nurses permission to care for other human beings. People who become nurses promise or agree to help all those human beings who need their services. Nurses, by virtue of their education, have the ability, the responsibility, and the obligation to help patients. The public trusts nurses to have the knowledge necessary to practice nursing, as well as the ethical commitment to fulfill the obligation of nursing.

A study of ethical behavior and decision making regarding ethical issues in nursing and health care is one of the most important aspects of your nursing education. You will be confronted almost daily with the need to make nursing decisions when there is no right or wrong answer. You will sometimes be caught in the middle. You will be able to see situations from both the patient's and the doctor's or institution's viewpoints. For example, you may intellectually understand reasons for cost-cutting measures but feel concern because you see the quality of care suffering.

A person can learn the knowledge and perform the skills assigned to nursing, but not everyone who has this knowledge and these skills has the personal traits that are so important to nursing. A nurse is someone who has internalized the concept of what it means to be a human being and accepts personal responsibility for relationships with other human beings. A nurse has an obligation to do good and not harm anyone and is committed to providing the same high-quality level of nursing service to all human beings.

✔ *A nurse has an obligation to do good and not harm anyone.*

Your interpretation of what it means to be human, your belief in what rights humans have, and your ideas of what is right and what is wrong are what make you the person you are. You cannot separate these values from the nurse you hope to become. A strong belief in the rights of people to be treated and respected as human beings must be the foundation of your relationships and interactions with your patients, with your fellow nurses, and with members of the health care team.

The NFLPN and the NAPNES have each developed a code of ethics for practical/vocational nurses. A code of ethics is a list of rules of good conduct for members of a particular group. Although laws establish the minimum behaviors of a group, ethical statements attempt to describe the ideals of that group.

✔ *A code of ethics lists rules of good conduct.*

The Code section of the Nursing Practice Standards for the Licensed Practical/Vocational Nurse (LP/VN), published by the NFLPN (see Appendix B), describes the ethical and moral standards for LP/VNs. NAPNES has also issued statements regarding ethical behavior and the practical/vocational nurse. The full NAPNES statement appears in Section A of Appendix C. Both of these statements identify those standards of behavior that reflect the high ideals of the practical/vocational nurse.

You will be provided with many opportunities during your educational program to acquire the knowledge, skills, and ethical behaviors expected of practical/vocational nurses. Your faculty will assist you in reaching your goal of becoming a nurse and learning the ethical behaviors that are expected. It is through their instruction and guidance that you will learn not only how to bathe a patient but also how to accept personal responsibility for what you do. You will learn to recognize that with responsibility comes accountability.

✔ *A nurse must maintain high ethical standards.*

You can continue to learn how to manage existing and emerging ethical concerns through books, journals, conferences, discussion groups, and Web sites.

A desire to help other human beings and a commitment to be responsible and accountable for your actions are the ethical foundations of your career as an LP/VN.

PERSONAL ACCOUNTABILITY

Being *responsible* means to accept being the cause of an action. For example, saying "I broke the window" indicates the acceptance of personal responsibility. Being held *accountable* means to accept the consequences of the action, for example, paying for the broken window. Being held accountable for what you do and how you do it can be the most rewarding part of your career in nursing. You can be proud of how you perform your nursing skills, you can feel great personal satisfaction about the knowledge you gain as you accumulate experiences in nursing, and you can accept the admiration of your peers because of your high ethical standards. Your patients will feel your concern for them as individual human beings, and they will remember the kind, caring nurse who helped them through a difficult time in their life.

UNETHICAL BEHAVIOR

Unfortunately, not all health care workers, nurses included, adhere to their code of ethics or base their practice on high ethical standards. You may see situations in which there is blatant disregard for basic human rights. You may hear patients referred to as "the bypass in room 212" or "the stroke in room 324." You may see members of the health care team ignoring a patient's questions or generally treating them without respect. You may find yourself working with people who chart procedures that were not done, don't wash their hands properly, or ignore standard precaution guidelines.

ETHICAL DILEMMAS

Box 10-1 includes examples of additional nursing situations in which ethics are involved. These are all situations in which there is no clear, single course of action. There is no yes or no answer.

These are situations that are all too common for nurses across the country. What are your options when you are assigned to work in a specialty area where you feel you are not competent to work? Do you refuse and get fired from your job, do you keep quiet and go to the assigned area, do you tell your supervisor why you cannot work on that unit, do you say that you are sick and go home, do you quit on the spot, or do you write a letter of protest? What do you do if this situation occurs frequently? What if nobody pays any attention to your fears of providing incompetent and unsafe care? What if you really need this job? You feel emotionally torn between what you believe is right for the patient and what you think you should do for the good of your employer. What you are facing is called an ethical dilemma.

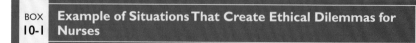

BOX 10-1	Example of Situations That Create Ethical Dilemmas for Nurses

- Working with a nurse who is a substance abuser
- Working in situations where the shortage of nursing staff compromises the quality of patient care
- Substandard performance by peers
- Medication and patient care errors
- Theft of supplies and equipment
- Inadequate access to health care
- Working in an environment where containing costs is more important than providing care
- Breaching confidentiality of patient information
- Disregard for the rights of individual patients to make their own decisions regarding health care
- Lack of adequate care for patients who are at the end of their life
- Working with or supervising unlicensed assistive personnel
- Unsafe activities related to charting, prescriptions, verbal orders, and security of computer data
- People being poorly informed about their treatment or treatment options
- Being assigned to work in a specialty area in which you feel you are not competent to work

✔ *Nurses face ethical dilemmas almost every day.*

An *ethical dilemma* is a situation in which there is a conflict or opposition between personal values, moral principles, laws, personal and professional obligations, and the rights of the individual and society. When you feel a conflict or opposition with what is being done or being planned, you are confronted with the need to make a decision about your concerns.

✔ *An ethical dilemma is a situation that often creates a conflict.*

What you choose to do is a difficult decision. If the majority of the people you work with frequently ignore the human rights of patients, your best decision may be to resign from that position. If the problem is limited to just a few people or one person, your nurse manager may also be concerned. Together, with tact and courage, you may be able to help that nurse perform his or her responsibilities at a level that reflects positively, not only on the nurse but also on all of nursing.

In most situations involving ethics, there is no one right or wrong answer and the best course of action may vary from situation to situation. To help you evaluate what, if any, action to take, general guidelines for dealing with ethical dilemmas can provide a framework for ethical decision making.

Ethical dilemmas of contemporary nurses are varied. They may be related to the more dramatic bioethical issues that are discussed later in this chapter, or they may surface in your daily practice of nursing.

Before taking any action on an ethical dilemma, you need to decide whether the problem is a legal one or an ethical one. To do this, you need to have a good understanding of the code of ethics, the nurse practice acts of the state in which you are working, and the policies and procedures of the health care facility in which you are employed. This will help you separate ethical issues from legal issues. For example, a nurse who is administering medications that have not been prescribed is breaking the law; a nurse who is giving substandard care is creating an ethical dilemma for you and for other staff members who believe that patients are entitled to a certain standard of care.

Some ethical dilemmas may have legal implications. For example, the nurse who is stealing drugs is not only breaking the law but also creating an ethical dilemma for the people with whom he or she works. Is your best course of action to report what you saw to your nurse manager, to your state board of nursing, or to a local law enforcement agency? Once you have decided that ethics is involved in the situation, several guidelines will help you decide on a course of action.

✔ *Follow guidelines when confronted with an ethical dilemma.*

Your first guideline in thinking about a specific ethical dilemma is to collect the facts. Did you directly observe the situation, or did you get the information from someone else? Did the situation happen once, or does it happen frequently? Was someone's life in danger? Was the quality of patient care compromised? Is the question one of what is right and what is wrong in relation to human beings, or is it a question of what you would personally prefer? These are questions you must answer clearly and factually for yourself.

The second guideline is to ask yourself what would happen if everyone acted or behaved in the manner in question. Your answer to this question may make the right course of action clear to you.

If your ethical dilemma is not resolved, a third guideline may provide further direction. In this step, you discuss your concerns with an authority. The authority is someone with extensive experience and knowledge that can help you separate the facts from the emotional components of ethical dilemmas. The discussion process may provide you with new insights, an appreciation of differing points of view, and perhaps even a better understanding of your own values (see Fig. 10-1).

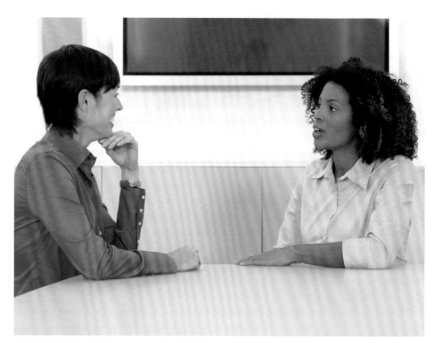

FIGURE 10-1. ● When you are faced with an ethical dilemma, it may help to discuss your concerns with someone who has extensive experience and knowledge.

✔ *Be sure you have all of the facts of the situation.*

✔ *It is sometimes difficult to separate ethical issues from personal beliefs.*

After collecting the facts, asking yourself what would happen if everyone behaved in a certain manner, and consulting an authority, you have to choose a course of action. You may decide to do nothing, or you may decide to pursue your concerns.

If you decide to pursue your concerns, often the best course of action is to discuss the issue with your immediate supervisor. This person is often in a position to deal effectively and positively with an ethical dilemma. If, after a reasonable time, you believe that your immediate supervisor has not taken the necessary action, you may decide to report your concerns to an authority higher up. Almost all organizations have organizational charts with lines of authority that you should follow in pursuing your concerns.

Because ethical behavior is difficult to define, particularly when specific situations may justify certain behaviors, an effective way to present your concerns may be through established institutional committees. The policy and procedures committee, the quality assurance committee, the nursing ethics committee, the patient relations committee, and similar committees may share your concerns. Volunteering to serve on one of these committees or telling your concerns to a member of that committee may be the most effective approach to dealing with some of your ethical dilemmas.

THE *Web*

The *Journal of Medical Ethics*, the Center for Practical Bioethics, The Center for Bioethics and Human Dignity, and McGraw-Hill Higher Education Bioethics Case Studies are just a few of the Web sites that provide case studies based on current ethical dilemmas.

BOX 10-2 · The Process of Ethical Decision Making

1. **Understand the components of ethical decision making.**
   - Religious beliefs
   - Personal values
   - Personal moral principles
   - Laws
   - Society's beliefs and expectations
   - Individual and group rights
   - Profession's code of ethics
   - Professional obligations
   - The obligation to not cause harm to anyone
   - The obligation to do good for everyone

2. **Describe the situation.**
   - Include as many aspects of the situation as you can think of.

3. **Describe the dilemma.**
   - Focus on the conflicts or opposition between one or more of the components of ethical decision making.

4. **Sort the information.**
   - Facts
   - Hearsay
   - Rumors
   - Emotional components of the situation

5. **List all possible courses of action.** Eliminate courses of action based on hearsay, rumors, or emotions—they are inappropriate.
   - Advantages and disadvantages of action A
   - Advantages and disadvantages of action B
   - Advantages and disadvantages of action C
   - Advantages and disadvantages of action D

6. **Make a decision.** Use the components of ethical decision making, facts of the situation, and advantages and disadvantages associated with each course of action.

Box 10-2 provides an overview of the process involved in making decisions regarding ethical dilemmas. Each person brings the components of ethical decision making to the situation. The dilemma occurs when there is a conflict or opposition within the components. It is essential in the decision-making process to separate the facts from hearsay, gossip, rumors, and the emotional components of the situation. All possible courses of actions, with advantages and disadvantages of each, are considered. An analysis of your findings can help you make the best decision possible.

When you make a decision to pursue an ethical dilemma, you must be prepared to accept the consequences of your action. It is possible that other people will not see the situation the same way you see it. You may be labeled a do-gooder, a perfectionist, or a whistle-blower. Or you may earn the respect of other people. Be sure of your facts and avoid making personal judgments about other people's behavior. Your motivation in pursuing ethical concerns has to be your desire to protect your patients' human rights and their right to adequate and safe nursing care.

An individual, a social, and a situational ethical dilemma are described in Box 10-3. Use the knowledge you have just gained along with the guidelines described in Box 10-2 to clarify your thinking.

BOX 10-3   Ethical Dilemmas Case Studies

AN INDIVIDUAL ETHICAL DILEMMA

Twenty-nine-year-old Brittany Maynard and her new husband were planning to have a family and enjoy their future together. Then, one day in January 2014, she was diagnosed with brain cancer. Just over 3 months later, her cancer developed into a glioblastoma multiforme tumor. She was given 6 months to live.

Brittany researched her disease and soon learned that she would most likely develop motor muscle loss and cognitive deficits, develop drug-resistant pain, and suffer personality changes. She investigated laws related to death with dignity in her home state of California and discovered that she had few options for care and any treatment she might get would destroy her quality of life.

Brittany and her family decided to move to Oregon where she could take advantage of the 1997 Oregon Death with Dignity Act. Brittany qualified for legal physician-assisted dying because she met the criteria of being mentally competent and having less than 6 months to live. She set November 1, 2014 as her date to die.

Discussion

Should terminally ill people have the right to choose when to die?
Should all states pass death with dignity laws similar to those in Oregon, Washington, Montana, Vermont, and New Mexico?
Who decides who meets the criteria to choose an end-of-life option?
Is there such a thing as a miracle or last-minute cure?
What would it take to get you to change your position on this topic?

AN ETHICAL DILEMMA FOR SOCIETY

Toby, a 52-year-old woman, was diagnosed with ovarian cancer in the spring of 2013. She had five cycles of chemotherapy, participated in a clinical drug trial for many months, had acupuncture and Reiki massage, followed a specialized diet, and drank an assortment of tea preparations. She tried several drugs and drug combinations to control the frequent chemotherapy-induced nausea and vomiting. Nothing worked, so after losing 20 pounds, she finally inquired about the use of medical marijuana.

She was issued a patient registry card and obtained the marijuana at a marijuana dispensary in her home state of Colorado. She choose the "Charlotte's Web" strain because it is effective in treating nausea but does not produce the psychoactive "high" typically associated with recreational marijuana use. She was able to control the nausea with two or three tokes three or four times a day.

Discussion

Should all states legalize the use of marijuana for medical purposes?
Does accessibility to medical marijuana increase accessibility for nonmedical use/abuse?
Is the composition of medical marijuana pharmaceutically consistent?
Does smoking marijuana have the same risks as smoking cigarettes?
Are there pharmaceutical preparations that are equally effective in controlling nausea?
What would it take to get you to change your position on this topic?

BOX 10-3	**Ethical Dilemmas Case Studies** *continued*

A SITUATIONAL ETHICAL DILEMMA

Robert is an 89-year-old man who has been living in a nursing home for the past 10 years. His two sons, three daughters, and ten grandchildren visit him often. He is in a wheelchair and tires very easily. He has coronary artery disease, diabetes, and severe osteoarthritis. It is painful for him to transfer from his wheelchair to the bed. He often tells his family that he just wants "to be done." His family and the nursing staff believe he is saying that he wants to die. Although the subject has been brought up a few times, he did not sign a living will nor did he appoint a medical power of attorney.

In the middle of the night, the nurse who was making rounds to the rooms noticed that Robert's breathing was irregular. She put on the overhead lights in the room, and he did not respond. She took his blood pressure, and it was quite low. She observed periods of apnea (no breathing), his hands and feet were cold to touch, and his lips were cyanotic. She was about to go the nurses' desk to call his doctor when he stopped breathing. She immediately went into the hallway and called "Code Blue" to her coworkers. She returned to Robert's bedside and prepared to begin CPR. Her coworkers placed a backboard under Robert's back, and they began CPR. Nothing was being done in a rush and there was no sense of urgency among the staff. After about 15 minutes, a call was made to 911 for emergency transport to the hospital.

Discussion

Should a "slow code" ever be an option?

Should a "slow code" be illegal and punishable by law?

Should the staff conduct a "slow code" when they are sure they know the patient's wishes?"

Who should decide how aggressive attempts to revive a person should be?

Should someone who is frail and ill be subjected to chest compressions?

What would it take to get you to change your position on this topic?

✔ *Be prepared to accept the consequences of your actions.*

ETHICAL ISSUES IN NURSING

Ethical issues in nursing care arise when the nurse believes he or she cannot provide the level of care that is appropriate and safe for the patient. Staffing shortages, time required to complete excessive paperwork and administrative tasks, cost-containment measures, managed care measures, and constant exposure to significant risks to personal health and safety are just a few situations that present ethical issues for nurses. When these situations are present in the workplace, the nurse has to choose between complying with the employer's requirements and with his or her own knowledge of what the patient needs.

Staffing shortages have a number of effects on patient care and create ethical dilemmas for nurses by

- Requiring each nurse to provide care for more patients than he or she can safely handle
- Having to leave care undone
- Having too little time for direct patient care
- Requiring nurses to work longer shifts each day and more shifts each week
- Reducing the amount of time the nurse can spend with a patient and the family

Excessive paperwork and administrative tasks have a number of effects on patient care and create ethical dilemmas for nurses by

- Having to spend between 25% and 37.5% or more of their time documenting care
- Having to take time to order supplies and complete some housekeeping
  duties and food service tasks
- Having to use valuable time to comply with various agency recording and
  reporting requirements

Cost-containment measures have a number of effects on patient care and create ethical dilemmas for nurses by

- Reducing the number, and sometimes the quality, of nursing staff members
- Adding unlicensed assistive personnel to the patient care team
- Requiring that nurses perform some duties for which they are not com-
  pletely qualified
- Depersonalizing care by increasing the use of protocols, care maps, and
  critical pathways
- Creating conflicts between the needs of the patient and the needs of the
  employer

Managed care measures have a number of effects on patient care and create
ethical dilemmas for nurses by

- Discharging patients too soon
- Substituting outpatient care for inpatient care
- Losing time while waiting for preapprovals
- Denying approval for treatments and diagnostic procedures
- Putting limits on how much can be spent on a specific illness
- Expecting families to care for seriously ill family members in the home

Constant exposure to significant risks to personal health and safety creates
ethical dilemmas for nurses who have to work by

- Having to live with chronic fatigue
- Being exposed to job-related injuries such as needlesticks and back injuries
- Living with the potential of a physical assault
- Being in an environment in which dangerous biological products abound
- Having to care for patients with contagious and infectious diseases

✔ *Regardless of your
personal beliefs, you are
expected to provide the
same quality of care to
everyone.*

Finding ways to balance what you believe is the right thing to do for patients
and what employers and insurance providers believe is acceptable has already
created and will continue to create difficult working conditions for nurses.

Other issues also create ethical dilemmas for nurses. Although you do have
the right as a nurse to refuse to assist with a procedure you believe to be morally
or ethically wrong, you do not have the right to refuse to provide nursing care for
the patient. For example, you may believe abortion is wrong, and you have a right
to refuse to assist with an abortion. You do not, however, have the right to deny
nursing care to the patient who has had an abortion. How you personally feel
about the patient's decision can in no way affect the quality of nursing care you
provide. You have, as a nurse, an obligation to provide nursing care.

✔ *Some of your patients
will make health care
decisions with which you
don't agree.*

If you have strong personal values associated with particular issues such as
abortion, genetic engineering, organ transplants, or other medical procedures,
you should not accept a position in a department or a health care facility in
which these procedures are routinely performed. The stress created between
your personal values and what you are expected to do will most certainly affect
your health, as well as your nursing practice. For example, if your personal values
oppose abortion, you should not accept a position in a doctor's office or clinic
that provides abortions.

BIOETHICS

As you work in the hospital and other health care facilities, you will also be involved in situations related to the ethical implications of biologic research and application. This is known as *bioethics*.

Part of being human is the right to make choices. Not that many years ago, choices related to health care were limited. Advances in science and technology over the past 50 to 60 years have created many more choices. Organ transplants and organ donations, advanced life support systems, genetic testing, stem cell engineering, and alternative methods of conception and contraception are examples of some of the bioethical issues confronting people today. No doubt the future will present us with bioethical dilemmas even more complex than those discussed in this chapter.

Although you may not be directly involved in making decisions about who gets an organ transplant or asking a grieving family to donate the organs of a deceased family member, you will probably be directly involved in caring for patients and families in these situations. For this reason, you should know something about these issues and you should continue learning about ethical issues that are yet to come.

Bioethics Committees

To attempt to make the best decision in situations related to a bioethical dilemma where there is no clearly right or wrong action, many health care facilities have created an ethics committee. Members of this committee may include doctors, clergy, community members, judges, lawyers, nurses, patients and their families, administrators, social workers, philosophers, and ethicists (people who study ethics). The work of this committee is to bring all available information and as many points of view as possible to a situation that presents a bioethical dilemma. The task of this committee is to make a decision about what action should be taken.

For example, a patient is in a persistent vegetative state. The family wants the doctor to "pull the plug," but she refuses. She also refuses to turn the care of the patient over to a physician who will do what the family wants. The family may decide to present their concerns to the health care facility's ethics committee.

Contemporary Bioethical Dilemmas

The following bioethical dilemmas are common in our society. Many of these are discussed in the media, in online discussion groups, and in television documentaries and dramas.

Reproductive Issues

The ethical issues related to birth control, abortion, and alternative fertilization are whether or not individuals have the right to control reproduction, and if so, what limitations, if any, should be imposed on them.

Limitations include questions regarding which methods are best, what age is appropriate, if methods should be available to married and unmarried people, whether parental consent for minors is needed, and if methods and information should be available through schools or public-supported clinics.

Birth Control

Birth control is the general term used to describe methods of controlling conception. The Planned Parenthood Web site lists 20 methods of birth control with some methods being more effective than others.

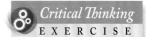

Critical Thinking EXERCISE

In two teams of two or three classmates, conduct a debate on the questions at the end of one of the scenarios in Box 10-3. One team should be for death with dignity, medical marijuana, or "slow code," and the other team should be opposed. Prior to the debate, collect as many facts as you can find, try to determine current public opinion, find out if there are any laws related to the situation, and apply the guidelines for making ethic decisions to the issue. Was your team able to change the other team's thinking? Did you change your thinking about the issue? What happens when an ethical dilemma goes unsolved?

✔ *There will be more and more bioethical dilemmas as medicine creates new treatments for diseases.*

Contraception prevents fertilization by blocking the union of sperm and egg by means of various devices such as condoms, spermicides, and oral contraceptives. When the use of contraception is stopped, fertilization is again possible.

Sterilization is either a surgical or nonsurgical procedure that is performed on men (vasectomy) or women (tubal ligation) to prevent reproduction. It is virtually permanent because neither procedure can be reversed with certainty.

Abortion

Abortion is the termination of pregnancy. Spontaneous abortion results from abnormalities in the fetus or in the maternal environment and occurs naturally. Therapeutic abortions are performed to protect the mother's life. An elective abortion is intentional and performed at the mother's request for personal reasons. Although elective abortions are legal, it raises numerous ethical issues. There is a major ongoing controversy regarding the right of women to have control of their own bodies, the rights of the father, whether and when a fetus is a human being, and whether a fetus has rights. The U.S. Supreme Court declared the legality of abortion in 1973, but the ethical and moral issues of if, when, and how abortions are performed continue to be debated. Your personal views will determine whether and to what extent you can comfortably assist in matters relating to abortion.

Alternative Fertilization

For some women who cannot conceive, medical techniques now provide the ability to bear children. In addition, men whose fertility was marginal can now father children, and people can have children through the services of surrogates (substitutes). These techniques involve artificial insemination, in vitro fertilization, and surrogate motherhood. All raise legal and ethical questions that remain unanswered. Your own views will be the basis for your decisions to participate in health care situations in which these issues are raised.

✔ *How, when, and where to dispose of frozen sperm and eggs continues to be an ethical dilemma.*

Artificial insemination is the medical implantation of donor sperm into a woman's uterus to fertilize her own egg and thereby conceive a child. The sperm can be that of the husband or another donor.

In vitro fertilization is a procedure in which sperm and egg are mixed outside the body in a laboratory dish and the fertilized egg is then implanted into a woman's uterus. The egg and sperm can be from husband and wife or from donors.

When a fertilized egg is implanted into the uterus of a woman who is not the wife, but who will carry the conceived child to term, or when a woman agrees to undergo artificial insemination for another couple, the woman is called a surrogate mother.

Womb Transplant

On October 4, 2014, a woman who had a uterus transplant gave birth to a healthy baby boy. This success opens up a new but still experimental alternative for thousands of women who are unable to have children because they lost their uterus. This procedure uses the woman's egg and partner's sperm to create an embryo through in vitro fertilization. The procedure and the antirejection medications are costly, and finding a suitable uterus donor can be difficult.

Genetic Issues

Human Genome Project

The Human Genome Project is a government-funded research project that began in 1990. The goal of the project was to determine the arrangement of the 100,000 or so human genes and to map the entire genetic script, all 3 billion bits of information, by the year 2005. On June 26, 2000—about 5 years ahead of schedule—government researchers and researchers from Celera Genomics jointly announced that they had developed a working draft of the genetic manual of the human body. The draft was slightly revised before it was totally completed in April 2003. It turns out that there are 20,000 to 25,000 genes, not 100,000 as originally thought. The result of this work to date is the identification of more than 6,000 disease genes that cause single-gene disorders in 1 out of every 200 births.

 THE *Web*

Recent developments about the Human Genome Projects are posted on their government Web site.

Genes are simply short segments of DNA that tell cells how to behave, and a genetic disorder is a disease caused in whole or in part by a variation or mutation of a gene. Variation or mutation of our genes causes 3,000 to 4,000 diseases including cancer, heart disease, diabetes, cystic fibrosis, Alzheimer's disease, and more.

Now that the human genome map is complete, researchers are focusing on the function of each gene and the role that faulty genes play in disease. This research will lead to improved diagnosis of diseases and a new approach to disease therapy.

It is likely that the major genetic factors involved in susceptibility to common diseases such as diabetes, heart disease, Alzheimer's disease, cancer, and mental illness will be uncovered in the next several years. For many of these conditions, altering diet, lifestyle, or medical monitoring could be beneficial for high-risk individuals. That discovery will open the door to wider availability of genetic tests to identify individual predispositions to future illness for just about everyone.

This newfound ability to probe our genes will no doubt have some negative consequences and raise ethical dilemmas. Debates about the ethics of issues listed in Box 10-4 have already begun. The Genetic Information Nondiscrimination Act of 2008 is intended to prevent discrimination on the basis of genetic information with respect to health insurance and employment. While this law does allay some fears that people have, there are still a large number of people who are concerned that their genetic profile will in some way lead to some type of discrimination.

BOX 10-4 Ethical Questions Related to Gene Therapy

What happens when
- The disease-causing gene is found before a cure or a treatment?
- Scientists learn to remove defective genes and replace them with other genes selected by the recipient?
- An insurance company decides to not insure people with certain genetic conditions?
- Employers will not hire people unless their "genetic map" matches certain company requirements?
- Parents want to use genetic engineering to create their "perfect" child?
- The cost of gene therapy is so expensive that only the very wealthy can afford it?

Genetic Screening

✔ It is possible for parents to make a decision to terminate a pregnancy based on genetic testing.

Genetic screening is done to confirm a suspected diagnosis, to predict the possibility of future illness, to detect the presence of a carrier state in unaffected individuals, and to predict response to therapy. It can be carried out on a fetus in the uterus, on a child, or on an adult (Fig. 10-2).

The decision to undergo genetic testing is a very personal one. For many, a pivotal consideration is whether there are preventive measures that can be taken if the test result is positive. For example, those who test positive for breast cancer can benefit from preventive measures such as screening for early detection and early treatment. In contrast, there are no preventive measures or cures for Huntington's disease. But a positive test for Huntington's disease might help an individual make lifestyle decisions, such as career choice, family planning, or insurance coverage. Testing a fetus for Down syndrome, hemophilia, Tay-Sachs disease, Duchenne's muscular dystrophy, and sickle cell disease or finding out if the fetus is a boy or girl can be done by a fairly simple procedure called amniocentesis. What parents decide to do with the information they gain from the amniocentesis may create a conflict of ethics with families, between husband and wife, and beyond the home into the community. Is it right to terminate a pregnancy for any reason? Is it right to terminate a pregnancy because the fetus has hemophilia but not right to terminate a pregnancy if the fetus has Tay-Sachs disease? Is it right to terminate a pregnancy because the fetus was of an undesired sex? These are the kinds of questions that can arise from genetic screening.

There are currently more than 25 companies offering a 1,000 or more direct-to-consumer genetic tests for individuals who want information about their specific genetic profiles. Examples include genetic tests for paternity, identification of members of your family tree, disease carrier status, inherited conditions, and probable responses to certain drugs. The costs of these genetic tests depend on the complexity of the test but range from about $100 for a simple test to more than $4,000 for a more complete personal profile. Some private companies even offer a genetic counselor to help clients cope with unusual genetic findings.

Critical Thinking
E X E R C I S E

On May 21, 2008, President George W. Bush signed the Genetic Information Nondiscrimination Act of 2008. This law prohibits discrimination in health insurance coverage and employment based on genetic information. Hospitals in the United States routinely test newborns for a number of genetic diseases that include PKU, type I diabetes, cystic fibrosis, and many more. As genetic testing becomes more sophisticated, additional testing might be included in the newborn assessments. What implications do positive test results have on the mental health of the parents? How might knowing the potential for developing diseases affect the child as he or she grows up? What do the parents tell the child about his or her condition? Use appropriate Characteristics of Critical Thinkers in Box 1-2 on pages 18–19 to develop your responses to these questions.

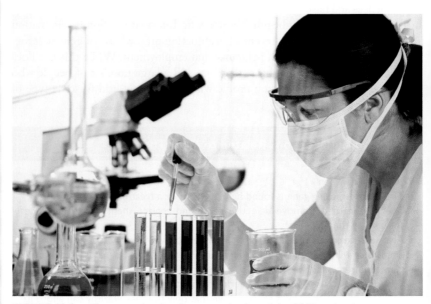

FIGURE 10-2. ● Gene tests involve direct examination of the DNA molecule.

Stem Cell Research

Embryonic stem cells are cells that are found in the developing embryo. Very simply put, these embryonic cells eventually develop into all of the tissues and organs in the body. They are believed by some researchers to offer promise in the development of medical treatments for a wide range of conditions including damage to the brain, spinal cord, skeletal muscles, and the heart. Treatments have been proposed for physical trauma (e.g., spinal cord injuries), degenerative conditions (e.g., Parkinson's disease), or even genetic diseases (in combination with gene therapy).

Pro-life advocates are strongly opposed to embryonic stem cell research because harvesting embryonic stem cells requires the destruction of the embryo, which they consider a human life. Pro-life advocates received support from President Bush (2001–2009) when he issued Executive Orders that did not permit taxpayers' money to be used for any human embryo stem cell research that destroyed human embryos.

Eight years later, President Obama issued an Executive Order that essentially overturned President Bush's position on human embryo research. In that March 9, 2009, speech, Obama said:

> Research involving human embryonic stem cells and human nonembryonic stem cells has the potential to lead to better understanding and treatment of many disabling diseases and conditions. Advances over the past decade in this promising scientific field have been encouraging, leading to broad agreement in the scientific community that the research should be supported by Federal funds.

Stem cell research is an issue that will continue to create an ethical dilemma and make the news headlines for years to come.

Organ Transplants

Since the first kidney transplant in 1954, the marvel of organ transplantation has become common. Kidney, liver, pancreas, intestine, heart, lung, cornea, skin, and bone transplants all occur several times a day in all parts of the country. As of September 14, 2015, a total of 122,521 people need an organ or multiple organs. From January through June 2015, there were 7,322 organ donors and 15,083 transplants were performed. It is obvious that more people are waiting for organs than there are organs available and that single donors are donating multiple organs.

 THE *Web*

The United Network for Organ Sharing oversees the national database of clinical transplant information and operates the computerized organ sharing system, matching donated organs to patients registered on the national organ transplant waiting list.

Transplants are expensive medical procedures that, in most cases, are only partially covered by private medical insurance or Medicare. Patients who have to pay 80% of their hospital bill might have a difficult time paying the balance (20%). The average heart transplant costs about $997,000 for the pretransplant treatment, procurement of the heart, hospital stay and surgery, and the immunosuppressant drugs after surgery. There are a number of charitable organizations that may be able to provide some financial assistance. In some instances, families conduct fundraising events to pay for the cost of the transplant. Foundations specific to the disease may offer additional financial or counseling support. Antirejection drugs that must be taken for a lifetime can cost $25,000 a year or more. Drug coverage for antirejection drugs through private insurance varies from no coverage at all to very high co-pays. Medicare-eligible patients may have limits placed on the number of years antirejection drugs will be covered. As new technologies and better drug therapies decrease the rate of rejection, the demand for organ transplants will most likely increase.

Who will get the few organs that are available? Who or what committee will make the decision? Is there a potential market in buying and selling human organs to the highest bidder? Who should pay the high cost of organ transplants? Should people who die younger than age 45 be required by law to donate their organs? These are just a few of the ethical questions people are asking about organ transplants.

Although there is no doubt that organ transplants and grafts save lives and improve the quality of life for a few people, some individuals are opposed to these procedures and research. These people raise questions about the cost of such procedures related to the benefit for society or the ethics of sacrificing animals for their transplantable organs (xenograph), or they may object to transplants for religious reasons.

Living donors, such as people who give one of their kidneys or a portion of their liver, have the satisfaction of knowing that their act has improved someone else's chances for a normal life. What happens if the donor's other kidney stops functioning or is damaged in an accident? Most organs used for transplant come from deceased persons. Some donors make arrangements for organ donation before death through an act of consent in their will, on a special donor card, or by authorization on their driver's license. Other donations are made with the permission of next of kin immediately after the donor's death. If the decision to donate organs is made during a time of extreme distress, what happens a week or month or year later when the next of kin who signed for the organ donation has second thoughts?

✔ *It costs about $997,000 for surgery and follow-up care during the first year after a heart transplant.*

Death

Determining when death occurs has been complicated by lifesaving devices and procedures. Respirators, heart and lung machines, and other assistive devices are able to keep patients alive who a few years ago would have died.

When death is in question, it is now defined on the basis of an electroencephalogram indicating the absence of brain wave activity. Death is legally defined as the irreversible cessation of brain function for a given period.

Although criteria have been established so that a person can be declared legally dead, it is now possible to continue a deceased patient's biologic functions. Therefore, the question of whether the patient is alive or dead is still at issue, especially in situations in which the removal of the life support system is requested by a next of kin.

Euthanasia

Sometimes called "mercy killing," euthanasia is the deliberate causing of someone's death by active or passive means. Active euthanasia is to cause someone's death by intentionally administering an agent that would bring about death. Passive euthanasia is to cause someone's death by withholding efforts to sustain life.

For example, in a health care facility, an act of active euthanasia could be the administration of a lethal dose of medication, whereas an act of passive euthanasia could be the withholding of a medication that the patient needs to stay alive. Active euthanasia is an unquestionably illegal act (murder) punishable by law. Passive euthanasia is not as well defined, but it is no less controversial. At what point in time is a decision made to discontinue feeding a patient? Who makes this decision?

Physician-Assisted Suicide

Oregon, Vermont, Washington, Montana, and New Mexico are the five states that allow physician-assisted suicide. Almost all of the other states in the United States are considering expanding legal end-of-life options for individuals living in that state. This legislation is not without controversy. Some say that this action is illegal and the physician should be prosecuted. Others say that a person who is terminally ill and mentally competent should have the right to end his or her pain and suffering. The Hippocratic Oath taken by doctors says that "I will neither give a deadly drug …nor will I make a suggestion to this effect." Is this a violation of a sacred oath? Does this provide a way for a family member to collect on a life insurance policy? Could a physician misuse this law? What if there is a cure for a terminal illness shortly after assisted suicide? These are just a few questions surrounding this controversial issue.

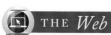 THE *Web*

Compassion and Choices is an organization that provides advice on legal ways to reduce end-of-life suffering.

Advance Directives

The Uniform Rights of the Terminally Ill Act (1985) allows people to anticipate their death and make an allowance to let it happen naturally by signing a living will. A living will is a document that testifies that the patient does not want heroic lifesaving measures instituted to maintain life when death would otherwise be likely. Living wills are not universally recognized as legal documents, but they do express the wishes, at the time of signing, of those who sign them.

A Health Care Proxy is a power of attorney that allows a person to make health care decisions for another. In most cases, the Health Care Proxy will use the person's living will as the basis for making end-of-life decisions.

The term *Ulysses Pact* is used to describe a situation in which the decision a person made in the past might not be the best decision for him or her in the future. For example, a person may have signed a living will 10 years prior to an automobile accident in which he or she sustained a brain and spinal cord injury and is now on life support. If new treatments are now available that might repair his or her brain and spinal cord and eliminate the need for life support, should the terms of his or her living will be carried out?

SUMMARY

In summary, learning to be a nurse requires more than passing written examinations and performing procedures correctly. It requires you to develop an ethical and moral commitment to provide the best nursing services you are capable of providing to every human being in your care. This commitment lives within you and cannot be turned on as you begin your nursing duties or turned off when you

✔ *It is sometimes difficult for nurses to accept the health care decisions their patients make.*

leave your patients at the end of your workday. This commitment pervades your life and influences all your decisions. The longer you are employed as a nurse, the stronger this commitment will become. Nurses who make this personal commitment to their fellow human beings are rewarded by great personal satisfaction; patients who receive nursing services from these nurses are rewarded by compassionate, personal, and competent care.

APPLY

Critical Thinking Skills

1. In the opening story at the beginning of this chapter, Jeannie used a 3 × 5 card to help her pass an examination. Does this action violate the NAPNES or NFLPN code of ethics? Could this behavior be harmful to a patient? Is Jeannie's behavior considered unethical? Explain your response.

2. Construct a list of what you believe to be basic human rights. Compare your list with that of one or two of your classmates. Do you agree or disagree on what constitutes basic human rights? Can you develop a list of basic human rights on which you all agree?

3. Think about your recent experiences in school or in your clinical facility, and try to identify an ethical dilemma. How did you handle the dilemma, and what do you think you might do if the situation happens again? Indicate why you believe your concern is an ethical one and not a matter of personal values. If you cannot think of your own situation, you may use one of these: cheating on tests, discussing confidential patient information in an elevator, and observing an employee taking a scrub suit for personal use at home.

4. Compare and contrast the NAPNES and NFLPN codes of ethics. How are they similar? How are they different?

5. In what ways might your personal values and spiritual and moral beliefs affect your ability to provide nursing care? If you think your values and beliefs might contribute to denying care, what do you think you should do?

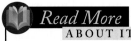

Read More

ABOUT IT

Burkhardt MA, Nathaniel AN: Ethics and Issues in Contemporary Nursing, 4th ed. Stamford, CT: Cengage Learning, 2013.

Corey G, Corey M, Corey C, et al.: Issues and Ethics in the Helping Professions, 9th ed. Stamford, CT: Cegagne Learning, 2014.

Guido GW: Legal and Ethical Issues in Nursing, 6th ed. Upper Saddle River, NJ: Prentice-Hall, 2013.

Pence G: Medical Ethics: Accounts of Ground-Breaking Cases, 7th ed. New York, NY: McGraw-Hill, 2014.

Pozgar GD: Legal and Ethical Issues for Health Professionals, 3rd ed. New York, NY: Jones and Bartlett, 2012.

Steinbock B, London AJ, Arras JD: Ethical Issues in Modern Medicine: Contemporary Reading in Bioethics, 8th ed. New York, NY: McGraw-Hill, 2012.

CHAPTER 11

Legally Responsible Nursing Practice

CHAPTER CONTENTS

LEARNING OBJECTIVES

When you complete this chapter, you will be able to:

1. Discuss the purpose of Good Samaritan laws.
2. List the two sources of laws and give examples of each.
3. Discuss the relationship between the nurse practice acts and the state boards of nursing.
4. Explain the association among responsibility, accountability, and legal liability.
5. Define the term *respondeat superior*.
6. Define the term *breach of contract*.
7. Define the term *tort* and give two examples of torts.
8. Illustrate the difference between a tort and a crime.
9. Differentiate negligence and gross negligence.
10. Discuss how nurses can assist in preventing malpractice claims.
11. Explain the purpose of malpractice insurance.
12. Give examples of crimes that may involve nurses.

Lito's phone rang a third time. He groped for the receiver.

"Hello?" he said drowsily.

"Lito?" a small voice asked. "Please help me. I'm sick." "Mrs. Thompson, is that you? I'll be right down," Lito said. He raced downstairs to his landlady's apartment.

Mrs. Thompson was lying on the floor next to her bed. Her eyes were closed. Lito dropped to his knees and put his fingertips on the pulse point on the side of her neck. "Mrs. Thompson? Can you hear me?" The sick woman's eyes opened weakly. Her mouth moved, but there was no sound before she lapsed into unconsciousness again. Lito quickly dialed the phone.

A shadow appeared in the open doorway as he waited for the call to go through. "What happened?" It was Milo Davis, the other tenant in Mrs. Thompson's building.

"I don't know, but she's unconscious," Lito said.

"I bet she didn't take her shot," Milo said, hurrying to the kitchen. He took a small bottle from the refrigerator and returned to the room where Lito was still holding the receiver.

"I'm calling an ambulance," Lito said.

"That's not necessary," Milo said. "She just needs her shot." He held up the bottle. It was a medicine bottle, but the label was smeared and unreadable. "She keeps the whatchamacallits in that drawer." He took a disposable syringe from the drawer and handed it to Lito. "Here. You do it." Lito shook his head. "No," he said without explaining further. He did not take the syringe.

"It's easy," Milo said. "I did it last year when this happened. Mrs. Thompson said you have lots of experience from the hospital, so you do it." "I'm a licensed practical nurse," Lito stated.

The man thrust the syringe at Lito. "Then do it!" he shouted angrily. "She might die!" At that moment Lito's call went through. He said there was an emergency and requested that an ambulance be sent immediately. Lito made Mrs. Thompson as comfortable as possible and waited. He monitored her breathing and pulse from time to time. Milo glared at him but didn't say another word. He also didn't administer the medication in the bottle.

When the ambulance was gone, Milo finally spoke. "How can you call yourself a nurse if you'll risk an old woman's life like that?" he snapped, brandishing the syringe like an accusing finger at Lito. "You're not a good neighbor, and you're certainly not a Good Samaritan. I don't know what you call yourself." With that he stalked out of the apartment.

Lito picked up the bottle and looked at the label. It was unreadable, but an expiration date was still legible. The date was over 2 years old. He held the bottle to the light. A suspiciously cloudy mass swirled inside the bottle.

After the ambulance took Mrs. Thompson to the hospital, Lito smiled as he remembered what Milo had said. "What I call myself is a good neighbor, a Good Samaritan, and a very good nurse," he said as if the man were still there. "And do you know why I'm a good nurse? I'll tell you. It's because I know what to do and when to do it, what I can do within the law, and when to ask for help."

Contemporary practical/vocational nursing is an active process in which you will interact with your patients to provide care in a one-to-one relationship that is based on their trust and your competency. Your duty is to do good and to avoid harm in accordance with the law.

Laws are rules of conduct derived from cultural values, moral practices, and ethical beliefs. In a democracy, they are made and enforced by the authority of the group to whom they apply.

✔ *Your duty as a nurse is to do good and to avoid doing harm.*

GOOD SAMARITAN STATUTES

The story of the Good Samaritan tells of a man who was beaten, robbed, and left to die at the side of the road. People walking by ignored him. But one man, a Samaritan, did not. He dressed the injured man's wounds and took him to safe lodging, without being asked and without being paid. Today, Good Samaritan laws protect people from prosecution who voluntarily go to the aid of others in an emergency. If the person providing emergency care does not act recklessly or does not intend to harm the victim, the Good Samaritan is almost always exempt from any legal action.

The laws vary from state to state, and you are responsible for finding out what the statute (law) in your state says. Generally, such laws require that people who render aid are expected to act as any reasonable, prudent person would in that situation. Nurses and other health care providers are expected to render care equal to that of another provider with the same level of skill, training, and experience. The intention of Good Samaritan laws is to encourage the giving of emergency care outside the hospital or health care facility.

✔ *A Good Samaritan act is done voluntarily and without payment.*

While all 50 states and Washington, DC have Good Samaritan laws, only a handful of states require people to help strangers in distress. It is very important to know the Good Samaritan laws of your state so that you do not risk losing your license as a result of your actions during an emergency. It is important to note that only in the most extreme cases have people been found guilty of breaking this law. Those who are found guilty under this law are usually those who did not assist someone in need when their assistance could have helped the victim. To act or not is an ethical decision you must make when faced with an emergency situation in a noninstitutional setting.

SOURCES OF LAWS

Laws come from two general sources. The first source is the government (federal, state, or local), and the second source is private. Laws that come from the government are termed *public (statutory) laws*. One type of public law, constitutional law, includes laws based on the Constitution of the United States, an individual state, or a subdivision within a state. Federal constitutional laws are based on the U.S. Constitution and its amendments. State constitutional laws, among other things, identify the legal relationships between the state and its counties, cities, townships, boroughs, municipalities, and villages. Municipal (city) constitutional law prescribes the form of government through which the city will operate and conduct its business.

Another type of public law, administrative law, creates federal, state, and local administrative agencies that have the power to make and enforce rules and regulations. Nurse practice acts are laws that are passed by state governments to control the practice of nursing in that state. A nurse practice act is an example of an administrative law and is discussed in more detail later in this chapter.

The last type of public law, criminal law, deals with offenses against the welfare or safety of the public. Criminal law includes minor offenses, misdemeanors, and felonies. An example of a minor offense is a traffic ticket. A misdemeanor includes indictable offenses that do not amount to a felony, such as perjury, battery, libel, conspiracy, and public nuisance. A felony is a more serious crime than is a misdemeanor. A conviction for a felony may make a person liable for the death sentence or for a life sentence in a federal or state prison. The federal government determines what constitutes a federal crime, and each state has the power to determine what it considers a crime.

Private law focuses on the enforcement of rights, duties, and other legal relations between private citizens. Laws related to enforcing contracts and laws related to torts, which are legal wrongs not included under contract law, are two divisions of private laws that are of particular interest to nurses.

Box 11-1 summarizes the major divisions within public law and private law. The examples included in this box are intended to help you understand the differences between the public law and the private law.

✔ *The two sources of laws are public and private.*

BOX 11-1   Sources of Law

PUBLIC LAW (ALSO KNOWN AS STATUTORY LAW)
Constitutional Law
Federal government (the U.S. Constitution and the Amendments)
   State government (the constitution of a state: many similarities to the U.S. Constitution)
   Local government (the constitution or similarly titled document that identifies the political structure and social responsibilities of local governing bodies)

Administrative Law
Federal (Occupational Safety and Health Administration)
State (State Boards of Nursing)
Local (city department of licenses and inspection)

Criminal Law
Federal (transportation of drugs between states)
State (murder of a citizen of the state)
Local (violation of a parking law)

PRIVATE LAW (ALSO KNOWN AS CIVIL OR COMMON LAW)
Contract Law (Implied, Oral, Written)
Written contracts (such as school loans)
Verbal contracts ("I will babysit for you on Saturday from 7:00 pm to 1:00 am")

Law of Torts (legal wrong not included under contract laws)
Negligence
False imprisonment
Confidentiality
Defamation of character
Consent
Assault and battery
Fraud

REGULATION OF NURSING PRACTICE

The basic law governing your practice as a licensed practical/vocational nurse (LP/VN) is the nurse practice act (an administrative law) that was passed by your state legislature. You will recall that after a bill is passed and signed, it becomes law, and that law is known as an act. A nurse practice act usually defines the legal functions, powers, and duties of the state board of nursing. It also identifies the membership of the board and how people become board members. A nurse practice act also defines terms such as nursing and the duties of the nurse practitioner, registered nurse (RN), and LP/VN. Laws governing licensure and legal titles are also included in nurse practice acts. Any changes in the nurse practice act must be made through the state legislature and must follow the same process as any other proposed law.

Nurse practice acts are administered by state boards of nursing or committees with a similar title. Members of the state board of nursing are RNs, LP/VNs, consumers, and others interested in the health and welfare of the citizens of the state. Such a board may be appointed by the governor of the state or elected by the people, and the majority of its members are usually RNs. Other members may include consumer representatives and LP/VNs. The board is headed by a salaried executive director, usually an RN who, with a paid staff, manages daily matters related to nursing in that state.

✔ *The state board of nursing enforces the nurse practice act.*

State boards have legal authority to interpret, implement, and enforce the laws governing nursing practice, education, and licensure. The state board of nursing issues rules and regulations, which are interpretations of the nurse practice act.

Disciplinary hearings for licensees and prosecution of violations of nurse practice acts are conducted by the boards. Keep in mind that the law of the state in which you practice nursing is the law that applies to you and that ignorance of the law is not an excuse for illegal acts. You must know the law and practice within it, and you are held responsible for your own acts as a nurse.

RESPONSIBILITY AND LIABILITY

Responsibility is the condition of being accountable for your actions. Whether you are a student or an employee, many of your responsibilities will be well defined in the written or verbal contract you enter into with your school or employer. But because nurses have a relationship with patients that includes touching, treating, collecting information, and providing personal services, you will have a number of other responsibilities that are not written and are not easily defined. These are responsibilities that come with the job.

Accepting responsibility for one's actions means that the individual who commits an act is the one who must explain the act and accept any consequences that follow. A student who borrows a library book and then loses it is responsible for what happened to the book and accountable for its replacement.

Liability is the legal obligation a person has to make good for the loss of, or damage to, something for which he or she is responsible. In the case of the library book, the student who lost it would be liable (obligated) to replace or pay for it.

✔ *Nurses are personally and legally responsible for their nursing actions.*

A person is always responsible and liable for his or her actions. As a nurse, you are legally responsible for the care you give or neglect to give your patients, as well as for your professional and personal conduct. Your best protection against charges regarding the performance of your duties, whether a legal action or a personal criticism, is to carry out your duties at or above the standards expected from someone with your education, ability, and experience. Even then, it is possible that a charge could be made against you, particularly in a social climate that fosters lawsuits.

LEGAL RELATIONSHIPS BETWEEN THE EMPLOYER AND THE EMPLOYEE

The legal relationship between the employer and the employee is fairly well defined. The employer has the right to hire employees and to direct and control the performance of work. An employee is a person who accepts wages as a result of services provided to the employer.

A legal term, *respondeat superior*, is used to describe the legal responsibility of an employer for acts of an employee. In other words, both the nurse who injures a patient and the nurse's employer can be held liable for the nurse's acts.

To protect themselves and their employees from potential legal problems, employers and institutions develop guidelines governing their operations. These guidelines, although based on laws, are not laws; they are policies that state what action is expected in specific situations. They are often more explicit than are laws in that they provide detailed procedures and clear directions. An example of a guideline (and in some states, a law) is the preemployment screening requirements for new employees. This screening could include a criminal background check, a child abuse check, and a check for alcohol and drugs. It is imperative that you become thoroughly familiar with your employer's guidelines for new and continuing employees.

✔ *A nurse's employer is legally responsible for an employee's actions.*

Because institutional and employer guidelines must reflect current conditions to be effective, they are changed periodically. Your duties will put you in daily contact with your employer's policies and procedures. You will be in an excellent position to know whether these guidelines are meeting the needs for which they were written and to suggest changes when they are not.

STANDARDS OF CARE

Standards of care are guidelines developed to identify appropriate levels of professional care. Nursing standards of care define the average degree of skill, care, and diligence that other nurses would provide under the same or similar circumstances.

✔ *Other nurses with the same job title are sometimes called to court to say what they would have done in the same situation.*

A *nurse practice act* is the state law that governs the practice of nursing. The rules and regulations issued by a state board of nursing are based on a legal interpretation of the nurse practice act. These rules and regulations define standards of care expected of professional and practical/vocational nurses.

A number of other organizations also develop standards of care. The Joint Commission, the Community Health Accreditation Program, and the American Osteopathic Association all include standards for nursing care in their accreditation guidelines. Many nursing specialty organizations such as the American Nurses Association, the American College of Nurse Midwives, and the American Association of Critical Care Nurses also publish standards of care.

The National Federation of Licensed Practical Nurses (NFLPN) and the National Association for Practical Nurse Education and Service (NAPNES) both publish standards of care that are specific to LP/VNs. Read Appendices B and C to learn more about the standards to which you will be held.

The policy and procedure manuals developed by health care facilities (the employer) identify acceptable standards of care and cover a wide range of topics from safety to specific nursing procedures.

It is important to be familiar with all laws, rules and regulations, accrediting agency and professional organization standards for nursing care, and your employer's policies and procedures regarding standards of care. Failure to provide the standard of care expected of a nurse in the same or similar circumstance can result in a malpractice suit or disciplinary action.

In the case of *Ferris v County of Kennebec*, a nurse was held liable for failing to provide the expected standard of care (Box 11-2).

BOX 11-2 Legal Issues Case Study

INTENTIONAL INDIFFERENCE EQUATES TO DEPLORABLE CARE

In the summer of 1996, Melissa Irene Ferris was arrested and placed in the custody of a county jail. She told them she was pregnant during the interview at the jail. On the evening of her 2nd day in jail, this woman experienced vaginal bleeding and complained to the facility's nurse, Nurse Sprowl, that she was having a miscarriage. She said she knew she was having a miscarriage because she had suffered one in 1991.

Sprowl took the woman's pulse and told her that her pulse rate indicated that she was menstruating and not having a miscarriage. The nurse then refused to fulfill the woman's request for sanitary napkins and ordered her to lie down. At first, the woman followed the nurse's order, but she could not continue to lie down because it made her feel worse.

The nurse made no further attempt at assessing the patient's condition, and the only other contact the nurse had with the inmate was to tell the woman that she would be transferred to another cell because she "refused to lie down and follow orders."

Ferris continued to complain of severe pain. Later that evening she was transferred to a smaller cell and had no further contact with Sprowl. On June 15, 1996, Ferris had a miscarriage in her jail cell. Approximately 6 months later, she filed a suit, and in October 1998, the case was moved to a federal court.

Federal court records indicate that Ferris claimed that the nurse (Sprowl) violated her Due Process and Equal Protections rights and her right to be free from cruel and unusual punishment under Maine and United States Constitutions (Count I), she negligently failed to provide medical treatment (Count II), and she negligently inflicted emotional distress (Count III). Count II was dismissed for a number of legal reasons. Sprowl was found guilty on Counts I and III.

According to the law, to justify a complaint for violations of Due Process and Equal Protections rights, "allegations must be sufficient to make a viable due process claim." This means that the plaintiff's medical condition must be serious, and there must be an effort to assess or treat the patient. If no effort is made to treat or assess a patient's condition, it may constitute deliberate indifference on the part of the caregiver. A definition of deliberate indifference is "where the attention received is so clearly inadequate as to amount to a refusal to provide essential care." This was the legal basis for Count I. The Court concluded that the nurse "should have understood that her failure to provide minimal care constituted deliberate indifference to [the patient's] serious medical needs."

The nurse's failure to respond to the inmate's complaints of pain and repeated requests for medical help led to a charge of guilty on Count III.

The nurse did admit that she knew she had an obligation to ensure that pretrial detainees received adequate medical care. The nurse also stated that "she believed that any reasonable person would agree that her treatment of [the patient] was not a violation of this standard; and, a reasonably prudent nurse would have treated the patient in the same manner."

- Is checking a pulse rate the way to determine a potential abortion?
- Would other nurses treat this patient the same as Sprowl treated her?
- What should the nurse have done in this situation? Would a nurse's lack of nursing experience excuse her actions?
- Should this nurse be fired from her job at the prison?
- Should this nurse loose her nursing license?

From the case of *Melissa Irene Ferris v County of Kennebec*, Civil No. 98-201-B.

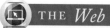

Critical Thinking
E X E R C I S E

Although it is still early in your nursing career, list at least four things the nurse in the case presented in Box 11-2 should have done for her patient. How do the NAPNES and NFLPN standards of practice relate to the actions of this nurse? What would you have done if you had witnessed the actions of this nurse, and why? Use appropriate Characteristics of Critical Thinking in Box 1-2 on pages 18–19 to develop your response to these questions.

✔ NAPNES and NFLPN standards are sometimes used in court to describe standards of care that should be provided by LP/VNs.

THE *Web*

Visit the Nurses Service Organization Web site to find legal case studies that provide descriptions of cases involving claims of malpractice.

LEGAL ISSUES FOR NURSES

Contracts

You will recall that private law deals with contracts and torts. A *contract* is an agreement between two or more parties. Contracts are either written or verbal promises in which something of value is exchanged. A verbal agreement to meet a friend is a social obligation and is not classified as a contract. A nurse who accepts employment, offered by an institution, a health care provider, or a patient, is entering into a contract. The value exchanged in this type of contract is money (from the employer) for services (nursing) (Fig. 11-1).

When entering into an employment contract, you should have a written agreement that defines hours and wages, length of the contract, benefits, vacation periods and lengths, length of sick leave, hours of work each week, insurance coverage, and job responsibilities expected by the employer. The employer, in turn, expects you to provide the services for which you will receive these benefits. These services are often understood to be those that are expected of anyone with the same education and license that you have.

Breach of contract is the term used to describe failure of one party to fulfill any or all parts of a contractual obligation. Breach-of-contract suits against nurses are most often suits in which damages are claimed. Damages are awarded to the plaintiff (complaining person) if it can be shown that he or she has suffered a financial loss. For example, suppose you agree to provide practical/vocational nursing services to one patient for 8 hours for $160.00. If you do not keep this contract, and the patient has to employ a practical/vocational nurse for $200.00 for that 8-hour period, the patient (plaintiff) may have a cause to act against you.

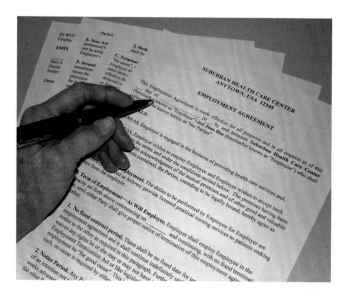

FIGURE 11-1. ● Read and understand your employment agreement before you sign it.

Torts

Tort is the French word for a "wrong." A tort is an injury or wrong committed by one person, a group, or an organization against another person or group of people. The three types of torts are strict liability, intentional, and negligence.

Strict Liability

Strict liability is the term used to describe an individual or a group of individuals whose actions, regardless of intent, negligence, or fault cause injuries to others. Examples of strict liability include manufacturers who sell dangerous or defective products that cause injuries. It also includes those who store chemical sprays, explosives, natural gas, and other materials that cause harm. Individuals who own wild and dangerous animals are subject to strict liability for injuries caused by those animals.

Cases of strict liability could be brought against manufactures of asbestoses, which is a product that is known to cause mesothelioma, and against manufactures of tobacco products, which are known to cause cancer; however, most strict liability cases are not related to medical care and treatment.

Intentional Torts

Intentional torts include injuries caused by willful, forceful, and aggressive behavior and include false imprisonment, violation of confidentiality, defamation of character, failure to provide informed consent, assault and battery, and fraud.

False Imprisonment

A nurse cannot confine or restrict a patient to a place against his or her will except in situations specified by law (e.g., when a physician orders it or in an emergency situation where the patient might harm himself or others). *Restraint* means the prevention of free movement by any means. Physical or verbal restraint without the consent of the patient or appropriate authority is *false imprisonment*.

To keep a patient confined anywhere by threat of reprisal ("I'll take away your television privileges"), by removing street clothes, by physical restraint (tying a patient to the bed), or by chemical restraint (administration of sedations) can all be acts of false imprisonment unless appropriate measures are followed, even when done in the patient's best interest.

Always record your efforts to inform a patient why restriction is being used. If the patient refuses, notify your instructor.

Patients with psychiatric problems are more likely to bring charges of false imprisonment, but any patient might do so, particularly if confused or uninformed of the reason for constraint.

Violation of Confidentiality

You are ethically obligated to treat information you have about your patients as confidential. Your intimate relationship with the lives of your patients gives you access to matters and information that in ordinary circumstances would be private. When the information you get is of a personal nature and when it has no direct bearing on the patient's treatment or well-being, this information is confidential and should be treated as such.

Unless the information you have suggests that harm would come to the patient or to others if it is withheld, you should respect its private nature. Normal exchanges of information with your supervisor and other members of the patient's health care team in the performance of your duties are not subject to

✔ *The Privacy Rule, a part of the HIPAA regulations, requires that medical information be kept confidential.*

this constraint. However, discussing a patient in public, whether confidential information is mentioned, may place a nurse in danger of being accused of breaking the principle of confidentiality. The so-called shoptalk (idly discussing or gossiping about patients with co-workers and others) should be avoided for this reason alone. Many regulations related to confidentiality are a result of federal legislation that was passed in August 1996.

THE *Web*

You can learn more about the Health Insurance Portability and Accountability Act (HIPAA) at the Health and Human Services Web site.

The release of information to anyone other than those persons directly associated with caring for the patient, without permission, is a violation of the patient's right to privacy and, in some cases, the law. It is generally outside the nurse's responsibility to provide information about patients to anyone, including the police, media, relatives, or visitors. Familiarize yourself with your program's, and later your employer's, standards on how patient information is to be handled and follow them.

Defamation of Character

✔ *Don't gossip about anyone to anyone.*

Making false or malicious (intentionally harmful) statements to someone that may harm another person's character or reputation is *defamation*, or *defamation of character*. When statements are made orally, they constitute *slander*; when written, they are called *libel*. Both are violations of law and ethics, and they can be causes for lawsuits.

You can protect yourself against accusations of slander or libel by restricting your verbal or written comments about patients (or anyone else) to nonjudgmental, objective statements of fact. Limit discussion about patients to the appropriate time and place, and make statements in terms that can be documented. Avoid idle comments and gossip, and when charting, limit your written remarks to accurate, objective statements.

Violating Informed Consent

✔ *Informed consent is not the same as consent.*

Informed consent is not a tort, but *violating* the principle of informed consent is. A fundamental right of patients is the right to make decisions regarding their own health care. This right means that patients can accept or reject health care. A patient who accepts health care is said to give consent. For consent to be legal, it must be both voluntary (freely given) and informed (the patient clearly understands the alternatives).

Voluntary, informed consent by the patient to treatment is required by law. The right to informed consent is also specified in the American Hospital Association's Patient Care Partnership brochure. This plain language brochure informs patients about what they should expect during their hospital stay with regard to their rights and responsibilities.

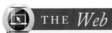

THE *Web*

Read the *Patient Care Partnership* brochure at the American Hospital Association Web site.

Consent is obtained from a patient either verbally or in writing, with written consent preferred. The physician is responsible for getting a patient's consent for certain procedures; the nurse is responsible for getting a patient's consent for nursing care.

If a patient seems unclear or poorly informed about a particular treatment, tell your instructor, so that the patient's physician or nurse manager can provide additional clarification. Once given, consent can be withdrawn by the patient. Withdrawal of consent may occur at the most unexpected times. Technically, you should ask for and receive consent from your patients before administering every nursing procedure. This isn't as cumbersome as it sounds because patients are expected to have a reasonable awareness of the nature of nursing care.

> ✔ *Patients have the right to refuse treatment without reprisal from the health care team.*

Nevertheless, you should always inform your patients about what you are doing and ask their permission to do it. The request and the response don't have to be direct; they can be implied. For example, if you tell a patient you are there to give a bath, and the patient says, "Yes, I'm ready for a bath," or words to that effect, direct consent has been given. If the patient does not say anything, but nods or otherwise indicates by actions that the procedure is acceptable, implied consent has been given. In both cases, you have consent to act. Conversely, if the patient says, "No bath today," or shakes his head saying "no," consent has been denied.

Obtaining direct or implied consent is always easier when the patient understands what is going on and why. Explain beforehand what you are doing and why it is necessary so that your patient can make an informed decision.

> ✔ *Always explain what you are doing and why.*

Consent for providing care for minor children is obtained from the minor's parent or legal guardian. It's a good idea to get the minor's consent as well, whenever possible. If care has been authorized by a legal guardian and a minor refuses it, inform your instructor before proceeding with treatment or withholding it. Consent for providing care for mentally incompetent patients must also come from a legal guardian.

In some instances, a person may be unable to make an informed decision, but is not legally incompetent. Intoxicated, unconscious, or confused patients are examples. It is not your responsibility to determine by whose authority consent can be given in such cases, but it is wise to know what the laws in your state are and what specific policy your employer or institution has regarding this situation.

Assault and Battery

One of the most common acts of nursing care, touching a patient, requires the patient's consent, whether the reason for touching is in her best interest or not. When direct or implied consent is not given, the potential for a charge of *battery*—touching another person without permission—is possible.

Permission to touch in a nursing care situation is generally implied, but you should always inform your patients about what you are doing. If permission to touch is refused and explaining the reason for touching fails to change the patient's mind, inform your instructor. Don't continue with the procedure.

> ✔ *Be careful of what you say and how you say it; joking or teasing might be taken seriously.*

Assault is the threat to touch without permission. A charge of assault can be brought even if the threat could not be carried out but the patient fears that it could. For example, telling a patient to take a prescribed medication or be faced with getting it by injection may get the patient to do as asked, but a charge of assault could be lodged.

Fraud

Fraud is intentional deception to prevent a person from receiving what is lawfully his. In a health care setting, a patient who has been charged for a service that was not performed has been defrauded. A nurse who falsely tells a patient that a medication has no side effects so that the patient will take it could be charged with fraud. It would be fraudulent to change a chart to cover up an error that, if discovered, could result in an action against the person who made the entry.

Negligence

Negligence includes the failure of a reasonable person to do something (or not do something) that a reasonable person in the same circumstance would do (or not do). The negligent person does not intend or plan to commit a wrongful act, but unreasonable carelessness causes harm or injury to someone. In health care, *negligence* is a general term describing neglect by a physician or nurse to apply the education and skills in caring for a patient, which other physicians or nurses customarily apply in caring for similar patients in similar circumstances.

✔ *Negligence is failing to perform your duties as any reasonable and prudent nurse would customarily do in a similar situation.*

Nurses who provide nursing services frequently find themselves in situations where their behavior could result in a lawsuit claiming negligence. Professional misconduct, lack of skill in performing duties, and illegal or immoral conduct can be the basis of a claim. Negligence also includes errors of omission and errors of commission. For negligence to be claimed, the nurse must have failed to do something that any reasonable and prudent nurse would have done in the same situation. In addition, some injury must result from the nurse's actions or failure to act. Typical acts of negligence by nurses include failure to protect patients from burns caused by water bottles, bath water, or compresses; failure to ensure that safety measures are in place and are fully operational so that patients do not fall; failure to make sure that wrong dosages or medications are not given; and failure to properly identify patients before performing treatments.

✔ *For a patient to claim negligence, some harm must have resulted from the nurse's actions.*

If an act is so atrocious that human life has been endangered or even lost, the action is usually called *gross negligence*. A charge against the person may be filed in criminal courts and criminal charges brought against the defendant. Crimes related to nurses are discussed in more detail later in this chapter.

Nurses commit acts of gross negligence when they perform duties beyond their education, experience, or legally defined limits. For example, if you administer a prescription medication without a physician's order and the patient dies as a result of your action, you may be guilty of gross negligence. You may be tried under private laws (tort) as well as under criminal law. Nurses must perform their duties as any ordinary, reasonable, and prudent nurse would in similar circumstances. Prudent nurses do not administer prescription medications without a physician's order.

✔ *Acts of gross negligence are often tried under criminal law.*

People who suffer injuries as a result of any of these torts have a legal option to sue those who cause their injuries. These law suits that involve health care facilities and health care professionals are called claims of medical malpractice.

Malpractice Claims

Charges of poor care, patient harm, and patient dissatisfaction do not usually end in malpractice claims and lawsuits, but when they do, they are often influenced by factors you should recognize.

The public is increasingly sensitive to the real or imagined impersonality of the American health care system. When health care is seen as a big and profitable business, patients within the system are more apt to enter a lawsuit for an alleged wrong. The fact that health care employers and providers carry liability insurance is used by people to justify claims against them. This is especially true of large claims against health care providers because many people believe that the insurance companies, not the health care providers, are the ones who pay the claims and the insurance companies can afford it. Also, frequent news stories of enormous judgments awarded in lawsuits may encourage some patients to initiate one to offset high medical care costs or even to solve financial woes.

Some patients are more likely to claim malpractice and bring a lawsuit than are others. Called "suit prone," they are quick to sue for damages whether the damages are real or the suit is justified. Some of the traits they exhibit include high levels of criticism, fault finding, hostility, uncooperativeness, and sensitivity to being offended. Success in earlier lawsuits in which they have been awarded damages (payment) may also encourage some patients to try again.

Use moderation when dealing with such patients. Work to meet their needs, rather than turn defensive or confrontational. Nurses who fail to respond to their patients' needs, who are insensitive and uncaring, or who exceed their own limits in providing care may encourage a lawsuit. Box 11-3 summarizes guidelines for avoiding malpractice claims.

Not all malpractice claims can be prevented, but many can be discouraged by strict personal and institutional adherence to high standards of care. In addition to providing high standards of care, attention to accurate documentation and being aware of areas in which nurses are often found negligent may help you avoid having to defend yourself in court.

> ✔ *Develop personal traits that foster patient satisfaction with your nursing care.*

BOX 11-3	**Guidelines for Avoiding Malpractice Claims**

- Maintain a healthy self-awareness of your competence to practice.
- Avoid allowing what you do to become so routine and unthinking that you perform your duties automatically.
- Find out what your strengths and weaknesses are, and deal with each according to its need.
- Capitalize on what you do well, and seek to improve those areas that need help through education, experience, or guidance from others.
- Don't hesitate to ask for advice from competent advisers.
- Don't accept assignments or perform duties that you are unsure of or for which you lack education, training, or experience.
- Evaluate assignments and establish priorities.
- Don't accept the role or duties of health care providers whose qualifications exceed yours.
- Don't "practice medicine" for friends and neighbors.
- Stay informed of your employer's procedures and policies.
- Exercise your right to refuse to do anything you are not qualified to do, that is unclear to you, or that is against stated policies, laws, nurse practice acts, and other legal restrictions.
- When you see a policy that is outdated, ineffective, or wrong, bring it to the attention of your instructor or an appropriate authority so that the policy can be changed.
- Maintain accurate, legible, consistent, and complete records in strict accordance with your employer's policies.
- Continuously observe the safety rules and regulations set by your employer.
- Be aware that some practices in one's personal life—use of alcohol or drugs, for example—or other behavior that reflects poorly on one's character may be used against one in a malpractice suit.
- Accurately document pertinent information.
- Avoid "shoptalk" and any breach of confidentiality.
- Always inform the patient and get his or her consent for nursing care.

Documentation

Documenting or charting your actions in your patient's medical record contributes to a legal record of the events that occurred (see Fig. 11-2). The importance of record accuracy, not only as an ongoing record of events but also as a lasting document that can be referred to later if the need arises, cannot be overstated. The care by which a record is kept protects the patient while under medical care and can be used to protect those who administered care in the event of a lawsuit later. In both cases, the level of protection is determined by how well the chart is kept. Anything that is not recorded on a patient's chart is presumed not to have happened, even if it did.

Entries on the patient's record must be factual, to the point, accurate, legible, and related to the patient's needs or plan of treatment. Personal opinions and feelings should never appear on the medical record. Saying that a patient is stubborn, uncooperative, dirty, and won't allow the staff to bathe him may be true, but the appropriate statement on the chart would be to say that the patient refuses to allow the nursing staff to bathe him.

✔ *Learn to think, act, write, and speak objectively.*

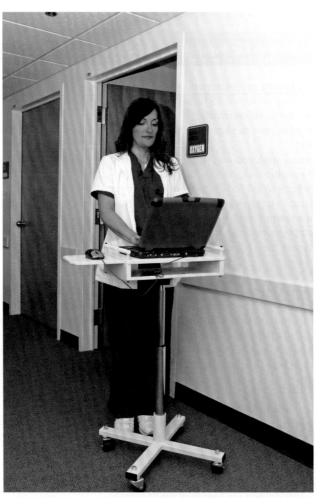

FIGURE 11-2. ● Patient charts are legal records of medical and nursing care. (Photo courtesy of IntegraCraft, Ltd.)

When charting on the medical record, it is also important to avoid including or implying reasons for errors in care. For example, it would be unwise to chart that the patient received 60 mg of codeine at 10:00 am and 60 mg of codeine at 10:15 am because the staff was very busy and the nurse who gave the medication at 10:00 am did not have time to record on the chart that she had given the medication. Recording the fact that the patient received two doses of medication within 15 minutes is appropriate; including or implying the reason is inappropriate.

Charts and charting procedures will be described to you by your instructor. Later, when you are employed, you will find that charting systems and procedures vary from one institution to another. Learn what is required and conform to that. Employers will expect you to be familiar with the charting process, but they will also recognize your need for time to learn the specifics of their system.

Be consistent when charting and use only agency-approved abbreviations and chart-correction procedures, so that any given entry always means the same thing whenever it is written and errors will always be corrected properly. Keep in mind that if the patient claims malpractice, the entries on the patient's medical record will be examined closely in court.

If you document your nursing actions on a computer, be sure that you do not leave the patient's chart on the screen so that others can read confidential information. Also be certain that your access code remains secure and do not share that code with anyone else for any reason.

✔ *Improve your charting skills through professional development programs.*

Delegation of Nursing Duties

Another area of increasing concern for nurses and one in which a claim of negligence is possible is the delegation of nursing tasks to unlicensed assistive personnel. In 2006, the National Council of State Boards of Nursing and the American Nurses Association jointly issued a document that provides guidelines on the licensed nurse's role in delegating nursing tasks. This document clearly indicates that the licensed nurse is accountable for the appropriateness of delegated nursing tasks. Inappropriate delegation by the licensed nurse may lead to legal action against him or her.

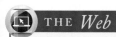 THE *Web*

Use the search term "Joint Statement on Delegation" at the National Council of State Boards of Nursing Web site to learn more about issues surrounding the delegation of nursing duties to others.

The best way for a nurse to avoid being sued for negligence is to constantly look for and correct situations in which a patient may suffer an injury. The nurse may be able to correct the situation immediately, or it may require the revision of a policy, procedure, or even a law to be resolved. Providing high standards of safe care requires nurses to be constantly involved in suggesting methods to improve the quality of care provided by health care facilities.

Malpractice Insurance

Malpractice insurance for nurses important in a society that is suit conscious. Paying for the defense of a lawsuit and paying any judgment that might be rendered are beyond the ability of most people. To protect their employees and themselves against any legal and financial consequences that could arise from provision of services, institutional employers carry malpractice liability insurance. However, because individuals are responsible for their own actions, it is still possible for an employee (e.g., you as a nurse) to be sued personally. This is true even in states where charitable immunity, the protection of nonprofit hospitals from legal liability, applies.

✔ *Having your own malpractice insurance policy is well worth the cost.*

A separate, personal malpractice liability insurance policy over and above your employer's policy is a wise investment that some would consider essential. There are at least three reasons why nurses should carry their own liability insurance policy. First, if you and your employer are codefendants and found liable and the cost of the settlement exceeds your employer's policy limits, you may be required to pay the excess out of your own pocket.

Second, your employer's insurance company may sue you if they believe they incurred a loss because of your actions.

Third, many employer policies are claims based rather than occurrence based. A claims-based policy covers claims made while the policy is in effect. If your employer discontinues the policy and a claim is made later (which often happens), you would not be covered. An occurrence-based policy provides coverage if the incident occurs within the policy period. If the policy is allowed to lapse and a suit is filed for an incident that occurred during the policy period, coverage would be in place.

For your personal protection against claims against you, make certain your employer carries a policy of liability insurance that covers you. Find out the exact nature and limits of the coverage it gives you. Then, with a knowledgeable insurance expert, determine what amount (dollar value) and type (occurrence or claims based) of personal coverage you should carry and purchase a policy accordingly. Since most policies cost less than $100 a year, purchasing a malpractice insurance policy can help protect you against a financial disaster.

Wills

A *will* is a legal statement of a person's wishes regarding the disposition of property after death. There may be times when patients ask you to help them prepare their wills. You should not accept the responsibility, but should refer the matter to your instructor or the nursing supervisor. An attorney is the appropriate person to help someone write a will, and the patient should be assisted to find one if so requested.

✔ *Nurses should not expect or accept gifts or money from their patients.*

On occasion, you may be asked to witness a patient's will. Not all institutions allow nurses to witness wills. Abide by the guidelines set by yours. If witnessing a signature is permitted, more than one witness will be required, which means that signing a will should be done only when other witnesses and the person whose will it is are present. Be sure the act of signing is accurately entered on the patient's chart, with particular attention to the time and date of signing.

Gifts

As a nurse, you should make it clear to patients and families that you do not accept gifts. It is legal to do so, but it is not ethical to accept gifts, and it is certainly not ethical to solicit them. However, at times, a patient may wish to give personal possessions as gifts to various people, including members of the health care team. This may be out of gratitude for care the patient has received or because he or she realizes that death is near. If the patient owns or has the right to dispose of the gift, and if the recipient accepts the gift, the act is valid within the law as long as the patient understands what he or she is doing and has not been coerced or deceived by anyone. Courteous refusal to accept the gift is the more appropriate response.

If a refusal is not accepted by the patient, particularly in times when the emotional climate is high, you should always protect yourself from any question about accepting a gift by having a witness present, informing your instructor or supervisor, and recording the patient's condition at the time.

CRIMINAL LAW AND NURSING

A *crime* is an offense committed against the public welfare or safety. You will recall that a tort is a legal wrong claimed by one person against another. Therefore, if you injure someone, the injured person is the one who prosecutes you. If you commit a crime, however, it is the state that seeks to prosecute you.

Criminal acts can be classified as minor offenses, misdemeanors, or felonies. Minor offenses include violations of traffic and parking regulations, and in some states, first time arrests for disorderly conduct, underage drinking, and shoplifting. A misdemeanor is less serious than is a felony and is generally punishable by a fine and/or 1 year or less in prison. Minor offenses are elevated to misdemeanors when they are the second offense. Felonies are the most serious grade of criminal act and include murder. A conviction of a crime can be grounds for denying, suspending, or revoking a nurse's license.

States have mandatory nursing licensure laws and practicing without a license is a felony punishable under public law. Those who may be arrested and tried include people who are practicing as nurses who were never licensed and nurses who have failed to renew their license.

Grossly negligent acts are considered crimes by many states. A nurse who restrains a patient against his or her will and without proper authorization may be charged with false imprisonment and prosecuted for committing a tort. However, if the same nurse becomes angry with a patient's behavior and restrains the patient with such force that circulation is impaired for a prolonged period, requiring the patient's hand to be amputated, the nurse would most likely be charged with a crime. To convict a nurse of a crime, the court would have to prove both a criminal act and a criminal intent.

Patient abuse is of great concern, particularly in long-term care facilities. Governmental regulations related to criminal background checks of long-term care workers and a national registry of those convicted of abusing the elderly are in operation across the country. Criminal abuse of the elderly includes physical abuse, such as withholding food and water, hitting, slapping and punching, and restraining with intent to imprison. Other abuses of the elderly such as sexual abuse, failure to provide a safe environment, and failure of a health care facility to provide care may lead to criminal charges.

In addition, other crimes in which nurses may become directly or indirectly involved include situations related to the right to die, violations of federal and state narcotic and controlled substance laws, fraud related to falsifying patient bills, robbery related to a patient's belongings, death because of lack of or incorrect nursing care, and murder.

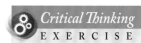

Critical Thinking
E X E R C I S E

You have been working in an assisted living facility for 3 years and have developed a close relationship with several residents. One day, one of your very favorite patients took a turn for the worse and told you she knew she was going to die. She said she wanted you to have her diamond and sapphire ring. You told her you could not take it, expressed your appreciation, and suggested she give it to one of her children or grandchildren. She kept insisting, so you told her you would think about it. What steps are involved in coming to a decision? What ethical and legal issues are involved in this situation? How will you feel in 5 years about whatever decision you make now? Use appropriate Characteristics of Critical Thinkers in Box 1-2 on pages 18–19 to develop your responses to these questions.

✔ *Nurses convicted of a crime will be investigated and may have their nursing license revoked.*

✔ *Most employers require criminal background, elder abuse, and child abuse checks, plus drug and alcohol screening prior to hiring.*

✔ *You are working hard to earn your nursing license; don't do anything that could ruin your life and your career.*

SUMMARY

In your nursing practice, you must practice within the law. You must be certain that your actions are based on your education, experience, standards of practice, and employer guidelines and not on emotional responses to sometimes difficult situations. You must think about what you are doing, why you are doing it, and whether a nurse with your similar education and experience would take the same or similar action that you intend to take.

As a licensed nurse, you must demonstrate high moral and ethical standards in both your professional and personal life. In your professional life, there are opportunities to misappropriate drugs, medical supplies, equipment, and blank prescription forms. In your personal life, there are opportunities to disclose protected health information, supply controlled and noncontrolled drugs to others, and dispense medical advice that exceeds your level of education. Maintaining high standards in all areas of your life will provide self-respect as well as the respect of your co-workers, your family, your friends, and your community.

So long as you practice within the law and maintain high moral and ethical standards, your nursing license will provide you with a lifetime of employment opportunities, a decent salary, respect, and most of all the satisfaction of helping people who are in need of comfort and care.

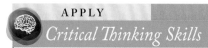

APPLY
Critical Thinking Skills

1. In the opening story at the beginning of this chapter, Lito didn't do what Milo wanted him to do even though Milo was very demanding and forceful. During your nursing career, it is quite likely that you could find yourself in a similar situation of being almost forced into doing something you don't want to do or that you know is illegal. For example, someone close to you may ask you to get drugs for him, someone else may ask you to supply prescription forms, or a peer may ask you to falsify patient records. Although you can always say no and explain why you won't do certain things, it is probably easier not to be asked. What behaviors and attitudes can you exhibit that would send the strongest statement of your personal values and ethics?

2. Obtain a job description for LP/VNs from your affiliating agency. Analyze how clearly the duties of the LP/VN are written.

3. Read your malpractice insurance policy if you have one. What acts are included and what acts are excluded? Is your policy claims based or occurrence based?

4. Ask your librarian to refer you to books and journals or visit Web sites that present summaries of malpractice suits. What similarities do you find in cases of negligence?

5. In addition to the suggestions presented in the chapter, what other actions by a nurse may reduce the possibility of a claim of malpractice?

6. Obtain and review the policy and procedures manual compiled by your affiliating agency. How do these documents define the standards of practice expected by this agency?

7. Imagine that you are driving to school and an automobile accident occurs in front of you. When you stop, you see that the driver of the car has hit his head on the windshield. What will you do and why?

8. Obtain a copy of the nurse practice act for your state. Analyze how these laws affect your practice of nursing.

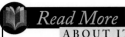

ABOUT IT

Burkhardt MA, Nathaniel AK: Ethics & Issues in Contemporary Nursing, 4th ed. Stamford, CT: Cengage Learning, 2014.

Grant PD, Ballard D: Fast Facts for Nursing and the Law, 1st ed. New York, NY: Springer Publishing, 2013.

Mathes M, Reifsnyder J: Nurse's Law: Legal Questions & Answers for the Practicing Nurse, 1st ed. Indianapolis, IN: Sigma Theta Tau International, 2014.

McTeigue J, Lee C: Legal and Ethical Issues for Health Professionals, 3rd ed. St. Louis, MO: WB Saunders, 2015.

Pozgar GD: Legal and Ethical Issues for Health Professionals, 3rd ed. Sudbury, MA: Jones and Bartlett, 2013.

Westrick SJ: Essentials of Nursing Law and Ethics, 2nd ed. Sudbury, MA: Jones and Bartlett, 2013.

Leadership and Followership Skills

LEARNING OBJECTIVES

When you complete this chapter, you will be able to:

1. Compare and contrast three styles of leadership.

2. Describe at least one situation in which each style of leadership is appropriate.

3. List at least 10 qualities of effective leaders.

4. Describe in a paragraph the characteristics of effective followers.

5. Given a fictitious situation, discuss possible solutions to resolving conflict.

6. Assess your leadership and followership skills.

"I never expected to feel the way I do today," Jamila said to her best friend Cindy. Cindy looked at Jamila and saw the tiredness in Jamila's eyes.

"What are you talking about? What's making you feel and look so bad?" Cindy asked. "Remember," Jamila said, "I told you I was scheduled for my 1-week team leadership experience this week." "Now I remember," said Cindy, instantly feeling that she should have recognized the symptoms. She had just finished her leadership rotation 3 weeks ago, and the experience was still fresh in her mind.

"How do you feel about being a team leader?" Cindy asked. "I always thought I was a leader until this week," Jamila replied. "Why is that?" asked Cindy. "Well, Cindy, a number of things happened, and I don't think I acted like a leader. Everything seemed so disorganized, and I just couldn't get all the problems resolved."

"Some of the team members complained about the assignments I gave them, and then two of them switched their assignments and didn't even tell me. I just feel like I wasn't in control. I was really looking forward to being 'the boss,' but it wasn't at all what I expected." "What did you expect?" asked Cindy. "Well," replied Jamila, "I read all the assignments and even went to the special seminar on developing leadership skills. I expected..." At that point, Ms. Jones, their clinical instructor walked up to Jamila and Cindy.

"How are you both doing?" asked Ms. Jones. "It seems to me that Jamila is trying to recover from her team leadership experience," Cindy said. Ms. Jones shared with them that in her many years of teaching experience, the team leadership assignment is often very difficult for students.

"Why is that?" they both asked simultaneously. "I think it's because 1 week doesn't give you enough time to profit from the mistakes that you make. The team leader assignment gave you an opportunity to explore the role and responsibilities of a nursing team leader. You are now more aware, as a result of your experience, of the skills that a good leader needs," said Ms. Jones. As Ms. Jones walked away, Cindy and Jamila looked at each other, and they both realized that if they ever wanted to be "in charge," they would need more preparation for that role.

A number of trends over the years have contributed to changing the scope of practice of licensed practical/vocational nurses (LP/VNs). The passage of Medicare and Medicaid legislation in 1965, the passage of the Affordable Care Act of 2010, and changes in the accreditation standards for health care agencies created an overall rise in the demand for licensed nursing service. Changes in how health care is funded, cost-cutting measures, and an increase in the number of people with health insurance has also contributed to changing the scope of practice by adding leadership positions to the LP/VNs job descriptions. LP/VNs now often function as team leaders, charge nurses, or care managers in settings where the patient or resident's condition is relatively stable. The requirements for this specialized nursing practice are outlined in the Specialized Nursing Practice section of the National Federation of Licensed Practical Nurses (NFLPN) "Nursing Practice Standards for the Licensed Practical/Vocational Nurse" (see Appendix B) and in the Managing section of the National Association for Practical Nurse Education and Service (NAPNES) Standards of Practice and Educational Competencies (see Appendix C). The LP/VN who is considering a specialized position such as a team leader is expected to have appropriate clinical expertise, have completed programs or courses of study designed to prepare for the position, and have personal characteristics that will contribute to successful performance.

✔ *Being a leader in patient care requires additional education and experience.*

One way to demonstrate clinical expertise is through national certification in a particular area of practice. The NFLPN Education Foundation offers two clinical certifications that would be appropriate for an LP/VN in a clinical leadership position. They are the *NFLPN IV Therapy Certification* and the *NFLPN Gerontology Certification*. NAPNES currently offers the *Certification-Long Term Care (CLTC)*, the *I.V. Therapy Certification (IVT)*, and the *Pharmacology Certification (NCP)* examinations and plans to add several additional national certifications over the next few years.

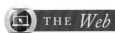 THE *Web*

Visit the NAPNES and the NFLPN Web sites to learn more about their certification programs for licensed practical and vocational nurses.

You can also prepare for a leadership position by learning from your clinical practice experiences and by attending formal learning activities such as seminars, workshops, continuing education classes, or employer-sponsored training programs. The content of these learning activities should be related to your area of clinical practice and to developing leadership skills.

A look at the personal characteristics of leaders shows that every leader is different in how he or she leads. But without a doubt, every leader has a mission or goal and a clear plan or idea of how to achieve that goal. Leaders are people who, because of charisma, focus and purpose, ethics, belief, knowledge, or other traits, are recognized by others as the person they want to follow.

If you believe you have a goal for high-quality patient care and want to be in a position to make that happen, and if you believe you have positive leadership characteristics, now is the time to begin developing the leadership qualities that will contribute to your opportunities for advancement in practical/vocational nursing.

LEADER AND LEADERSHIP DEFINED

A *leader* is a person who, through leadership skills, is able to get others to follow his or her plan to achieve specific goals. *Leadership* is the process that helps a group of people achieve those goals.

✔ *A leader is responsible for guiding the group to achieve its goals.*

The person responsible for leading the nursing team is called the care manager, the head nurse, the charge nurse, or the team leader.

Some of the specific goals of a nursing team leader could include
- Providing a safe environment for staff and patients
- Providing excellent nursing care
- Working as a team
- Minimizing nursing and medical errors

- Establishing pleasant working relationships among nurses, patients, families, physicians, and other members of the health care team
- Sharing knowledge and experience
- Communicating accurately and effectively
- Motivating each team member to achieve his or her maximum potential
- Promoting an interest in incorporating new nursing skills in nursing practice
- Developing a creative problem-solving environment

Although a team leader might have many other goals, this list provides an overview of some goals that can be accomplished through leadership and the efforts of the team members.

A job title does not make a person a leader. You have probably known or will know supervisors, nurse managers, or team leaders whom you would describe as leaders and others in the same positions whom you would not identify as leaders. Leadership behaviors are very different from manager behaviors. (Managers and managing are discussed in the next chapter.) Leaders have followers and create a vision, motivation, standards, and values that followers accept. Not everyone would be a good leader. Take the "Leadership Self-Assessment" on pages 253–254 to determine your feelings about leading others.

LEADERSHIP STYLES

Researchers have studied leaders and leadership skills extensively and have generally found that effective leaders use various styles, have diverse personalities and personal qualities, and handle people in dissimilar ways.

Authoritarian Leader

✔ *The authoritarian leader usually dictates what the work is and when and how it is to be done.*

The *authoritarian* or *autocratic leader* is one who is primarily concerned that tasks are accomplished. This type of leader has little concern for people and rarely involves staff in the decision-making process. The authoritarian leader often uses techniques such as coercion, threats, punishments, and constant observation to keep team members under control. An authoritarian leader issues directives and orders, determines rules for workers, and independently makes decisions that affect the entire team.

Permissive Leader

✔ *The permissive leader provides little direction to workers.*

The *permissive* or *laissez-faire leader* provides little or no direction or control for the team. This type of leader assumes that the staff is self-directed and will do what needs to be done correctly and efficiently without supervision or direction. The permissive leader often has a personal need to be liked by everyone and, for this reason, avoids blame for team actions by giving responsibility to individual team members.

Democratic Leader

✔ *The democratic leader encourages participation in decision making.*

The *democratic leader* encourages staff participation and often consults and collaborates with staff. This type of leader believes that team members have knowledge and skills that can contribute to better decisions for the team and the organization. The democratic leader respects team members, and interactions between team members and the leader are open and trusting. Democratic leaders accept responsibility for the actions of team members and consider themselves an integral part of the team.

| ASSESS YOURSELF | **Leadership Self-Assessment Activity** |

This self-survey will provide you with feedback as to your feelings of leading others. Rate yourself on a scale of 1–5, with 5 being a definite YES and 1 being a definite NO. Be honest about your answers as this survey is only for your own self-assessment.

Circle the number that you feel most closely represents your feelings about the task

	NO				**YES**	
1.	1	2	3	4	5	I enjoy working on teams.
2.	1	2	3	4	5	I am able to speak clearly to others.
3.	1	2	3	4	5	I enjoy relating to others on an interpersonal basis.
4.	1	2	3	4	5	I am good at planning.
5.	1	2	3	4	5	I can interpret rules and regulations.
6.	1	2	3	4	5	I feel comfortable asking others for advice.
7.	1	2	3	4	5	I enjoy collecting and analyzing data.
8.	1	2	3	4	5	I am good at solving problems.
9.	1	2	3	4	5	I am comfortable writing memos to others.
10.	1	2	3	4	5	I can delegate work to others.
11.	1	2	3	4	5	I am effective at handling employee complaints.
12.	1	2	3	4	5	Giving directions is comfortable for me.
13.	1	2	3	4	5	I know how to develop goals and carry them out.
14.	1	2	3	4	5	I am comfortable at implementing new techniques.
15.	1	2	3	4	5	I enjoy appraising performance and giving feedback.
16.	1	2	3	4	5	If I made a mistake, I would admit it and correct it.
17.	1	2	3	4	5	I am able to resolve conflict in the workplace.
18.	1	2	3	4	5	I believe in diversity in the workplace.
19.	1	2	3	4	5	I thrive on change.
20.	1	2	3	4	5	One of my greatest desires is to become a leader.

SCORING

Score the survey by adding the numbers that you circled: _____

A score of 50 or higher indicates a desire to become a leader and a perceived ability to perform the tasks required of a leader.

A score of 50 or less indicates a general dislike of wanting to become a leader or a perceived inability to perform the tasks required of a leader.

BUT, no matter what your score is, your commitment, desire, and determination are the biggest indicators of your ability to become a leader.

Use this assessment to help you determine what skills and abilities you can continue to improve (strengths) and what skills and abilities you need to develop (opportunities for growth).

What are your strengths?

What are your opportunities for growth?

continued on page 254

RELIABILITY AND VALIDITY

Since this survey is a learning tool used in training programs such as leadership development, rather than a research tool, it has not been formally checked for reliability or validity. However, since I have received feedback from various sources and have been updated numerous times, I believe it to be a fairly accurate tool.

Copyright 1998 by Donald Clark. Created January 27, 1998, and updated December 30, 2007, from http://nwlink.com/~donclark/leader/self.html

Situational Leadership

It should be evident that one style will not work in every situation. It is often necessary to use different styles in different situations. During an emergency such as a fire in a patient's room, the authoritarian style of leadership is most effective and most appropriate.

A democratic style would probably be the most appropriate style to use in the day-to-day operation of a nursing unit. A leader using this style would incorporate the opinions and expertise of the staff when making decisions affecting policies and the operation of the patient unit.

A permissive style would be most appropriate in a situation in which all team members are experienced, skilled, self-directed, conscientious, and trustworthy. A group of professionals working on research projects might effectively work with a permissive leader.

As you can see, different situations require different leadership styles. This is called *situational leadership*. Situational leadership theorists believe that effective leadership occurs when the leader's style matches the overall situation. The overall situation includes the leader (style and expectations), the followers (knowledge and skills), and the events (work requirements) that are occurring. The leader is expected to consider all three when selecting a style or combination of styles of leader behavior.

Caution should be exercised when changing your prevailing style as a leader. Everyone agrees that certain situations demand certain styles; however, frequent changes in leadership style are detrimental. Leaders who are democratic one day, permissive the next, and authoritarian the 3rd day create an environment of chaos and confusion for their team. Your prevailing style should be one that fits your personality and the personality of your team.

Figure 12-1 illustrates that the most effective leadership style, for most situations, falls within the darker shaded area. The situation combined with staff skills, knowledge, capabilities, and personalities may require the leader to add some of the characteristics of the permissive or authoritarian leadership styles to his or her democratic style. For example, all staff members on a certain nursing team are skilled in performing their duties, and they have personalities that work well together. But almost all of the team members arrive 10 to 15 minutes late for work almost every day. This causes the previous shift to have to wait for them to arrive. Facility policies are very clear on the requirement to arrive for work on time. This situation has been discussed individually and with the team as a whole on several occasions, but the problem was not resolved. At this point, the democratic leader may decide to incorporate some authoritarian style and clearly outline to the staff the requirement of being on time and the actions that will be taken for continued lateness.

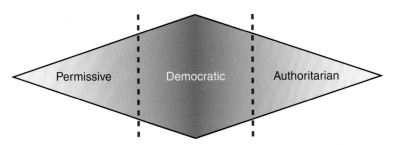

FIGURE 12-1. ● Democratic leaders occasionally display permissive and authoritarian behaviors to some degree.

In addition to finding a leadership style or combination of styles that is effective and comfortable, a good leader must also develop an interpersonal behavioral style that fosters cooperation and harmony within the nursing team.

TYPES OF BEHAVIOR

As there are styles of leadership, there are also styles of behavior. Knowing the characteristics and consequences of different styles of behavior will increase your awareness of your own behaviors and perhaps offer insight into changes that would enhance your ability to be a leader.

Passive Behavior

The word *passive* means not taking part in something. People who exhibit *passive behavior* avoid conflict and do nothing in situations in which an action is required. They do not contribute ideas and suggestions to improve the work of the nursing team, do not encourage patients to participate in their care, and rarely, if ever, express how they feel about a situation.

People who are passive often blame others, say "Yes" when they mean "No," and work extra shifts when they are physically unable to do so. Passive people who are scheduled to work on a requested weekend off will work. They will never confront the situation or express their feelings to the person responsible. Over time, passive people become angry and hostile because they feel hurt, used, and abused by others. They pay a high price for not expressing feelings, needs, and wants.

✔ *Passive people rarely express their true thoughts and feelings about a situation.*

Aggressive Behavior

Aggressive behavior is almost the opposite of passive behavior. Other words that mean the same are pushy, forceful, hostile, and combative. People who are behaving aggressively ignore the rights and feelings of others. They are focused only on their own needs and feelings and often act and speak before thinking.

✔ *Aggressive people demand that they get what they want.*

People who use aggressive behaviors often get their own way at the expense of others. They, like those who are passive, are ineffective nursing team members. They make statements such as "My way or no way," "I refuse to take care of Mr. Doe," and "You are incompetent." When assigned to work on a weekend they requested to be off, the aggressive person might say, "Before I'll work next weekend, I'll quit. Then you'll see."

Assertive Behavior

Assertive behavior is that in which you express your needs and feelings without attacking someone else. An assertive person uses statements that begin with "I"

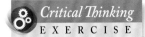

Critical Thinking
E X E R C I S E

Select at least three people you know who are in leadership positions. They could be a teacher, a pastor, a scout leader, a parent, or perhaps a coach. As you think about the people you chose, identify some of the leadership traits they have in common. Then, identify some of the leadership traits that make them very different. Analyze the differences among the three people and identify what you learned from your analysis.

Use appropriate Characteristics of Critical Thinkers in Box 1-2 on pages 18–19 to develop your analysis of leadership styles.

to describe his or her own feelings or needs. An example of assertive behavior with a supervisor is as follows: "I requested next weekend off over 2 months ago, and I see on the schedule that I am assigned to work. I cannot work that weekend." If you are assertive, you may not get the response you want from your supervisor, but you have openly and honestly expressed your feelings. Your supervisor may have made an error and may apologize and correct the situation; your supervisor may explain the reasons you were scheduled to work that weekend; or your supervisor may offer other solutions to resolve the problem. The assertive approach allows discussion and compromise; the aggressive approach leaves no options for the person making the statement. The passive response is actually no response, and by avoiding any response at all, the person has no options but to work as scheduled.

Assertive statements such as "I do not want to hear gossip about others," "I do not share your views about (related to prejudices or people)," and "I expect you to respect my right to not hear yours" or "I find it very distressing when you criticize me in front of others. If you have something critical to say, please say it in a private place" will help you avoid accumulating the anger, hostility, and resentment that passive and aggressive behaviors encourage.

Learning to be assertive rather than passive or aggressive takes a conscious effort. Being assertive means

- Asking for your rights but not at the expense of others
- Expressing needs and feelings that are of significant importance to you
- Being honest and truthful with yourself and others
- Not deliberately hurting others
- Making statements that begin with "I"
- Being sure that what you ask for is what you want
- Taking responsibility for your request
- Not being self-centered and selfish

Learning to incorporate assertive behaviors with sensitivity, honesty, and flexibility will go a long way toward making your working relationships productive and pleasant.

QUALITIES OF EFFECTIVE LEADERS

In addition to applying an effective leadership style and using principles of assertive behavior, good leaders possess many other more personal qualities that make them successful (Fig. 12-2). An effective leader is much easier to recognize than to describe. From your own experiences, you can no doubt identify team leaders, nurse managers, and supervisors who are effective leaders and others who are not. Becoming an effective leader does not happen naturally; it takes study, experience, and work to develop the necessary personal qualities.

Now is the time, early in your career, to begin studying and practicing the personal and interpersonal qualities of an effective leader.

Effective leaders are emotionally mature. They do not have temper tantrums, pout, complain, or find fault. They do not speak loudly or joke inappropriately in the presence of patients or their visitors. An emotionally mature leader is even-tempered, tolerant, and patient and maintains a businesslike atmosphere everywhere, especially in patient care areas.

Effective leaders are open-minded and willing to listen to the suggestions of others. The open-minded leader looks for better methods and safer procedures and frequently asks for others' opinions.

✔ *Assertive people let others know what they want and expect.*

✔ *A good leader knows how to lead without being dictatorial.*

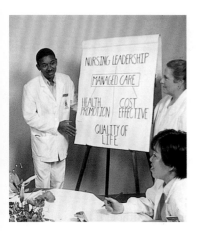

FIGURE 12-2. ● Becoming an effective leader requires study, experience, and the development of a number of personal and interpersonal qualities. (From Craven RF, Hirnle CJ: Fundamentals of Nursing: Human Health and Function, 5th ed. Philadelphia, PA: Lippincott Williams & Wilkins, 2007:111.)

Effective leaders are fair. This means that a leader does not allow personal friendships and favoritism to cloud relationships with staff. The leader respects each member of the nursing team and expects everyone to make a maximum contribution to patient care.

Effective leaders are consistent in enforcing policies that regulate staff conduct. On rare occasions when an exception can be justified, staff members are given an explanation for the exception.

✔ *A good leader respects those he or she is leading.*

Effective leaders are assertive. They respect the rights of others as well as their own rights. They express how they feel about a situation by using statements that begin with "I." They expect staff members to meet the needs of the patients they are serving.

Effective leaders are responsible. They accept responsibility for the actions of their staff members and, when indicated, defend those actions to their superiors. When a staff member is at fault, they try to help that person make positive adjustments rather than dismissing the individual from the team.

Effective leaders are courageous. After making a decision, the leader changes the decision only when it is clear that the original decision was a poor one. The courageous leader can admit to having made a poor decision and can offer a sincere apology to an individual or individuals who have been offended.

Effective leaders have the ability to teach. The leader who has a desire to share knowledge and skills with others is well on the way to becoming a teacher. Patience, tolerance, and praise are qualities that enhance any teaching–learning situation.

✔ *A good leader develops leaders while leading.*

Effective leaders have developed excellent problem-solving abilities. The effective leader defines the problem, gathers the facts, analyzes the information, proposes several solutions and the consequences of each, makes a decision, and evaluates the effectiveness of that decision.

Effective leaders have excellent clinical skills. They recognize that they "set the standard" of care and serve as role models for staff members. The effective leader offers workable suggestions and techniques to manage difficult nursing care situations.

Effective leaders are critical thinkers. They welcome different viewpoints and are creative in finding solutions to problems. They collect all the facts about a situation from every available resource, they weigh all of the possible solutions, and they take responsibility for their actions. Critical thinkers learn from their mistakes and use what they have learned when faced with similar or new situations.

<table>
<tr><td colspan="2">BOX 12-1   Leadership Qualities</td></tr>
<tr><td>Emotionally mature</td><td>Skilled problem-solver</td></tr>
<tr><td>Open-minded</td><td>Clinically proficient</td></tr>
<tr><td>Fair</td><td>Critical thinker</td></tr>
<tr><td>Consistent</td><td>Sensitive and objective</td></tr>
<tr><td>Assertive</td><td>Flexible</td></tr>
<tr><td>Responsible</td><td>Capable of using humor</td></tr>
<tr><td>Courageous</td><td>Positive role model</td></tr>
<tr><td>Teacher</td><td>Capable of profiting from experience</td></tr>
</table>

✔ *A good leader knows the needs of the team.*

Effective leaders are sensitive as well as objective. Although they enforce the rules and regulations of the employer and the unit, they are aware of the special needs and abilities of the people they are leading. They interact with each member of their team as a unique human being with a vast array of personal needs, cultural differences, and interests.

Effective leaders are flexible and match their style of leadership to the situation. During an emergency, an effective leader is decisive and gives direct orders to the team members. In the daily routine, the effective leader follows a fairly well-established and consistent style of leadership. An effective leader who is making long-range plans may encourage suggestions from members of the nursing team and incorporate their recommendations into the plan.

✔ *A good leader considers leadership an opportunity for service.*

Effective leaders have a sense of humor. Adding appropriate humor to an embarrassing, difficult, or tense situation often defuses the tension and allows everyone to relax. When relaxed, people can think more clearly, make better decisions, and work more effectively.

Effective leaders often select a role model who exemplifies the qualities of an effective leader. By observing the role model's personal and interpersonal relationships with staff members, the inexperienced leader can identify some of the personal qualities that contribute to effective leadership skills.

These are just a few of the personal qualities of an effective leader. These qualities may not come naturally, but you can develop them if you make an honest effort to incorporate them into your life and your nursing career. Do this by being aware of what they are, by observing them in yourself, by noting how they change as you practice them, and by making corrections when your actions do not produce the results you want.

It is important to know that leaders, no matter how much education or experience they have, make mistakes. Learning from your mistakes is a quality that will probably contribute most to your development as a leader. Being the leader of a patient care team is a tremendous responsibility but one that can provide equally tremendous rewards. Box 12-1 summarizes the qualities of an effective leader.

LEADING AND TEAM BUILDING

Having an effective patient care team doesn't just happen. An effective leader creates an environment that encourages team members to work together to do their best so that patients receive the best care possible (Fig. 12-3).

One of the ways the leader can do this is by being a positive role model for the team members. Being a positive role model includes everything from your professional appearance to your desire to provide the best possible care for your

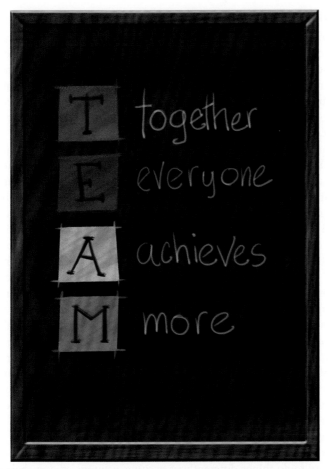

FIGURE 12-3. ● Positive relationships among team members improve patient care.

patients to your commitment to the nursing profession. Consistently dressing appropriately and being involved in committees, professional organizations, and continuing education programs are all behaviors that you would want from your team members.

To build an effective team, the leader must be able to motivate the team members to achieve their goals. This is easiest when the team members are involved in setting the goals. If one of the goals of the team is that they have no work-related injuries for 1 month, it is likely that all of the team members will work to make that goal a reality. Rewards such as a staff party, a monetary bonus, time off with pay, a recognition banquet, award pins, and so forth often reinforce the motivation to achieve a defined goal.

Building an effective team also requires coaching. It is as important to let the team members know when they have done a good job as it is to let them know when they have not. Praise of good work is highly valued by team members.

Other ways of building an effective team include recognizing the individual strengths and weaknesses of the team members. Capitalizing on an individual's strengths gives opportunities for increased self-esteem. Coaching an individual on how to overcome a weakness will help that individual achieve his or her maximum potential. Even if this results in losing a team member to a promotion, you have the satisfaction of knowing that you were able to help someone else grow in his or her career.

✔ *Part of the leadership role is to build a team just as a coach builds a team.*

HANDLING CHANGE

As a leader, you will no doubt be faced with the necessity of coping with change yourself and explaining changes to your team members. In health care settings, changes involve policies and procedures, staffing patterns and schedules, work conditions, salary and benefit packages, new equipment, job responsibilities, patient care protocols, government regulations, accrediting agency regulations, and many other things that will affect your work and how you do it.

✔ *Know that change is a way of life.*

You and your team have three options when you are confronted with change. You can resist change, you can accept it, or you can avoid it. If a change is unacceptable to you, your best action is to avoid it through resignation or transfer. Suppose, for example, that you have been working in an operating room of a hospital that does not perform abortions. The hospital is sold, and the new owners hire a physician who will begin performing abortions in the operating room in 2 months. You are morally, religiously, and ethically opposed to abortions. In this situation, your best action may be to resign or to request a transfer to another area within the hospital because it is highly unlikely that you will be able to convince the new owners not to make this change.

Resisting change requires a great deal of personal energy and can take its toll on your physical and mental health. People often resist change because they fear that they will lose their jobs, or that change will require more work for them, or because they do not understand the change. As a leader, it is important for you to make every effort to be involved in planning changes, getting facts related to the change from the source, and interpreting for your team the effects of the change on them.

✔ *Learn the reasons for proposed changes in your work environment.*

How you as a leader handle proposed or real changes will directly influence how your team members handle change. If you accept change and view it as an opportunity to do things differently, as exciting, as progress, as a challenge, and as a way to learn new things, then your team members may also be less resistant to the change. The more involved you and your team members are on your employer's committees, in professional organizations, in continuing education, and in the politics affecting health care, the more able you are to influence decisions that will change your work environment.

✔ *The leader's attitude toward change can be contagious.*

HANDLING CONFLICT

It would be rare to find a nursing team that does not experience conflict. This conflict may be between staff members, between the staff and the leader, or a combination. Team members often look to the leader to resolve team conflict. Unless the leader takes action, conflict will rarely resolve itself. Avoiding the situation or denying that a problem exists will not resolve the issue.

Using the problem-solving approach outlined in Chapter 2, the leader should identify the problem and consider possible solutions. It is often advisable to discuss the problem and proposed action with a supervisor or other nurse manager whom you respect and who can maintain confidentiality of information. Discussing the problem and getting feedback from someone whose judgment you trust often helps you clarify the problem and evaluate your proposed solution before you act.

Once you have chosen a course of action, follow it through to the end. Don't change your mind (unless you are obviously wrong), and don't be influenced by the opinions of others.

Keep disciplinary sessions private and professional. Shouting or threatening will not accomplish a solution. If necessary, involve your supervisor in the session. Have your facts straight, listen to what the individual or team members have to say, clearly state what action will resolve the problem, and specifically identify what you expect in the future.

When conflicts cannot be resolved and you are no longer an effective leader, it may be necessary to request a transfer or to resign from your position. Having effective leadership skills does not guarantee success. To be an effective leader, you must have effective followers as well as an organization that supports your goals as a leader.

FOLLOWERSHIP QUALITIES

A leader cannot be a leader without followers. The success of any patient care team depends to a great extent on the knowledge, experience, and attitudes of the followers.

Followers contribute to the success or failure of a leader. A person with excellent leadership skills will fail miserably if members of the group are not good followers. Box 12-2 lists some characteristics of good followers. An effective follower is one who is competent in performing his or her job responsibilities, has experience, has a positive attitude toward the role of the leader, and will help the leader achieve nursing team goals. A good follower will assist the leader by offering suggestions, giving information, willingly complying with assignments, asking for constructive criticism, and following policies and guidelines of the employer.

On the other hand, a follower who denies his or her incompetence, complains about assignments, withholds important information, rejects constructive criticism, and fails to abide by employer policies and guidelines hinders a leader's effectiveness.

Occasionally, a person in a follower role will take on an informal leadership role with peers. The informal leader has significant power within the group and is in a position to contribute to the leader's effectiveness or destroy the leader. When you are in a follower role, it is important that you avoid behaviors that prevent the leader from leading. If the leader is ineffective, the situation should be handled either through the employee grievance procedure or through a supervisor.

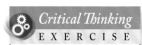

Critical Thinking
E X E R C I S E

For a little over 2 years, you have been the team leader on 2 West in an assisted living facility that opened about 3 years ago. You have worked with the same team since you became the team leader, and everyone works well together and gets along fantastically. Most of them socialize together outside of work. However, you thought you noticed some tension between two of your staff members last week, and today you have no doubt that you are right. The two of them are engaged in a shouting match in the laundry room. Their argument can be heard in every patient room on 2 West. What is your immediate response, why this response, and what do you think their response will be to you? After the shouting has stopped, what are at least four courses of action you could take? What effect might your decision have on the remaining team members?

Use appropriate Characteristics of Critical Thinkers in Box 1-2 on pages 18–19 to develop your responses to these questions.

BOX 12-2	Followership Qualities

Competent	Shares information
Experienced	Willingly accepts assignments
Positive attitude	Asks for constructive criticism
Offers suggestions	Follows policies and guidelines
Loyal to the group	Supports team decisions

✔ *A good follower avoids actions that would sabotage the leader's effectiveness.*

DEVELOPING LEADERSHIP SKILLS

Not everyone wants or should be in a leadership position. It is as important to the nursing team to be a positive team member as it is to be an effective team leader. If you have the desire and interest to be a leader, do all you can to be effective. If you find that you have no desire to be a leader, do all you can to be a supportive follower. The task of learning to be an effective leader is never finished, and there is always room to improve your leadership skills. Change can occur when you realize that your skills are not what you want them to be. Ask peers or supervisors to help you be more aware of your behaviors as a leader. Ask them to point out behaviors that do not enhance your effectiveness as a leader; then, take some calculated risks that include behaviors that are new to you. If you frequently forget to recognize and praise excellent work, remind yourself to look for opportunities to do this. If your team is not working well together, schedule a team meeting to find ways of creating a more pleasant working environment. If you are insensitive to your team members' needs, try to develop a better awareness of their problems and concerns.

✔ *Remember to say "Please," "Thank you," and "Great job!"*

Reading journal articles and books on leadership skills can provide insight into your own leadership strengths and areas that could be improved. Completing online continuing education programs and attending workshops and seminars can also provide opportunities to learn and practice new leadership skills.

 THE *Web*

> Mind Tools, LTD. is a commercial Web site that provides many interactive self-assessments and online training courses related to leadership and management skills.

You can also get information about leadership skills from additional Web sites by typing in the address of your favorite search engine and searching for "nursing leadership."

SUMMARY

Whether you prefer being a leader or a follower, it is important that you learn as much about each role as you can. It would be rare to find an individual who possesses all the leadership skills discussed in this chapter. However, to be effective, a leader must know what skills are important and work to acquire as many of these skills as possible. Continue learning about your own strengths and about how you can improve your skills. Don't be afraid to admit when you make mistakes, and don't be afraid to compliment your staff when they earn it.

It would also be rare to find individuals who possess all the followership skills discussed in this chapter. Good followership skills are as important to the team as good leadership skills. Team members must work to develop "following" skills that enhance the leader's effectiveness.

Good leaders who have good followers have the potential to provide excellent patient care in a pleasant working environment. Both leaders and followers can feel satisfaction in knowing that together they made a patient's stay in a health care facility as comfortable as possible.

APPLY
Critical Thinking Skills

1. In the opening story at the beginning of this chapter, Jamila and Cindy both realized that they would need more preparation if they ever wanted to be "in charge." After reading this chapter, what are three or four things they could do to prepare for this "in charge" role?

2. Use a search engine or your school library to develop a list of some journals and organizational Web sites that publish articles on leadership and management.

3. Select one or two leadership qualities that you think are important, and practice incorporating these in your relationships with your peers.

4. Interview a nursing leader in your clinical affiliation and ask the following questions:

   How long have you been a leader?
   What education did you have for your position as a leader?
   What advice would you give to someone who wanted to be a team leader?
   What is the most difficult part of your job as a leader?
   What is the most rewarding part of your job as a leader?

5. Get five or six of your classmates together and role-play the following situation: You are the team leader and your classmates are the team members. The team members tell you that they want you to schedule a team meeting to discuss their lunch assignments. Currently, you make the lunch assignment by 10:00 am and lunch is 30 minutes. Your team members want lunch times assigned by 7:30 am and they want 45 minutes for lunch.

Read More
ABOUT IT

Alfaro-Lefevre R: Critical Thinking and Clinical Judgment: A Practical Approach, 5th ed. St. Louis, MO: Saunders, 2013.

Dahikemper TR: Anderson's Nursing Leadership, Management, and Professional Practice for the LPN-LVN in Nursing School and Beyond, 5th ed. Philadelphia, PA: FA Davis, 2013.

Huber DL: Leadership and Nursing Care Management, 5th ed. St. Louis, MO: Saunders, 2014.

Kelly P, Tazbir J: Essentials of Nursing Leadership & Management, 3rd ed. Clifton Park, NJ: Delmar, 2013.

Marquis BL, Huston CJ: Leadership Roles and Management Functions in Nursing, 8th ed. Philadelphia, PA: Lippincott Williams & Wilkins, 2014.

Sullivan EJ: Effective Leadership and Management in Nursing, 8th ed. Upper Saddle River, NJ: Prentice-Hall, 2012.

Yoder-Wise PS: Leading and Managing in Nursing, 5th ed. Revised Reprint. St. Louis, MO: Mosby, 2014.

Yoder-Wise PS: Nursing Leadership and Management Online for Yoder-Wise Leading and Managing in Nursing—Revised Reprint (User Guide and Textbook), 5th ed. St. Louis, MO: Mosby, 2014.

Management Skills

LEARNING OBJECTIVES

When you complete this chapter, you will be able to:

1. Describe the personal qualities and educational and experience requirements of a manager of a patient or resident unit.

2. Apply beginning skills associated with managing care for a group of patients.

3. Apply beginning skills associated with ordering supplies and equipment.

4. Continue developing effective communication skills.

5. Integrate knowledge of your state nurse practice laws, employer policies, job descriptions, and staff capabilities when making management decisions.

6. Describe some of the general responsibilities of the charge nurse for maintaining a safe environment.

7. Maintain an environment that eliminates or at least minimizes the risk of illness or injury to patients.

8. Create an environment that encourages visitors to spend time with a patient.

The entire class seemed to be talking at the same time, but an immediate hush fell over the room when Ms. Donnelly, the teacher, entered. "I could hear you talking all the way down the hall," Ms. Donnelly said. "What is causing all the excitement?" For a few moments, no one said anything until Jackie raised her hand. "Yes, Jackie?" "Well," said Jackie, "we were just talking about that assignment you gave us on management. We think that every manager we were assigned to observe has a different style." "Can you be more specific?" asked Ms. Donnelly

"Our assignment was to observe a nurse manager and to write down how he or she makes patient assignments, keeps supplies, evaluates performance, manages time, and communicates with others. I was comparing my notes with Roberto, and our two managers seemed to be quite different. For example, the manager I observed made patient assignments in the afternoon for the next day, and Roberto's manager didn't make assignments until about an hour after the shift started. My manager had plenty of supplies on the utility room shelves, and they were organized and easy to find. Roberto said that his manager didn't have many supplies and that the utility room was a mess."

"What you and Roberto found was what I had hoped you would find," said Ms. Donnelly. "There are many different styles of management, and you have given us two examples of how different styles could affect the staff. Managing a patient unit is a complex task. Management skills can be learned and, with experience, these skills should improve. Our class today will explore what you found during your observation, how certain management behaviors can affect the staff, and what you need to know to prepare for a position as a manager."

Management is the coordination of all of the activities associated with delivering nursing services. Although nursing services are offered in many different types of health care settings, licensed practical/vocational nurses (LP/VNs) are most often offered management positions in long-term care facilities, assisted living facilities, boarding homes, group practice offices, and rehabilitation centers, to name a few. As the health care system changes, as new laws are passed, and as more people obtain health insurance and seek health care, LP/VNs will probably be offered management positions in more and different types of health care settings.

✔ *Management is the coordination of all activities associated with delivering nursing care.*

In this chapter, you will learn about some of the qualities and skills nurses need to be successful managers.

PERSONAL QUALITIES OF MANAGERS

Being a good manager requires a combination of management and leadership qualities. Leadership qualities are the subject of Chapter 12, and if you have not already done so, you should read that chapter now.

A person can be an excellent leader and a poor manager or a poor leader and an excellent manager. The skills and behaviors for each are very different. The

| BOX 13-1 | **Qualities of an Effective Manager** |

Outstanding clinical skills
Outstanding communication skills
Organized
Punctual
Knows and follows the rules
Adheres to schedules
Solves problems quickly
Anticipates staff needs for equipment and supplies
Prevents situations from becoming problems
Works well with others
Finds ways to streamline work
Gets broken equipment fixed promptly
Delegates work assignments according to skills and ability

✔ *Leadership qualities and management skills are essential for success.*

most effective person to be the "boss" is the one who has developed the qualities of both an effective leader and an effective manager.

An effective manager needs to develop behaviors and traits that will enable the staff to do their work as efficiently and effectively as possible. For example, the effective manager must be organized and able to create order out of chaos. The patient care unit can become a very busy place, and left to its own, it can become so chaotic that patient care suffers. The effective manager uses organizational skills to develop priorities, direct the work, and keep the work flowing in a positive direction. Box 13-1 summarizes some of the other qualities of an effective manager.

A good manager must make efficient use of available time. Much of how you manage your time, whether at work or at home or in school, is a matter of habit. Complete the self-assessment test "How Well Do You Manage Your Time?" on pages 268–271 to get an idea of how you currently manage your time. You may find that there are some things you can do now to change habits that waste time.

Hundreds of self-help books are available that can help you learn to manage time more efficiently. Practicing time management skills now will help you when you are responsible for managing the care of a group of patients.

✔ *Experience can be an excellent teacher.*

Being a manager of a patient unit is a position of great responsibility and one that requires preparation. Experience and education are two things that anyone who hopes to become a manager must have.

Working as a staff nurse provides opportunities to observe other managers in action. You will see what works and what does not work in various situations. You will develop an understanding of your job as well as of the job of others on your team. You will be able to think about what you might do in certain situations. You will learn about the complexities of the patient unit through the variety of experiences you will accumulate over a period of time.

EDUCATION

In addition to experience both in clinical practice and in observing other managers, preparation for a management position requires additional education. Continuing education courses, mentoring programs, professional journals, formal courses at a college or on the Internet, distance learning courses, and certification programs in clinical specialties all contribute to developing the skills that a good manager will need.

ASSESS YOURSELF   How Well Do You Manage Your Time?

Answer these 26 questions as honestly as you can. You should get an idea of how well or badly you manage your time, as well as which habits are your worst time-wasters.

1. When you are faced with a task that requires careful attention to detail, how are you likely to react?
   a. I hate highly detailed work. I avoid it as much as possible. I'll gloss over the details and try to get the "big picture" quickly.
   b. I love highly detailed work. I could spend my life doing it. In fact, when I have such work to do, I'm likely to stretch it out because I enjoy it so much.
   c. I fall between the two extremes. I can do highly detailed work, but I know when to wrap it up and get on to other things.

2. Do you generally put in longer hours than do other people who work at jobs similar to yours?
   a. Yes, just about all the time
   b. Yes, frequently
   c. Occasionally
   d. Rarely or never

3. Is it very important to you to feel popular with coworkers?
   a. Yes
   b. Somewhat
   c. Not really

4. Would you be more likely to agree or disagree with this statement: "If you want a job done well, you usually have to do it yourself."
   a. Agree
   b. Disagree

5. When you plan to meet someone at a specific time, do you usually arrive when you said you would?
   a. Yes
   b. I'm occasionally late
   c. I'm often late
   d. I'm just about always late

6. When an important decision has to be made at work, you generally prefer to make it
   a. On your own
   b. In conjunction with others at a meeting or brainstorming session

7. Are you a pack rat? Do you have trouble throwing things out even when you know there's virtually no chance you'll ever need them again?
   a. Yes
   b. Somewhat
   c. No

8. Do you have trouble saying no to people?
   a. Yes
   b. Sometimes
   c. No

9. Do you worry a lot?
   a. Yes
   b. Yes, but probably no more than most people
   c. Some, but not much
   d. No, hardly at all

10. Do you take up various interests, sports, or hobbies only to abandon them before you've achieved any real competence in the area you've chosen?

   a. Yes, frequently

   b. Sometimes

   c. Not usually

11. Do you often make false starts at work, beginning projects and then not finishing them?

   a. Yes

   b. No

12. Are you a perfectionist?

   a. Yes

   b. No

13. If you have two tasks to do and one is easy while the other is difficult, which one will you try to do first?

   a. The difficult one

   b. The easy one

14. When you have several things that need doing, do you have trouble setting priorities and deciding which are the most crucial?

   a. Yes, a lot

   b. I have some trouble doing this.

   c. I have little or no trouble setting priorities.

15. Do you often try to do more than one thing at a time (such as studying or reading reports while you watch television)?

   a. Yes

   b. Occasionally

   c. No

16. Do you usually get things done on time?

   a. Yes

   b. No

   c. Sometimes yes, sometimes no

17. When faced with a task, do you usually set a deadline for yourself, even in instances where no official deadline has been imposed?

   a. Yes

   b. Sometimes

   c. No, I usually assign it a lower priority and do it when I have time

18. Do you tend to leave things until the last minute?

   a. Yes

   b. Sometimes

   c. No

19. Would you be more likely to agree or disagree with this statement: "I find I often underestimate the amount of time I need to get things done."

   a. I agree

   b. I disagree

continued on page 270

20. How's your attention span?
    a. Very good. I can concentrate for long periods of time without getting distracted.
    b. Pretty good. I can concentrate when I really have to, but if I'm not under heavy pressure, my concentration sometimes slips.
    c. Pretty bad. It takes a great deal of effort for me to stay focused, and I can concentrate only for brief periods.
    d. Very bad. I am easily distracted despite my efforts to concentrate, and I have a hard time completing tasks.

21. Would you say that, deep down, you really know what you want out of life?
    a. Yes
    b. No

22. Do you feel you never really have enough time to do all the things you need to do?
    a. Yes
    b. Sometimes I feel like that
    c. Not usually

23. Do you often work on holidays and weekends, and postpone or cancel vacations because you have too much work to do?
    a. Yes
    b. No

24. By the end of the day have you usually accomplished the things you set out to do when you began the day?
    a. Yes
    b. Not always, but most of the time
    c. No
    d. I don't generally set an agenda for my day. I take things as they come.

25. Is the area where you do your primary work messy and disorganized?
    a. Yes
    b. Somewhat, but it's not badly disorganized
    c. No

26. Which of the following statements most closely reflects your decision-making style?
    a. I often make impulsive, spur-of-the-moment decisions.
    b. I don't make a decision until I have every possible relevant and useful fact at hand.
    c. I'm between the two extremes.

SCORING

For each of your answers, find the assigned point value below, and add all the values. The highest possible score is 130, the lowest is 26.

1. a = 1, b = 2, c = 3	**10.** a = 1, b = 3, c = 5	**19.** a = 1, b = 5
2. a = 1, b = 2, c = 4, d = 5	**11.** a = 1, b = 5	**20.** a = 5, b = 5, c = 1, d = 1
3. a = 1, b = 3, c = 5	**12.** a = 1, b = 5	**21.** a = 5, b = 1
4. a = 1, b = 5	**13.** a = 5, b = 1	**22.** a = 1, b = 3, c = 5
5. a = 5, b = 4, c = 2, d = 1	**14.** a = 1, b = 3, c = 5	**23.** a = 1, b = 5
6. a = 5, b = 1	**15.** a = 1, b = 3, c = 5	**24.** a = 5, b = 5, c = 1, d = 1
7. a = 1, b = 3, c = 5	**16.** a = 5, b = 1, c = 2	**25.** a = 1, b = 3, c = 5
8. a = 1, b = 3, c = 5	**17.** a = 5, b = 3, c = 1	**26.** a = 1, b = 1, c = 5
9. a = 1, b = 2, c = 4, d = 5	**18.** a = 1, b = 3, c = 5	

96–130 points: You are extremely thrifty with your time. You manage it well and don't get sidetracked easily into doing things you didn't plan to do. You are probably extremely good at setting priorities, and you don't let minor things take up major portions of your time. You are not necessarily one of those people who seem to have something scheduled for every minute of every day. Such people, though they seem efficient, often are the biggest time-wasters. They look busy because they manage time poorly and consequently are always on the verge of being swamped by the things they have to do. Actually, people who score high on this psychograph often look like time-wasters. This is because they organize their priorities so well that they have plenty of time left over to do as they like. The executive who spends large chunks of time on the golf course or the tennis court is often the most effective type of manager. He knows how to delegate work so he doesn't get bogged down in minor details that his subordinates should handle. Those in this high-scoring category may sometimes appear to be chronic daydreamers. But their daydreams are not wasted. Someone like Albert Einstein may have looked like he spent large amounts of time puttering around and daydreaming, but it would be hard to argue that he didn't use his time productively.

61–95 points: You are about average when it comes to wasting time. When something is really important, you'll usually get it done on time and in good order, but in other areas of your life you tend to be lackadaisical about organizing your time. Things you would like to do get put off because you never seem to have time; noncritical work assignments keep slipping further and further down in the growing pile of paperwork on your desk; the dreams of accomplishment you once had seem to recede further and further from your reach. If you don't get organized, you'll find your life has sped by without you ever doing the things you most wanted. Look at any answers you chose that carried point values of 1 or 2. These are your weak areas; start working on them.

26–60 points: You are a spendthrift when it comes to time. You very rarely get full value for the time that slips through your fingers at an alarming rate. However, because time-wasting is basically due to bad habits, you can do something about it. To improve your habits in using your time, work on these areas: concentration, setting priorities, and keeping a time diary.

Copyright 1998, Allies Consulting. Adapted with permission from Allies Consulting, San Rafael, CA.

 THE *Web*

> Go to the Cumulative Index to Nursing and Allied Health Literature (CINAHL) Web site to search more than 1,300 journals for full text of articles on management of nursing care.

If your goal is to someday become a manager of a patient or resident unit, you need to develop a plan to help you reach that goal. Ask good managers what steps they took to prepare for the role of manager or discuss your goals with a school counselor. Learn as much as you can about what experience and personal characteristics made other people successful managers. Develop a written time line that describes what you will do to reach your goal and by when. Keep a portfolio that documents all of the knowledge and skills you have gained through educational programs and clinical experiences.

Certifications

One of the most common ways to document the knowledge and skills you gained through education and experience is to complete the processes required to receive national certification in a specialty area. National certification indicates that a person has, on a written exam, by experience, or both, demonstrated extensive knowledge and skills related to a clinical specialty. LP/VNs can apply

✔ *A good manager has strong clinical skills.*

for a number of national certifications with more certification exams being added every year.

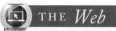 THE *Web*

A few of the certifications available to LP/VNs can be found on the Web sites of the following organizations:
National Association for Practical Nurse Education and Service
    NAPNES Certified in Long-Term Care (LPN, CLTC or LVN, CLTC)
    NAPNES Certified in Pharmacology (LPN, NCP or LVN, NCP)
    NAPNES Certified in I.V. Therapy (LPN, IVT or LVN, IVT)
National Federation of Licensed Practical Nurses
    IV Therapy certification
    Gerontology certification
Development Disabilities Nurses Association
    Certified Developmental Disabilities Nurse (CDDN)
Prepared Childbirth Educators, Inc.
    Breastfeeding Counselor Certification (CBC)
    Childbirth Educator Certification (CCE)
National Board of Certification of Hospice and Palliative Care Nurses
    Certified Hospice and Palliative Care Nurse (CHPLN)
National Alliance of Wound Care
    Wound Care Certified (WCC)

One must be careful when applying for a special certification. There are many organizations that offer certifications for nurses; however, not all certifications have value. If you aren't sure about the value of a certification or the organization offering it, check the creditability (worthy of confidence) of the organization.

One way to check the credibility of an organization is to find out if it is accredited by the National Commission for Certifying Agencies (NCCA). NCCA is an organization that promotes excellence in competency assessments for practitioners. You can think of NCCA as an accrediting agency for certification programs similar to the Accreditation Commission for Education in Nursing that accredits nursing schools. Membership in NCCA is expensive, and this is one reason why some agencies that offer well-known and highly valued certifications are not members.

THE *Web*

The Institute for Credentialing Excellence Web site provides a list of the organizations that are accredited by NCAA.

✔ *Certification in a specialty improves your credibility.*

Another way to check the credibility of an organization that offers certifications is to determine if it is a professional organization. NFLPN, NAPNES, State Boards of Nursing, and the National Council of State Boards of Nursing (NCSBN) are all examples of professional organizations. Certifications offered or endorsed by professional organizations are almost always highly valued.

The final way to check the credibility of a certification is to ask respected nursing educators, nurse managers, and directors of nursing. Nurses in these positions are quite likely to know which certifications have value and which do not.

Certification from a respected organization can significantly improve your credibility when you say, for example, "I am very knowledgeable about wound care." A certification in wound care will back up your verbal statement. A specialty certification will give you opportunities for employment in a variety of practice settings; the employer will sometimes require it; and it may provide an increase in salary or salary supplements in your job. A certification most of all presents evidence to your employer or potential employer and patients that you are committed to providing a high level of clinical care.

Now that you understand the personal qualities and the educational and clinical experience requirements for the position of a manager of a patient unit, you can begin to learn about managing a patient care unit.

LEVELS OF MANAGEMENT

The first level of management is the team leader, charge nurse, or manager of a patient care unit. The next level is supervisor, clinical specialist, or assistant director of nursing. The third level of management is chief nurse executive, vice president for nursing, or director of nursing. Each level of manager has specific duties that are generally written in a job or position description.

LP/VNs are most often first-level managers responsible for a specific patient unit. It is important for LP/VNs who are considering applying for a management position to know the nurse practice law and the scope of practice permitted in the state in which they work. Most states require that LP/VNs work under the supervision of a registered nurse, a primary care provider, or a dentist.

✔ *Many LP/VNs work as first-level managers.*

In addition, an LP/VN who is considering a management position should have 1 year or more of full-time clinical experience as a staff nurse. During this time, the nurse must use every opportunity to learn as much as he or she can about the care and treatment of patients in his or her area of practice. Strong clinical skills provide the foundation the nurse manager will need as he or she solves clinical problems and assesses and evaluates staff performance.

MANAGING PATIENT CARE

The effective manager (team leader, charge nurse, or patient care manager) combines strong clinical skills with high-quality leadership and management skills to direct patient care on a day-to-day basis. Managing day-to-day patient care includes
- Assessing staff capabilities
- Diagnosing patient needs for nursing care
- Planning and delegating patient care
- Implementing assignments
- Evaluating performance

✔ *Know the skills and abilities of each of your staff members.*

Assessing Staff Capabilities

The first step in directing patient care is to assess staff capabilities. To do this, you will need to know the functions all team members are legally permitted

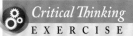

Critical Thinking
E X E R C I S E

You are the manager on 1 East. You know the abilities and personalities of your staff and have been making assignments and delegating duties to them for nearly 2 years. Today, you just found out that one of the seven members of your staff was injured in an automobile accident and will be unable to work for some time. Your supervisor assures you that she will send a replacement. You do get the replacement, but how do you know what this person can do? How do you verify this person's skills? What right do you have in asking to see this person's license and continuing education documentation? Is this really any of your business? What actions would you take and why? Use appropriate characteristics of Critical Thinkers in Box 1-2 on pages 18–19 to develop your responses to these questions.

✔ *Know the nursing needs of all of your patients.*

✔ *Know which team member is most qualified to meet the needs of the patient.*

to perform, their educational preparation, how long they have been working in their positions, and what technical and interpersonal skills they have.

The functions your staff is permitted to perform are defined by the nurse practice laws of your state and are also outlined in job descriptions developed by employers. The purpose of the nurse practice laws has been previously discussed and must be adhered to by all licensed nurses.

Job descriptions are written documents that outline what is expected from employees in each job title. Job descriptions for a typical nursing team would include separate descriptions for job titles such as LP/VN manager, staff LP/VN, certified nursing assistant, unlicensed assistant, and unit secretary. Although they are not employees as such, volunteers may also have job descriptions.

Knowing the educational preparation of your staff for their positions helps you decide how to best use them on your team. For example, if a new certified nursing assistant joins your staff, it is helpful to know whether this person completed a 75-hour or a 480-hour training course. The person who completed the 75-hour course will probably have less experience and fewer skills than the person who completed the 480-hour course. Having this information will help you decide how to best use this person on your team.

You will also need to know how long your team members have been working in their positions. Those who have several years of experience should be capable of working at a level that requires less supervision than those who have been in their positions for a short time.

Knowing the technical and interpersonal skills of your staff is also important. There may be those on your team who cannot perform all of the tasks listed in their job description. You have a responsibility as a manager not to assign tasks to someone who is incapable of performing them. Some staff members will have excellent interpersonal skills and would be able to work with anyone; others may work better when assigned to work with those with whom they get along.

Diagnosing Patient Needs for Nursing Care

The second step in directing patient care is to diagnose the particular nursing care needs of patients on your unit. Does the patient need care that can be provided only by an LP/VN, or can a nursing assistant meet a particular patient's care needs? At this point, you might also consider the personality of the patient. Although all nursing staff members should be able to meet the needs of any patient on your unit, it sometimes improves communication between the patient and the nurse when personalities are well matched.

Planning and Delegating Patient Care

The third step in directing patient care is to plan and delegate patient care. The plan is generally communicated through a written assignment sheet or assignment board. The assignment sheet includes the staff members' names, their break and meal times, room numbers of patients to whom they are assigned, and any other general duties that staff members are expected to complete during their time on duty.

When making assignments, it is important to be as fair as you can to every member of your team. Be sure the work is divided as evenly as possible and that patients who are physically or emotionally difficult to manage are not always assigned to the same person. Your experience as a staff nurse will make you aware of how physically difficult it is to care for an overweight, unresponsive patient day after day.

To delegate patient care means to assign some or all of the responsibility you have for the care of patients on your unit to someone else. You have a legal responsibility as a licensed nurse to delegate tasks according to applicable state laws, staff capabilities, and patient needs. It is important to exercise extreme caution when delegating tasks to unlicensed assistive personnel (UAPs) and others whose position is not well defined by law or by practice.

Because the delegation of nursing duties is of so much concern to nurses and to the public, in 2006, the National Council of State Boards of Nursing (NCSBN) and the American Nurses Association (ANA) jointly issued a statement on the delegation of nursing duties. Most state boards have also issued guidelines similar to those included in the NCSBN/ANA statement on the delegation of nursing duties to UAPs.

THE *Web*

The NCSBN and the ANA Joint Statement on Delegation can be viewed at the National Council of State Boards of Nursing Web site. Your state board of nursing guidelines for delegation of nursing duties can be viewed at your state board of nursing Web site.

✔ *When delegating duties, always apply the five rights of delegation.*

Contained in the NCSBN/ANA document is a list of the five rights of delegation (Fig. 13-1). These five rights are as follows:
1. Right task
2. Right circumstances
3. Right person
4. Right direction/communication
5. Right supervision/evaluation

Memorize these rights and apply them in every situation in which you have to make a decision about assigning tasks and duties to others.

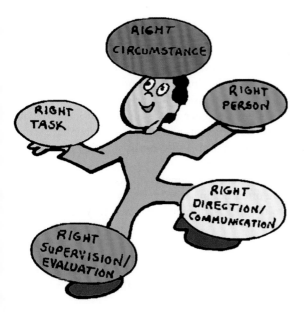

FIGURE 13-1. ● The five rights of delegation.

Before delegating any of your duties as a licensed nurse, whether in a management or staff position, you should completely understand the importance of proper and legal delegation of duties. If in doubt, ask a trusted supervisor for direction and advice.

Implementing Assignments

The fourth step in directing patient care is to post the written assignment sheet. The assignment sheet must be completed and available to staff at least 15–30 minutes (or as your employer policy dictates) before the shift begins so that staff members can determine their priorities and organize their workday. Giving verbal directions along with written assignments avoids confusion and misunderstanding between staff members and the manager.

✔ *Know how to communicate assignments to your staff.*

On occasion, it may be necessary to change an assignment. When this happens, the manager must verbally tell the staff member of the change as well as change the written assignment sheet. An effective manager would also explain why the change was necessary and acknowledge how the change affects the staff member.

Evaluating Performance

The fifth step in directing patient care is to evaluate the performance of your nursing staff. This is done through informal and formal evaluations.

Informal Evaluations

Informal evaluations are those that occur almost daily. As you supervise the work of your staff, you might ask yourself the following evaluation questions about each staff member: Do patients have any comments on their nursing care? Are procedures being done properly? Are assignments being completed on time? Are break and meal times being followed?

✔ *Use tact and firmness when handling difficult situations.*

If you find it necessary to discuss poor performance with a staff member, do so in a private place. Try to determine the cause of poor performance, and if the team member is lacking necessary knowledge or skills, provide information that will help improve performance. Otherwise, suggest that a certain quality of patient care is expected and that you expect everyone to provide that quality.

For example, suppose you see a nursing assistant piling dirty linen on a chair in a patient's room. The time to confront this breach in procedure is when it occurs. A verbal discussion (informal evaluation) with the nursing assistant should be all that is needed to correct the situation and prevent it from happening again. Remember: Conduct such discussions in a private place.

✔ *Be objective when evaluating the work of others.*

If a staff member is behaving in a manner that is unsafe and inappropriate, discreetly move the person away from patients and visitors, or call or have someone call for assistance from your supervisor. This difficult situation requires tact and sensitivity on the part of the manager.

Don't forget to acknowledge excellent judgment or exceptional patient care when it occurs. Managers are often dealing with so many different issues and problems that they forget to tell their staff members when they have done an outstanding job.

Formal Evaluations

Formal evaluations are written and include an assessment of an employee's overall performance over a period of time, usually a year. The form on which an evaluation is written is developed by the employer. These formal evaluations may be the basis for an increase in salary, so being fair and objective is of utmost importance.

Unless you keep some kind of journal or written notes, chances are that when the time comes for the annual evaluation, you will remember only what that employee did in the last few weeks. Written notes encourage a more objective evaluation and also allow you to furnish dates and specific events on which you base your comments. An employee may have been early for his or her shift for the past 11 months and late six times in the month before the evaluation. Writing on the evaluation that the employee is frequently late would not be a fair statement. It would be more objective to say that the employee was never late for 11 months and was late six times in the past month.

The first-line manager is expected to contribute to the evaluation of staff members. The manager should be familiar with the evaluation form and should make every effort to be objective when writing an evaluation. First-line managers should document both positive and negative staff behaviors with examples. When standards of performance are clearly understood by management and staff, evaluating performance is more objective. Managers must keep subjectivity and personal bias out of the evaluation process. It is possible to like a staff member but not the person's job performance, just as it is possible to dislike a staff member but to recognize that the individual's job performance is outstanding.

A written evaluation is always reviewed with the staff member. The staff member should be told in advance about the date and location of the review. You should find a quiet, private place for this conference. During this time, you can discuss the staff member's strengths and areas for improvement. Give the staff member an opportunity to respond to the evaluation and to your comments. The evaluation should end on a positive note with goals for the future.

As you evaluate performance of your staff and quality of nursing care each day, you also collect information that will assist you when you begin the same process the next day. Experience as a manager will provide valuable lessons in developing skills that contribute to quality patient care.

MANAGING THE UNIT

In addition to managing patient care, the team leader, charge nurse, or patient care manager has many other functions that contribute indirectly to patient care. These functions are related to the operation of the patient care unit and include ordering supplies and equipment and maintaining a safe environment.

Ordering Supplies and Equipment

Supplies and equipment essential for patient care must be available to your nursing staff. Responsibility for having necessary supplies and equipment on the patient unit belongs to the unit manager, or you may delegate (assign) this responsibility to a member of your staff. Regardless of whose responsibility it is to order supplies and equipment, you must periodically check to be sure they are being ordered properly.

All supplies, including drugs, must be put away promptly. Storage spaces must be kept neat and orderly so that items needed in an emergency can be located quickly. Equipment must be kept clean and in working order. Requests to repair equipment must be followed up on until repairs are completed.

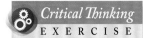
Critical Thinking EXERCISE

As the manager on 6 North, you are required to give your staff members an informal but written evaluation every 6 months. After you complete the evaluation, review it, and have it signed by your staff member, it goes to your supervisor. Part of your job rating is based on the quality of your evaluations of your staff. Your dilemma is this: You have an employee who does a really good job and deserves an excellent rating, but your supervisor has told you that he believes this person is incompetent and lazy. What are you going to do to give this person a fair evaluation and at the same time get a good evaluation for yourself? How many options do you have, and what might be the outcome of each option? Use appropriate characteristics of Critical Thinkers in Box 1-2 on pages 18–19 to develop your responses to these questions.

✔ *Having adequate supplies and proper equipment contributes to quality patient care.*

The manager is also responsible for being sure equipment and supplies are not wasted and that they are being consistently charged to the patient for whom they were used. Every patient care unit or department has an operating budget. The manager needs to know what that budget is and should periodically evaluate the level of spending. Correct billing of patients is extremely important to the financial health of the agency.

Maintaining a Safe Environment

Health care facilities are complex. They are filled not only with people in constant activity but also with all sorts of equipment, machines, and electronic devices. A wide variety of combustible materials, including flammable liquids and gases, are everywhere. As a manager, you are responsible for seeing that unsafe situations are corrected. Although not everything that needs fixing can be fixed immediately, certain measures can be taken to prevent further damage or even injury to people in that environment. The potential for an accident or a fire is never far away. Patients, dependent on you and others for their physical safety, are in the middle of it all.

Learn the fire and safety regulations of the facility you serve. Know the locations of all exits. Personally check where fire extinguishers are kept so that you know where to get one if needed. Require your staff to know the location of fire extinguishers, how to check pressure gauges on fire extinguishers, and how to use them. Be sure they know how to sound an internal fire alarm and when to call the local fire department. Review evacuation procedures and discuss the possibility of having a mock fire drill with your nursing supervisor.

If you do smell smoke or see flames, immediately follow the procedure set by your facility's regulations. Don't attempt to put out a fire without first informing the staff and sounding the required alarm. Don't panic. Your patients will need you if an evacuation is necessary.

Mention any safety problem, no matter how small, to your team leader. A loose wire, a lamp that sputters, a peculiar smell, a loose bed rail, a slippery spot on the floor, and a machine that feels hot but shouldn't are all significant enough to report.

✔ *Accept personal responsibility for creating a safe environment.*

Other aspects of patient safety may be less apparent, but just as important. Be sure the patient has an identification bracelet on the wrist. Check the name on the bracelet to be sure you are administering medications or treatments to the right patient. Be sure that medical supplies are removed after treatments or procedures are completed. A needle or other potentially dangerous piece of equipment left in the patient's bed or room can cause serious injury.

Know whether it is required that bed rails be up for a particular patient. If they are to be up, be sure they are up when you leave the patient's room. This is especially true for children in cribs. If the height of the bed is adjustable, be sure it is in the low position before you leave the patient. Use locking devices to ensure patient safety (see Fig. 13-2). If restraints are ordered to prevent a patient from injuring himself, be sure they are snug but not too tight. Check the patient frequently to be sure restraints have not constricted circulation.

✔ *Most accidents can be prevented.*

Clean up spills when they occur. Not only might a spill cause a patient to slip and fall, but also nurses and others may fall. Close doors and drawers when you are finished. Many an injury has been caused by tripping over open cabinet doors or bumping into the corner of an open door. Remove broken chairs, wheelchairs, and similar equipment from your unit to prevent inadvertent use. Require your staff to keep the medication room or medication cart locked when not in use.

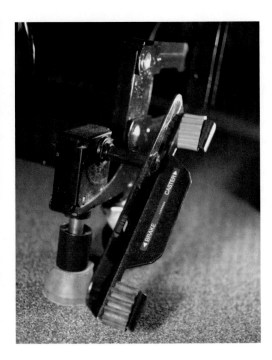

FIGURE 13-2. ● Locking devices are intended to improve patient safety.

There are many opportunities in the health care facility for accidents to occur. Use common sense, look around you, and accept personal responsibility for correcting situations that could lead to accidents and injury. Don't wait to be told to take action. If a situation is beyond your ability to correct (e.g., a frayed electrical cord), be sure you report it to your instructor or other appropriate person. Then, be persistent so that the situation that needs correcting is not forgotten.

✔ Make "Safety First" a rule on your patient care unit.

Violence in the workplace is a concern among health care workers. The Bureau of Labor Statistics reported 518 murders and nearly 2 million assaults in the workplace in 2010. About two thirds of these crimes occur in health care settings. Over 50% of the nursing population is affected by violence in the workplace. Drug and alcohol addiction, frustrations, anger, rage, increased stress due to staffing issues, and decreased insurance coverage can contribute to violent outbursts from staff, patients, and visitors.

With experience, common sense, and a concern for the safety of your patients and staff, you will develop a habit of looking for situations that are unsafe. As the manager, you must accept personal responsibility for correcting these situations.

 THE *Web*

The National Institute for Occupational Safety and Health Web site provides information on hospital violence including a section on safety tips for hospital workers.

MANAGING COMMUNICATION

As you learned in Chapter 3, good communication skills are essential in nursing. You will want to be sure you understand information you are receiving, and you will want to be clear in information you are sending.

✔ On April 14, 2003, all health care providers were required to implement the medical privacy rules of HIPAA.

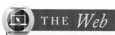

You will also want to be sure you are not communicating protected health information to those who have no need to know the information. On April 14, 2003, all providers of health care were required to implement the medical privacy rules of the 1996 federal law known as the Health Insurance Portability and Accountability Act (HIPAA). This law very clearly requires that everyone who has access to patient information keeps that information confidential. It also requires that health care providers (hospitals, doctors, dentists, nurses, pharmacists, etc.) inform patients of their privacy policies and practices in writing. When you accept employment in a health care facility, you will be required to complete a training program in which your employer will teach you the specific policies and procedures that their organization has developed to guide employees in complying with these privacy rules.

THE *Web*

For more information about confidentiality of health care information, visit the HIPAA regulations Web site.

Communicating With Visitors

Visitors

Most patients in a health care facility welcome visitors, but some have no visitors. For those without visitors, you and your coworkers become substitutes for the family, relatives, and friends who might otherwise stop in to see them.

The presence of visitors can have a major effect on the patient's recovery. The effect can be positive or negative. As an objective but concerned party in the patient's welfare, you can influence what that effect will be by creating a positive relationship with your patient's visitors. By being open, friendly, courteous, kind, and otherwise responsive to the visitor's concerns, you will instill a feeling of trust.

✔ Visiting hours are usually described in the patient's admission package.

Being friendly does not mean that you give up your authority when the patient's best interest is in question. You must remain firm and persuasive when visiting hours are over, when a distraught visitor would do more harm than good, if a scheduled procedure requires visitors to leave the room, and in other situations in which your duties supersede visitors' wishes. Yet you must demonstrate your authority in a pleasant way, even when the visitor resorts to unpleasantness.

Always respect your patient's privacy. If your duties can wait until visitors leave, avoid disturbing them. On the other hand, if nursing care is required, you may have to ask the visitors to leave the room. When it is necessary to ask visitors to leave, tell them how long you will be and suggest a comfortable place where they can wait. When you are finished, you can let the visitors know that they can return to the patient's room.

Consult with your instructor or facility guidelines regarding policies on visiting hours, when a patient can receive visitors, how many visitors are allowed, and other restrictions.

✔ HIPAA regulations limit the kinds of patient information you can provide to visitors.

The HIPAA regulations prevent you from giving protected health information to a visitor or even a member of the family. What you know about a patient's diagnosis, laboratory results, plan of treatment, or even the patient's room number is essentially confidential and not to be shared with anyone without the patient's written permission. You can tactfully suggest that these kinds of questions are best answered by the patient's primary care provider.

On occasion, visitors may become disruptive to the unit. As the manager, you must attempt to elicit their cooperation .If you are unsuccessful, you should immediately notify your nursing supervisor and ask for assistance.

Communicating With Supervisors

Your relationships with nursing supervisors can be positive and beneficial to you. It is important to recognize that your nursing supervisor is ultimately responsible for the quality of nursing care that you and your staff provide. You should view your supervisor as a resource person to whom you can go for advice and assistance in managing your patient unit.

To maintain a good working relationship with your nursing supervisor, you must keep him or her informed of problems or incidents that occur on your unit. Problems that may seem small and insignificant to you may turn out to be major problems to the institution. You must also report your errors and the errors of your staff to your supervisor and complete a written description of any negative incident that occurs on your unit.

✔ *Your supervisor is a source of advice and assistance.*

When you communicate with your nursing supervisor, it is important to present the facts of the situation clearly, concisely, completely, and objectively. It is unfair to the supervisor, who will probably have to make a decision related to a situation, to present only what you want the supervisor to know.

Your supervisor is, like you, in a management position. Just as your subordinates will not always like or understand all your decisions, you will not like or understand all the decisions of your supervisor. You must do your part to contribute to creating a relationship with your supervisor that is positive and productive, not negative and destructive.

Communicating With Primary Care Providers

Communicating with the patient's primary care provider is an essential part of management in nursing (Fig. 13-3). As in communicating with your supervisor, you should keep the primary care provider (doctor, physician assistant, nurse practitioner, etc.) informed of changes in the condition of his or her patient. You must be able to clearly and concisely describe the facts you are reporting.

If a primary care provider's treatment or medication order is unclear or questionable, it must be verified with the primary care provider. You are not expected to blindly follow orders that you believe could be harmful to your patients. It is

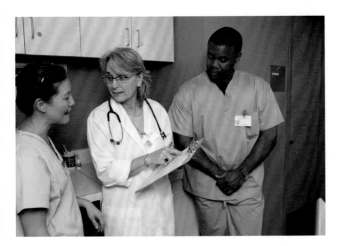

FIGURE 13-3. ● Share important information about your patients with their primary care providers.

important to use tact and good communication skills when requesting verification from the primary care provider.

You, through your staff, are in a position to provide valuable information about patients to their primary care providers. The nursing team spends a great deal of time with patients and consequently has information that may influence the methods a primary care provider chooses in treating patients. Sharing that information through verbal communication with primary care providers can make an enormous contribution to the total plan of care for patients. Thus, the team leader, charge nurse, or patient care manager must establish effective methods of communication with primary care providers.

Communicating With Other Departments

A significant amount of your communication will be with other departments within your facility and with agencies and organizations outside your facility. You may need to call the dietary department to report a missed meal tray or to request a special meal; you may need to call the rehabilitation department to reschedule a patient's appointment; you may need to call the dialysis center to clarify an order on the patient's chart; you may need to call a hospital to arrange for admission of one of your residents.

Whatever the reason for contacting another department or facility or for being contacted by them, you must apply all of the elements of good skills in communication. Being courteous and polite on the telephone will go a long way toward establishing an effective working relationship with these other departments. Be sensitive to the fact that you are not the only person asking for something. Be patient, and if the delay in response time seems to be extraordinarily long, question the delay with tact. Be careful to avoid blaming anyone, especially the person who happens to answer the telephone. Review Chapter 3 for more details on how to communicate effectively with others.

✔ *Work to maintain effective relationships with other departments and facilities.*

SUMMARY

Managing patient care is a tremendous responsibility, but with that responsibility can come equally tremendous rewards. You can enjoy the satisfaction that comes from working with your team, your supervisor, and primary care providers to provide the quality of nursing care that you could never achieve alone.

APPLY

Critical Thinking Skills

1. In the opening story at the beginning of this chapter, the two students were talking about the differences between the nurse managers they observed. In addition to those discussed in this chapter, what additional characteristics, traits, or behaviors are important for nurse managers and why?

2. Obtain the job or position descriptions for members of the nursing team in your clinical affiliation. Analyze each to determine the minimum education, experience, and skills required for the position.

3. In addition to the responsibilities of the patient care manager discussed in this chapter, list some of the other duties that might be assigned to this person.

4. Suppose you are the charge nurse of a 20-bed unit in an extended care facility, and one of the nursing assistants has not been coming back from her break on time. Outline what you would do and why.

5. While evaluating the quality of patient care, you notice that a bed rail is broken. What would you do first and why?

6. During your clinical experience, listen carefully to a conversation between a nurse and the nurse's supervisor. Analyze the conversation for its effectiveness in communicating information, ideas, or both. Was the purpose of the conversation understood by both the supervisor and the nurse? Was mutual respect evident? Was the conclusion of the conversation satisfactory to both parties? Were any comments made by either party after the other left?

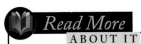

Read More
ABOUT IT

Anderson MA: Nursing Leadership, Management and Professional Practice for the LPN-LVN, 5th ed. Philadelphia, PA: FA Davis, 2013.

Belker LB, McCormick J, Topchik GS: The First Time Manager, 6th ed. New York, NY: AMACOM, 2012.

Cherry B, Jacob SR: Contemporary Nursing: Issues, Trends, & Management, 6th ed. St. Louis, MO: Mosby, 2014.

Covey SR: The 7 Habits of Highly Effective People: Powerful Lessons in Personal Change. New York, NY: Simon & Schuster, 2004.

Kennedy L, Foust, J: Communication for Nurses: Talking With Patients, 3rd ed. Burlington, MA: Jones & Bartlett Learning, 2014.

Marquis BL, Huston CJ: Leadership Roles and Management Functions in Nursing: Theory and Application, 8th ed. Philadelphia, PA: Lippincott Williams & Wilkins, 2014.

Sullivan EJ: Effective Leadership and Management in Nursing, 8th ed. Menlo Park, CA: Prentice-Hall, 2012.

Yoder-Wise PS: Nursing Leadership and Management Online for Yoder-Wise Leading and Managing in Nursing—Revised Reprint (User Guide and Textbook), 5th ed. St. Louis, MO: Mosby, 2014.

MOVING *Forward*

Beginning Your Nursing Career

LEARNING OBJECTIVES

When you complete this chapter, you will be able to:

1. Compile a list of places, other than hospitals and nursing homes, where an LP/VN could be employed.
2. Describe some activities that ease the transition from student to employee.

LEARNING OBJECTIVES *continued*

3. Explain the value of self-assessment before deciding on what type of nursing position to apply for.

4. List several sources of information on available nursing positions.

5. Prepare a chart that compares the fringe benefits of different positions.

6. Write a letter of application.

7. Prepare a personal résumé.

8. Write a letter of resignation.

9. Name and give the purposes of the nursing organizations to which LP/VNs usually belong.

10. Describe the influence of the political process on health care.

11. Compare the advantages and disadvantages of union membership.

"We're nearing the end of our year together so I'd like to say a few things that I hope you'll remember. I've enjoyed being your instructor for almost a year now. But I'm not speaking as your instructor today. What I have to say is coming from the heart of someone who cares about nursing and cares about each one of you."

"Sixty years ago, nurses wore starched white uniforms and nursing caps, stood when a doctor entered the ward, provided all of the personal care a patient needed, and gave all of the medications and treatments that were ordered. They were not asked their opinions about a patient's response to treatment, and they did not have aides to assist them. When I became a nurse about 30 years ago, nursing was quite different from what it was then. We wore white uniforms, but caps were optional. Those of us who were lucky had nurse aides and orderlies to assist with patient care. We were beginning to be respected for our knowledge and skills by the physicians with whom we worked. We documented our nursing care on paper charts. Some of us were just beginning to be legally permitted to start IV's on the patient unit. And most of us worked in a hospital.

In the years since I graduated, I have seen many, many changes. Computerized medical records, digital radiography, single-dose medication administration systems, short hospital stays, technology everywhere, outpatient surgery, patient barcodes, disposable medical equipment, and ethnic, cultural, and gender diversity on the nursing team are just a few changes I have experienced. And more of my classmates work in health care setting outside a hospital than in a hospital.

Had I not kept up with these changes through continually learning new ways of doing things, I wouldn't be here teaching this class today. And that's the 'message' in what I want to say to you today."

"There's no way that all of us on the staff could fully prepare you for the many choices you will face. There are simply too many. You've been busy enough learning what we could teach you. The other things you will have to know—the choices you will be making—are going to be up to you. Once you graduate, you'll be on your own. Oh, we'd love for you to come back anytime, and you know you're always welcome. But out there, out in the world of nursing practice, you won't have someone to remind you to finish an assignment, to practice a procedure until perfect, or to read up on something you're uncertain of. Those things and many more will be expected from you, including things you haven't even heard of yet, just as my class hadn't heard of laparoscopy surgery."

"Now, just for a moment, let me pretend I'm one of you. This is what I would say: 'But, Mrs. Fuller, if we haven't heard of something, how are we supposed to know what to do?' Yes, it sounds funny, but isn't that what you were thinking? I thought so. So listen now to the answer."

"Nursing is dynamic, growing, and ever-expanding. It will never again be what it is today, and what it becomes tomorrow will also change. Nursing moves into the future automatically. Nurses do not. I'll say that again. Nurses do not automatically keep up with nursing. Nurses move into the future by listening, watching, and preparing for it."

"All of you are ready for graduation because you have prepared for it, day by day, for almost a year. Those of you who will be in nursing's future have to begin preparing for it, day by day, starting today."

"Thank you class—you've been wonderful."

Today's newly graduated practical/vocational nurse has options undreamed of by those who completed their programs just a few years ago (Fig. 14-1). Finding that first job requires thoughtful preparation on your part, and it also requires knowing what career opportunities are available.

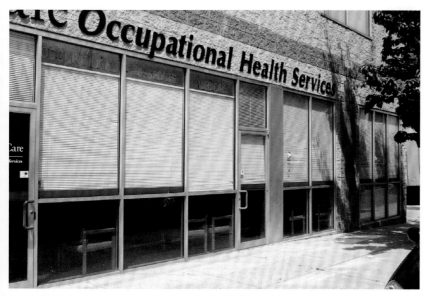

FIGURE 14-1. ● Employment opportunities for LP/VNs continue to expand.

CAREER OPPORTUNITIES IN NURSING

Just as you probably evaluated your educational options before you chose your nursing school, you must also evaluate your employment options. Selecting your first nursing position will be an important decision and one that should be made very carefully.

The employment opportunities for licensed practical/vocational nurses (LP/VNs) extend beyond those provided by hospitals and nursing homes. As private businesses and government agencies respond to the growing needs of a complex society, more areas where nursing care is needed are opening. You have an opportunity to look for the type of nursing that best meets your personal interests, needs, and capabilities.

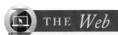

THE *Web*

Use the Internet to find Web sites that list job opportunities in the area in which you want to work.

Hospital Nursing

In no work setting has there been more change than in hospitals. Today, people are rarely admitted to hospitals for diagnostic studies or procedures, such as removal of gallstones. Mothers and their babies leave the hospital after 2 days—not 3 to 5 days as they did just a few years ago. With so many "short" procedures being done on an outpatient basis and with much shorter lengths of stay in the hospital, many hospitals have decreased the number of inpatient beds as well as the number of staff, including nurses. Patients who are admitted to hospitals now are much sicker, and many require a level of care that can only be provided by highly trained registered nurses (RNs).

✔ *According to the American Hospital Association, in 2000, there were 6,300 hospitals with more and 1 million staffed beds. In 2012, there were 5,723 hospitals with 920,829 staffed beds.*

Although employment opportunities for LP/VNs in inpatient units in acute care hospitals may be declining, there are opportunities for employment for LP/VNs in other areas of hospitals. LP/VNs often work in hospital-based clinics, outpatient same-day surgery units, operating rooms, radiology units, hospital-based long-term care units, or a home health department that is a part of the hospital. If working in a hospital is your career goal, you should look beyond the traditional patient care unit for opportunities for employment.

Hospital work schedules are generally set in three 8½-hour shifts. For example, there can be day (7:00 am to 3:30 pm), evening (3:00 to 11:30 pm), and night (11:00 pm to 7:30 am) shifts. Some health care institutions offer 12-hour shifts with full benefits for an employee who works between 24 and 36 hours a week. The institution sets shift, weekend, and holiday rotations, time off, and other scheduling procedures. Scheduling may vary from one institution to another to accommodate staffing needs and personal needs of employees.

Community and Public Health Nursing

Nurses who work in community or public health care experience a very different nursing setting. There, nursing is provided to patients under the administration of established health care programs. These programs are operated and funded by voluntary agencies or local, state, or federal government agencies.

Nurses employed in public health may work inside community health centers with patients who come to the center, or they may work outside the center, traveling to the patient's home to give care there. The nursing staff of a city's Department of Health clinic, for example, may provide in-clinic immunizations, prenatal care and counseling, and other services to individuals who visit the clinic, or they may give the same services at a person's residence.

The LP/VN in public health will work under the direction of an RN or other qualified supervisor. Among the qualifications for this work is the ability to work independently and responsibly when away from the health center.

✔ *Employment opportunities for LP/VNs are increasing in community and public health agencies.*

Office Nursing

An especially challenging opportunity for an LP/VN is that of the office nurse. As the employee of a physician, dentist, or other health care provider, an office nurse may be responsible for a variety of duties in addition to nursing duties.

In a small office, the nurse may be the receptionist, secretary, lab assistant, bookkeeper, and supply clerk. He or she may perform preliminary patient examinations and routine treatments, oversee a waiting room full of patients, assist with treatments, schedule appointments, and collect payment for the visit.

✔ *Nurses work in the offices of doctors, dentists, veterinarians, researchers, podiatrists, and other health care providers.*

In larger offices, the nurse may only have nursing duties, with other staff members completing clerical and scheduling tasks. Flexibility, adaptability, self-direction, and excellent communication skills are important assets for office nurses.

Private Duty Nursing

The private duty nurse works directly for a patient. Nursing care may be given in an institution, at the patient's home, or at another place requested by the patient. The patient is the nurse's employer and pays the nurse directly. A self-employed, private duty nurse is responsible for handling taxes, licenses, and other financial matters relating to self-employment.

✔ *The private duty nurse provides comprehensive care to one patient.*

A private duty nurse in an institution is subject to the institution's policies and direction and is responsible to the physician or other authority in charge of a patient's care. In a home setting, although working under the direction of the patient's physician, the nurse must have the skills and knowledge needed to function without direct assistance from others.

Home Health Nursing

The principle of home health nursing is to provide nursing services in the patient's home. Although many agencies provide these services, the best known are the visiting nurse societies and associations.

The home health nurse or visiting nurse goes to the patient's home and provides a variety of nursing services for the patient (see Fig. 14-2). This position also requires that the nurse teaches family members to care for their relative. The usual length of a home visit ranges from 30 to 90 minutes, depending on the needs of the patient and family.

✔ *According to the National Association for Home Care and Hospice, in 2014, there were more than 33,000 agencies providing home care services to more than 7 million individuals.*

It is far less costly to care for patients in their homes than it is to care for them in a hospital or nursing home. Most patients also prefer to be at home in familiar surroundings. For this reason, the number of nurses employed in home health nursing agencies has steadily increased since 2000.

Nurses who provide nursing care in the patient's home must have excellent clinical skills as well as good communication and teaching skills. They often have to be creative in improvising equipment and supplies and must be able to accurately document each visit. Home health nurses must be self-directed and able to prioritize work to benefit the client.

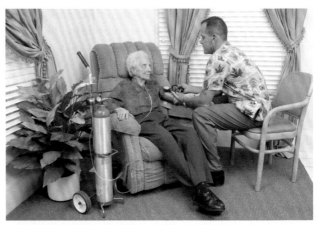

FIGURE 14-2. ● The number of nurses who choose home health nursing is increasing.

Industrial/Occupational Nursing

Factories and manufacturing plants have had limited in-plant nursing services for years. Generally oriented to first aid with an emphasis on accident prevention, health services were established in response to the influence of labor unions. Today, as business and industry provide more services for their employees, nursing opportunities in the industrial sector are increasing.

> ✔ Industrial and occupational nurses must be skilled in first aid and emergency care.

With a concern for good health now a national issue, many companies have developed health-oriented programs that address more than on-the-job accident prevention and treatment. Companies provide physical exams, screening tests, diagnostic surveys, wellness programs, nutrition counseling, fitness areas, and a variety of other health-related programs.

Industrial and occupational nurses need an ability to assess the learning needs of employees and to plan and conduct programs to meet those needs. They must also be skilled in handling emergency and first-aid situations.

Hospice Nursing

The hospice movement is dedicated to making the inevitable death of terminally ill patients dignified and humane. It provides compassionate care and understanding in settings that are comfortable and familiar.

> ✔ The National Hospice and Palliative Care Organization reports that more than 1.7 million people received hospice services in 5,500 hospice programs in 2012.

Nurses who work with dying patients require specialized training as well as a good understanding of themselves and of their patient's unique place in the world. The nurse in a hospice setting must also be able to interact with the patient's family, yet not interfere with the patient's and family's personal relationships and business.

Hospice care is based on a philosophy that can be implemented in a variety of settings. Most hospice services are provided in the home; however, they can also be provided in hospitals, long-term care facilities, and other health care settings.

School Nursing

School nursing, like nursing services in business and industry, has expanded from the delivery of simple first aid, immunizations, and health screenings to a comprehensive program of prevention, treatment, and education. Depending on the size and philosophy of a school district, a school nursing department can be small or extensive. A single nurse may serve a number of schools, or each school may have its own nurse. The RN in a school or schools functions independently and is generally under the authority of a physician appointed by the school district's board of education. LP/VNs assist the RN with routine screening programs and daily activities associated with school nursing.

School nurses have to enjoy being around and working with children. They often provide health-related instruction in the school and work with families to improve health care for the children.

✔ School nurses can be role models for children.

Nursing Homes

The rise in the number of elderly Americans has accounted for a significant increase in the need for nursing and convalescent homes to care for older people who are unable to provide for themselves at home but who do not require hospitalization. The need for nurses to staff these institutions has increased accordingly.

A nursing home may be privately endowed or funded by local or state money. It may be a for-profit or not-for-profit institution, and it must be licensed by the state in which it is located. Services provided may range from simple custodial caretaking to complete medical and rehabilitative care. In general, nursing care is supervised by an RN who is responsible for the overall care of residents under the direction of a physician on call. LP/VNs are often employed as charge nurses, and they direct day-to-day delivery of nursing care.

✔ About 39% of licensed practical and vocational nurses work in nursing care facilities.

Veterans Administration Hospitals

The Veterans Administration's (VA's) hospital system is the nation's largest, and its hospitals are some of the biggest. They are federally operated hospitals that care for veterans of the U.S. Armed Forces. Many of the VA hospitals are affiliated with schools of medicine and nursing.

A wide range of job experience, potential for travel, and other benefits are associated with employment in VA health care facilities. The VA lists job openings on their VA Careers Web site.

✔ In 2014, there were more than 152 VA medical centers and nearly 1,400 community-based outpatient treatment centers providing care to more than 8.3 million veterans each year.

Other Employment Opportunities

LP/VNs often work in shelters for the homeless, boarding homes, group homes for people who are mentally challenged, prisons, outpatient psychiatric clinics, neighborhood health clinics, day care centers for children and older adults, and rehabilitation facilities. Although the roles of LP/VNs vary from setting to setting, they are in a position to provide a variety of health care services from giving medications to performing nursing skills to teaching people how to prevent illness.

LP/VNs also work for insurance companies and in managed care businesses. In these positions, their responsibilities may include coding treatments and procedures, doing physical examinations for insurance policies, and reviewing medical records.

✔ LP/VNs work in a wide variety of settings.

Many companies that sell medical equipment and supplies find that hiring LP/VNs is cost-effective for them. They find it easier to teach someone who knows about health care how to sell a product than to teach someone who knows how to sell a product about health care.

Getting that first job may not be easy, but being aware of the many, many places where you could work will certainly increase your chances of success.

EMPLOYER EXPECTATIONS

Regardless of where you choose to work, employers have certain general expectations of their employees. Knowing what employers expect of employees in any work situation will help you understand and accept your new role.

Employers expect you to have a theoretical basis for what you do and for you to understand the care you give, how to give it, what is expected from it, and what the effects of that care will be, so that, if necessary, additional action can be taken. Your nursing skills and how well you perform them will be expected to be comparable with other nurses who have the same level of education and experience. An employer will expect you to complete your assignments within a reasonable period of time.

Employers expect a nurse who does not know how to perform a skill, or who needs help, to ask for assistance. Employers will expect you to function within the law and according to the job description for your position.

Employers expect you to contribute to the organization by participating in conferences, serving on committees, and maintaining the skills required of the position. Employers expect you to support their philosophy and implement their organization's objectives. They expect you to be loyal to the organization and fair in your relationships with them.

✔ *Employers have clearly defined job expectations.*

Employers expect you to know how to keep records of your activities. Because medical records are so important to patient care and are legal documents, skills in documenting your activities are definitely expected. Although most employers allow time to learn their specific system, once the system is learned, you will be expected to keep accurate, legible, and technically and grammatically correct records.

Employers expect you to assume responsibility for your work. This includes specific obligations spelled out in the hiring agreement and other implied obligations such as honesty, promptness, and commitment to the job.

As you begin your career in practical/vocational nursing, your skills and abilities may not yet match all of your employer's expectations. Making the transition from being a student to being a productive employee who is able to meet an employer's expectations can be a difficult process.

TRANSITIONAL CHALLENGES

If you decide to become an employee in the institution where you were assigned for clinical experience, the transition may be relatively easy. If you decide to accept a position in an institution that is unfamiliar to you, the transition may be more difficult. In either case, some transitional challenges will confront you as a beginning nurse. Being prepared to meet these challenges will help you adjust to your first job as an LP/VN.

There are many differences between being a student nurse and being a graduate practical or vocational nurse. When you are a student, the conditions under which you are learning are controlled to provide maximum educational benefit to you and your classmates. Your clinical assignments are selected to contribute to your educational development.

Your clinical instructor is legally responsible for your performance in the clinical area and is there to help you resolve problems and answer questions.

As a graduate, you will receive assignments based on the needs of your patients and employer. You will be responsible and accountable for your own actions. And you will be expected to carry out your assignments within the allotted time.

✔ *Expect to experience some difficult times as you make the transition from student to staff member.*

Making these adjustments from student to employee may be difficult. You will not always have the same amount of time to spend with your patients as you had when you were a student. Your workload and the pace at which you will be expected to carry out your assignments will be increased. Some experienced members of the nursing team may help you during this transition period; others may not.

Expect to have mixed feelings—some very positive and others less so. You will be excited to finally have the chance to put what you have learned to actual use, but you might also be a bit nervous about it. You may feel that there is more work than you can handle. You may have difficulty adjusting to the leadership and management styles of your supervisor. But remember, you successfully made similar adjustments when you began your nursing program, and you can do so again.

Some techniques that help ease the transition from student to employee include being honest about your limitations but not shirking your share of the work. If you find that you are getting behind schedule, let your supervisor know. You may want to ask an experienced nursing team member for suggestions on how to better organize your work. Observe how experienced nurses organize their schedules so that assignments are completed on time. You might ask your supervisor to evaluate your performance on a daily or weekly basis and use that information to improve your practice. Take every opportunity you can to learn more about your patients' medical conditions and their nursing needs. Admit your mistakes and learn from them. Be prepared to put in the extra time needed to complete your assignments. In a surprisingly short time, you will make the adjustment and feel the satisfaction that comes from being accepted as a contributing member of the nursing team.

SELF-ASSESSMENT

Now that you have reviewed some of the career opportunities in nursing, employer expectations, and transitional challenges, you should assess yourself. Self-esteem and sound skills lend encouragement and confidence to one's outlook and tasks, whereas lack of self-esteem and poor skills can undermine one's confidence. The ability to make an objective analysis of yourself will help point out areas of strength and areas that need improvement. The key is to see yourself as you are without the influence of your beliefs or wishes about how you would like to be. Accurate self-assessment is not always easy, but the rewards make the effort worthwhile.

✔ *An honest assessment of yourself will help you find a job that matches your personality and lifestyle.*

A review of your clinical strengths and weaknesses is an important consideration when thinking about the type of nursing you would prefer to do. If you seem to have a special ability to work with older people, you may consider employment in long-term care. If you enjoyed your clinical experiences with children, perhaps being a school nurse may be the best place for you to begin your career.

You should assess your personal health and physical condition. If you have a health problem or physical condition that limits your activities, you should avoid seeking a position that would adversely affect your own health.

You should assess your work habits, how you prefer to dress, and other personal characteristics. Working in a situation that requires you to behave very differently from the way you usually behave can cause a great deal of stress and personal conflict.

Finally, you should assess your personal and interpersonal characteristics. The self-assessment titled "What Are Your Personal and Interpersonal Characteristics?" on page 296 lists some traits that generally contribute to successful job performance. After you complete the assessment, ask someone who knows you well to fill it out as he or she sees you. Compare the responses. The results are not scientific, but they will give you an indication of your self-perception and how others may see you. Use them to alter those aspects of yourself that may need changing. Evaluations from instructors during the course of your program can also be used to help assess yourself.

ASSESS YOURSELF	**What Are Your Personal and Interpersonal Characteristics?**

Personal Characteristics	Always	Usually	Never
1. I accept responsibility for my work.	_____	_____	_____
2. I welcome criticism.	_____	_____	_____
3. I tell the truth.	_____	_____	_____
4. I don't waste time.	_____	_____	_____
5. I am patient with myself.	_____	_____	_____
6. I like solving problems.	_____	_____	_____
7. I am organized.	_____	_____	_____
8. I know my own limits.	_____	_____	_____
9. I am comfortable with rules and regulations.	_____	_____	_____
10. I accept change.	_____	_____	_____
11. I do not have to be told what to do.	_____	_____	_____
12. I do more than I'm asked.	_____	_____	_____
13. I control my emotions.	_____	_____	_____
14. I have a good sense of humor.	_____	_____	_____
15. I ask for help when I need it.	_____	_____	_____

Interpersonal Characteristics	Always	Usually	Never
1. I enjoy working with others.	_____	_____	_____
2. I am a good listener.	_____	_____	_____
3. I don't mind sharing credit with others.	_____	_____	_____
4. I am patient with others.	_____	_____	_____
5. I keep promises.	_____	_____	_____
6. I like meeting strangers.	_____	_____	_____
7. I like being in charge.	_____	_____	_____
8. I like talking about work with colleagues.	_____	_____	_____
9. I am tolerant of others' mistakes.	_____	_____	_____
10. I treat everyone as an individual.	_____	_____	_____
11. I go out of my way to help coworkers.	_____	_____	_____
12. I like being a part of a group.	_____	_____	_____
13. I keep judgments of others to myself.	_____	_____	_____

FINDING A POSITION

The job-seeking process should be started 1 or 2 months or more before your graduation. You should review all of your clinical assignments and determine which area of nursing you prefer. For example, if you prefer the long-term care environment, you probably should not look for a position in a surgical department in a hospital.

✔ *The first step in finding the right position for you is to decide what type of nursing you want to do.*

As your graduation approaches, check your list of potential employers from time to time. Ask about the present hiring situation, whether it has changed from the last time you inquired, and what the future looks like. Begin to cultivate relationships with people who are employed at the health care facilities where you believe you would like to work.

According to the U.S. Department of Labor, as many as 80% of all jobs are obtained through personal contacts. Networking, the deliberate effort to make connections among people for a variety of interests, including employment opportunities, is a popular method of making personal contacts. Networking may be casual, as when a group of health care workers meets from time to time over coffee to talk, or it may be more formal, as when groups meet with the specific intention of exchanging information. Look for networking opportunities in your program, among graduates, and among others in the health care field in your community.

You will also learn about employment opportunities by talking with and listening to fellow students, your instructors, and others associated with your program. When you hear something that sounds interesting, make a note to yourself to follow it up with an inquiry.

✔ Most jobs are found through personal contacts.

If your program has a placement service, it can be an invaluable resource. Use it to get information about your local employment market before you are ready to begin applying for a job. Stay in touch with employment developments in your area through the placement service. When the time comes to begin making serious inquiries and applications, you will be up-to-date.

Most schools have a "Job Opportunities" bulletin board where notices about employment opportunities are posted. Make the board a regular stop and watch for new offers to appear.

Other good sources for job listings are the Web sites of local health care facilities. Most of the larger facilities list vacant positions and post the job application on their Web site. Newspapers, nursing publications such as Nursing Spectrum, and job announcements mailed to your home also include listings of job opportunities.

You might also use the Internet to locate job openings. You can find hundreds of jobs by inserting "LPN or LVN jobs" in the search box of your favorite search engine. Job listings on the Internet will give you access to information about local, national, and international jobs.

Some communities have employment agencies, and larger cities have placement agencies that specialize in health care personnel. Either kind of agency is a good resource, but agencies that specialize are likely to have more listings and better contacts with employers. If you register with an agency, your name will be available when applicants are needed to fill newly opened positions. Commercial employment agencies charge for their services, usually a percentage of the first year's salary. In some cases, the employer may pay this charge; in other cases, it is paid by the employee (i.e., you). Ask what the fee is and who will pay it before signing an agreement with an employment agency.

The Application Process

You can apply for a job informally by personally visiting prospective places of employment, or more formally (and preferably) by submitting a postal or e-mail letter of application with an accompanying résumé. A letter ensures that the prospective employer has a written record of your interest; a résumé provides the prospective employer with an outline of your qualifications.

✔ Your application is your "first impression" to prospective employers.

Large institutions with many employees often have personnel or human resources departments where it is appropriate to "walk in" to fill out an application. Also, some employers who advertise may invite walk-ins. More and more large institutions are relying on their Web site to obtain applications for employment.

The Letter of Application

A letter of application should be simple and direct. Its objective is to introduce you, announce your interest in employment (naming the position being applied for), briefly state your qualifications, and express your availability. It should be printed on good-quality white paper in standard business letter form. It should be no more than one page long. It should be free of grammatical and spelling errors. Figure 14-3 is an example of an application letter.

The Résumé

The word *résumé* means summary. Your résumé should include a summary of your previous education and work experience. Like your letter of application, your résumé presents you to your prospective employer. Neatness, clarity, legibility, and organization reflect similar personal qualities. Although you may wish to write your own résumé, the general availability of résumé writing services and computer programs makes the task much simpler.

Many employers expect to receive your résumé via e-mail, from an electronic bulletin board, or through the use of an electronic application form. Or they might even ask for the address of your Web page to see your e-portfolio. If you need assistance, there are many Web sites that will teach you how to prepare and submit an electronic application and résumé.

✔ *Consult with a professional or use reference books or the Internet to get help in preparing your letters of application and your résumé.*

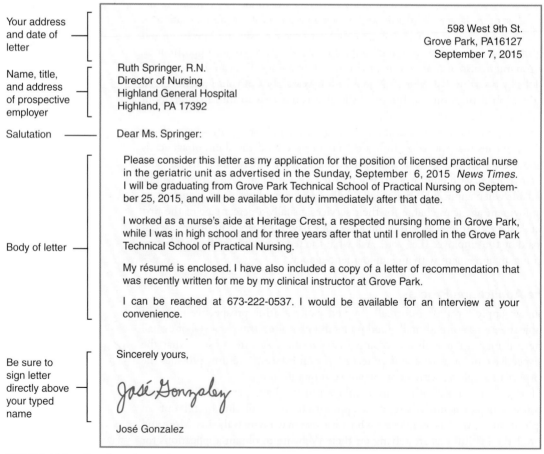

FIGURE 14-3. ● Sample application letter.

Whether you prepare your own résumé or have someone prepare it for you, it must be typed and should follow a standardized format. If you're doing your own, get some advice from books or other publications or from the placement office at your school. Don't simply prepare a "homemade" résumé; it will stand out, but not in the way a good résumé is intended to. Figure 14-4 is an example of a solid résumé.

The following categories of information should be included on your résumé:

- Name, address, and telephone number
- Immediate goal
- Career goal
- Education
- Licenses
- Experience (work and volunteer)
- Memberships and honors
- Reference availability

Sandra Melanie Lewis, L.P.N.
1038 University Avenue
Boulder, Colorado 80302
303-555-0537

Immediate Goal:
Employment as a licensed practical nurse in the geriatric section of a major area hospital

Career Goal:
To provide quality nursing care for older adults in long-term care

Education:
2015: Arapahoe Hospital, Boulder, Colorado: L.P.N.
2013: Boulder High School, Boulder, Colorado: H.S. Diploma

Licenses:
Certified Nurse Assistant, State of Colorado, 2012
Licensed Practical Nurse, State of Colorado, 2015

Experience:
2012–2015: Certified nurse aide at Boulder Nursing Home, Boulder, Colorado
    2012–2013 Part time while in high school
    2013–2014 Full time for one year after high school
    2014–2015 Part time while in practical nursing school
    Duties included assisting residents with activities of daily living, personal hygiene, and social activities.

Memberships and Honors:

2009–2013	Health Occupations Students of America (HOSA) Club
2009–2013	Boulder County 4-H Club
	Club Secretary 2010–2012
January 2013	Boulder Nursing Home employee of the month
July 2014	Hopkins Pharmaceutical Company scholarship winner

Availability:
Immediate

References:
Available on request

FIGURE 14-4. ● Sample résumé.

It is a matter of courtesy to ask people whose names you want to give as personal references for their permission. This should be done prior to an interview so you will be able to provide the interviewer with names, addresses, and telephone numbers if requested during the interview.

The Online Application

The online application usually requests information already contained in your current letter of application and resume. Some Web sites allow you to cut and paste information from your documents into the online application, while others allow you to upload your existing documents. Some prospective employers include an online test (e.g., drug dosage calculations) to be completed along with the application. Some Web sites ask you if you want to make your online resume visible to employers other than the one you have chosen.

Whether you apply in person, by mail, by e-mail, or online, be certain that all of the information is correct, there are no spelling errors, and the documents are properly formatted and that you have followed all of the prospective employer's directions for applying.

The Interview

We have all heard the warning, "You never get a second chance to make a good first impression." Psychologists, writers, and seminar leaders caution that we only have from 7 to 17 seconds of interacting with strangers before they form an opinion of us. Whether this finding is completely accurate, it underscores the fact that when you go for a job interview, you should assume that your appearance and how you present yourself will make an important first impression on the interviewer.

✔ *Prepare for the interview by role-playing the interview in front of a video camera.*

If you have done your "homework" and have taken the time to learn as much as you can about the employer you're seeing, you'll have a good idea of what the interviewer is looking for in an applicant and how you can prepare yourself to meet those expectations. In general, a few simple guidelines will be sufficient:

- Dress appropriately. You are applying for a job. This means that what you wear should be businesslike. You should present a serious, capable image that is neither frivolous nor too casual.
- Be well-groomed. Combed hair, clean skin, and an overall appearance that shows you take good care of yourself will also signal to an employer what kind of care you are likely to give patients.
- Be pleasant and polite, but avoid forcing an unnatural charm. Act like yourself, not someone you aren't.
- Don't be too concerned about nervousness. Most interviewers expect this, particularly in new entrants to the job market.

The interviewer will no doubt ask you questions that cannot be answered with a simple "yes" or "no." Some of the following are typical questions that might be asked during a job interview:

- What are your strong points?
- In what areas do you need more experience?
- What clinical experiences did you enjoy the most while you were in school?
- How do you feel about rotating shifts (working weekends, holidays, overtime, etc.)?
- How do you feel about working on a unit to which you are not regularly assigned?

- How well do you think you get along with others?
- Why do you want to work for us?
- What are your long-term career goals?
- Where do you see yourself 5 years and 10 years from now?
- What would you like to tell me about yourself?

Being prepared ahead of time to answer these and similar questions will demonstrate that you are very interested in your career and in obtaining a position with that employer.

A number of questions are illegal to ask during a preemployment interview. Questions about your age, marital status, citizenship, birthplace, national or ethnic origin, religion, number of children, living arrangements, sexual preference, and spouse's employment are illegal questions. Rather than telling the interviewer that the question is illegal, be prepared to tactfully respond to such inquiries. If an interviewer asks about your spouse's occupation, you might respond by saying, "My decisions about my career are independent of anyone else, and from everything I know, I believe this would be an excellent place to work." Your local Equal Employment Opportunity Commission can provide further guidelines on illegal preemployment questions.

The Americans with Disabilities Act of 1992 provides the legal support that helps people with handicaps or disabilities not directly related to job performance have equal opportunities for employment. If you have a handicap that does not interfere with job performance and if you expect an employer to take reasonable measures to accommodate your handicap, be prepared to clearly explain what special equipment or supplies you will need to perform your job.

✔ *If you need special accommodations because of a disability, be prepared to clearly explain what you need from the prospective employer.*

You will show your interest in the employer if you ask questions, but be sure to ask them at appropriate times. Although it is acceptable to inquire about wages and benefits, for example, it is not appropriate to ask about them before the subjects come up. Normally, this would be well into the interview. The early part of the interview should focus on the employer, the position offered, its requirements, and your own qualifications for the job. Offer to review your portfolio or to leave an electronic version of your portfolio with the person who interviews you.

Prepare a list of good questions ahead of time to avoid the possibility of "going blank," which could be interpreted as lack of interest. When given the opportunity to ask questions, you can ask about issues such as staff-to-patient ratios, educational opportunities, orientation programs, and others that apply directly to you.

✔ *Even though you don't get the money in your pocket, the benefits provided by your employer can represent a significant amount of money.*

Avoid asking questions about information that may have been provided in written form unless you need clarification. Most employers provide prospective employees with a fact sheet that answers many of the following questions.

Some questions to investigate include the following:

Vacation, Sick Leave, Holidays, and Leave of Absence
- How much time for each of the above is provided?
- Does the time provided increase with length of employment?
- Is the time off with or without pay?
- How many and which holidays are included?
- How is a leave of absence granted?
- Is job status affected by a leave of absence?
- How does a leave affect seniority?
- What are the specific guidelines for family and medical leave?

Insurance, Credit Union, and Pension
- Are insurance and pension plans group or individual plans?
- How soon after employment begins do plans become effective?
- What does each plan offer?
- Who is eligible?
- What are the conditions of eligibility?
- Who pays insurance premiums? How much (full or percentage)?
- Are payments automatic (payroll deducted) or voluntary?
- Are employees eligible to join a credit union?
- Is interest charged for credit union loans? How much?
- Is interest paid to credit union members? How much?

Work Environment
- Is the facility convenient to public or private transportation?
- Is safe parking provided? Is it free or paid?
- Are uniforms required? If so, what kind and who provides them?
- Is the facility clean and safe?
- Is equipment and care delivery up to date?
- Do present employees exhibit good morale?

Preemployment Requirements
- Is a physical exam required, and if so, who performs the exam and who pays for it?
- What immunizations, vaccinations, and blood tests are required and who pays for them?
- Is drug testing required and is it randomly repeated?
- Is fingerprinting required?
- Are child and elder abuse background checks required and who pays for them?
- Are there any skills tests required for this position?
- Is a consumer report requested?

Miscellaneous
- What are the work hours, shifts, and rotation schedules?
- Are meals provided, either free or at employee discounts?
- Is there a cafeteria? What are its condition, service, and fare?
- Does the facility have an orientation program or in-service education program?
- Does it offer advanced educational opportunities at outside institutions?
- Who pays tuition and costs for advanced education programs?
- Is there a union, and if so, what are the annual dues?

If you are applying for a nontraditional position (i.e., not in a hospital or long-term care facility), there are things you need to know in addition to those previously mentioned. Is there any flexibility in the starting and quitting time? If travel is involved, what is the rate of reimbursement? Will you be expected to be away from home overnight, and if so, how often?

The Job Offer

When all of your employment investigation has been done, letters of application written, résumés sent, and interviews completed, one or more of the prospective employers may offer you a job.

Review each offer before accepting or rejecting it to make sure the choice you make is the one you want. If you've already made up your mind that you will accept, do so. If you're uncertain, tell the employer that you will make your decision by a specific date and time.

At this point in your career, at the outset of your practice, you must be as sure as possible that your chosen employer is what you want. Nursing administrators generally recommend that you stay at least 2 years at your first job. The first 6 months or so will be spent learning organizational skills, work routines, expectations, and attaining proficiency in nursing skills. The next 18 months provides practice and experience so that you are no longer considered an inexperienced and newly graduated nurse. New graduates and even seasoned nurses who voluntarily change jobs every year or two is a red flag to most employers. The hiring and orientation process is expensive, and most employers will avoid spending money to hire someone who has a history of staying with an employer for a short time.

It is far better for you to take time at the beginning to ensure that the job being offered is what you want than to find out after you're hired that it's not, and then to have to face resigning and beginning anew. Avoid "closing the door" to a first job on the basis of unrealistic demands. Although the perfect job may be waiting for you, it's more likely that you will have to make some compromises.

✔ *When you accept your first job, plan to stay a minimum of 2 years.*

EVALUATING POSITIONS

Considering whether to accept a position includes weighing all of the information you have about each job offer before making a decision. Investigate each employment opportunity on its own merits, paying close attention to all its parts. These include the job description, salary, benefits, work hours, and many other matters that will directly influence your working life and often your whole life. For example, poor working conditions can make you unhappy, and unhappiness often follows you home.

Specific items to consider when comparing and evaluating employment opportunities are included in the following five sections. You may wish to add items of personal concern to the list.

Wages

Your earning power is determined by your credentials on the one hand, and by what the job market offers in the form of salary on the other. Ideally, you should earn the maximum salary or wages possible for your level of education and experience, with salary or wages increasing with your level of experience. However, pay rates vary for a number of reasons.

Generally, regional salaries and wages will be similar because employers are competing for the same prospective employees. Where rates vary, other inducements may be offered to make up the difference. Frequently, the inducements (benefits) are as important as the salary or wages alone (sometimes more so).

✔ *It is a good idea to get advice about the financial aspects of employment from a professional.*

Be cautious when you see above-average salaries or wages for a position you believe you are qualified for. There is usually a good reason for salaries or wages to be noticeably above a regional average. The position description may call for responsibilities and competencies beyond your qualifications, or the wages may be offered because of high staff turnover resulting from difficult working conditions. In the cost-conscious health care field, money that does not have to be spent seldom is.

Carefully study the salary ranges in your area and learn why those that vary do so. Find out what the maximum starting salaries are, what maximum salary can be earned from each employer, how long it takes to reach the maximum salary, and what conditions you have to satisfy to qualify for maximum earnings.

Also, find out what a prospective employer's wage increase policies are. Some may give automatic raises, others may give merit raises, and still others may not give raises at all. Learn how long it takes to qualify for an increase and what is needed to qualify, such as additional education, length of service, or other requirements.

Hours and Shifts

Your intention to work full time or part time, as well as your willingness or ability to work different shifts, will have a great bearing on which employment opportunities to consider. The general rule is that employers set the conditions to maintain continuity of services. You may find some flexibility even in those instances, however.

Hospitals and other health care agencies that provide round-the-clock nursing services devise schedules in a variety of ways, but they are usually based on shifts, generally three 8½-hour or two 12-hour shifts per day. Many employers either require or offer rotating shifts. Also, work schedules are often rotated so that all employees have the opportunity to have some weekends and some holidays off.

✔ Be sure you understand what your work schedule will be before you accept a job.

Your personal circumstances will dictate which schedules you can work. Be certain before accepting a position that you will be available for the hours and shifts being offered or required.

Mandatory overtime is the term used to describe the situation in which an employer mandates direct caregivers (including nurses) to work overtime. Nurses are concerned because they believe being required to work overtime when they may already be tired puts the patient at risk. Employers say they have to mandate overtime because insufficient nurses are available to work the shift. Fifteen states have restrictions on overtime for nurses, and sixteen states have enacted laws regarding mandatory overtime. Several additional states are considering restrictions or legislation related to mandatory overtime. Before accepting a position, be sure you know your state regulations and laws regarding mandatory overtime for LP/VNs as well as the prospective employer's policy on this subject.

Employer Reputation

Your evaluation of potential employers should include knowing their reputation for upholding high standards. Good and bad reputations are earned for a reason. Learn your prospective employer's reputation and how it was acquired. Don't accept hearsay. Someone may praise or belittle an institution for totally unjustifiable reasons.

Find out for yourself. Ask the opinions of those who have worked or received care there. Ask health care associations and societies about their members. Also ask the employer; those with good reputations will provide verifiable references, whereas those who have something to hide won't provide such references.

Opportunities for Advancement

Although it may be early in your career to think of advancing beyond the immediate goal of earning your license as an LP/VN, there may come a time in the future when you'd like to continue your education in nursing. Leave this option open by looking at employment opportunities with employers who offer or encourage employee advancement.

Benefits

Benefits include a wide range of items. Some benefits, such as vacation time, may be considered basic, whereas others, such as day care facilities for an employee's children, may be less standard. Look closely at the benefits package of each employer you are considering. Benefits can be a decisive factor in choosing a position.

A high salary without certain benefits may result in a lower overall income for you, whereas a lower salary or wage with good benefits may net you more. Some benefits to look for are insurance plans (life, health, vision, dental, and prescription), overtime pay, pension plans, reimbursement for tuition, employee credit union, in-service educational programs, meals, and vacation, leave of absence, and holiday policies.

These are just some of the things you need to consider when evaluating offers of employment. Your personal circumstances will no doubt include the need to have answers to additional questions.

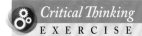
Critical Thinking
EXERCISE

You have had five interviews for jobs in long-term care facilities. The two positions that you really want are at National LTC Facility and at Westwood Nursing Home. When you get home from shopping, you have messages from both facilities offering you the job you interviewed for. They both want your decision by 12:00 noon tomorrow. Because you are equally interested in both positions, you decide to base your decision on which position to accept on the value of the benefits package. Use the information in Table 14-1 to evaluate the major benefits of each employer. Which is the best financial package for you and why? Use appropriate Characteristics of Critical Thinkers in Box 1-2 on pages 18–19 to develop your responses to these questions.

TABLE 14-1	**Typical Benefit Packages**	
	National	Westwood
Salary	$20.00/hour[a]	$42,400/year[a]
Personal illness	10 days/year	10 days/year
Health benefits	Employer pays 10% of salary for premiums	Employer pays 80% of premiums[b]
Dental	Premium paid by employer	80% of cost paid by employer
Vision	Premium paid by employer	80% of cost paid by employer
Prescription	Premium paid by employer	80% of cost paid by employer
Vacation	1st year = 7 days 2nd year = 10 days 3rd year = 15 days 4th year = 20 days	12 days/year
Tuition reimbursement	100%	100% for an A 90% for a B 80% for a C 0% for less than C
Pension plan	401(k)	401(k)—employer matches employee contributions
Continuing education	With approval, employer will pay 100% of the registration costs for two conferences each year.	$200 annual continuing education allowance
Sign-on bonus	$1,500 at the end of 6 months $1,500 at the end of first year	$400 each month for the first year of employment
Life insurance	Equal to salary	Equal to salary for the first year then + 10% for each additional year up to 10 years

[a]Full-time employees work about 2,020 hours/year.
[b]Premiums are $400/month.

ON THE JOB

Once you are hired, a new round of learning begins. You'll be learning your employer's routine, your specific duties, the names and faces of coworkers and patients, and scores of other details. Your confidence in yourself and your competence will get you through the rough parts, and understanding from the people you're working with will help to smooth the transition. You can expect some highs and lows, but you should always know that in a surprisingly short time, the insecurity of being new will be replaced by poise and self-assurance.

✔ *Most people feel apprehensive when starting a new job.*

However, confidence in yourself alone will not guarantee satisfactory performance. Your own standards should be high, perhaps even higher than those your employer sets, so that your work will never come into question and your ability will never fall short of what's expected.

Accept the responsibilities you are given. Do your work to the best of your ability with interest and commitment. Be punctual and reliable, and if illness or other circumstances prevent you from reporting to work, notify your employer as soon as possible. Show a willingness to learn by asking questions when you are uncertain, and be equally willing to share when someone comes to you for help. Abide by the regulations set by your employer, and if you have serious differences with them, seek to correct the situation through proper channels. Don't snipe, gossip, or complain about something that upsets you; do something about it, but in the appropriate manner. You are not only working for your employer but also working with your employer to provide the service that is the basis for economic security for both of you.

Nurses learn early in their careers that personal problems and concerns must be left at home. When you go to work, you must leave your personal problems behind. Positive personal characteristics such as honesty, courtesy, good humor, compassion, and understanding are valuable assets that are appreciated by employers and patients alike.

✔ *Nurses must consistently demonstrate professional behaviors and attitudes.*

Politeness in person or on the phone, in greeting people who are new to you, or in your relationships with those you see regularly is also important. Showing good manners on any occasion, whether in an employee cafeteria or in a patient's room, helps to set an example and a tone that inspires similar behavior from others.

Avoiding gossip about your institution or its staff is more than desirable; it is essential. Backbiting, grousing, complaining, and speaking ill of anyone or anything not only poisons others' attitudes but darkens your own viewpoint. Use caution when talking about personal work issues. Others may not share your views, and it is not fair to impose your views if they are negative.

You will always be working directly or indirectly with others. How closely you work together will vary. Some people will have authority over you; others will be under your supervision. Some you may rarely see, whereas others may be at your side constantly. Good relationships with others will depend heavily on what you do to keep them good. In general, what you put into a relationship is what you get out of it.

There may be times when you witness care or are asked to deliver care that is below the standards of good nursing or health care. Your first obligation is to your patients. If the care you see is truly substandard and can be verified, you should act to prevent it. Report the situation to your supervisor. Don't act on your own to correct the situation because the possibility exists that you're not seeing all the factors involved. Health care at any level always includes the potential of serious consequences, the worst being the possibility of death.

Dealing with people will be the major part of your work. However, in the process of providing care, you will also be responsible for such things as dressings, medications, instruments, machines, and a long list of supplies. They belong to your employer and are expressly for use in the delivery of services to patients. Their misuse or misappropriation for a staff member's private use, without permission, is unethical and illegal.

To avoid problems over the use of equipment and supplies, abide by your employer's regulations regarding them. Fill out the forms that may be required. Make accurate counts when taking inventories or requisitioning supplies. Return unused items to their proper place. File reports regarding breakage or failed equipment. In short, do everything you are supposed to do regarding use of facilities and supplies.

✔ *Employees are expected to be judicious in their use of supplies and equipment.*

Health care facilities of every size are continuously battling increasing costs. Any loss, no matter how insignificant it may seem—taking a set of linens or a towel, procuring wound dressing materials for use at home, or using medications for personal use, for example—raises costs. When an employer's costs are excessive, cost-cutting procedures, including staff cuts, may become necessary. Your job will depend on your employer's ability to pay you. How you use your employer's facilities, equipment, and supplies will affect that ability.

With your career aspirations in mind, take advantage of opportunities to advance. If you need additional classes, in-service training, or experience, accept the added effort, knowing that no advancement is possible without it.

RESIGNATION

There may come a time when you decide to leave your position. This decision should never be made without careful study. A brief upset or disagreement with someone is certainly not grounds for leaving, although a long period of inability to get along in an institution or with staff members may suggest the need for a change for the better.

✔ *When resigning, always give a minimum of 2 weeks' notice in writing to your supervisor.*

If you decide to resign, always do so in the manner set forth by your employer. If no prescribed form is established, write a letter of resignation. Give ample notice (2 weeks is standard) so that your employer can find a replacement for you. No matter what the circumstances of your departure, don't infuse the situation with ill will. You will be looking for another job, if not immediately, then at some time in the future. Your employer's recommendation will be invaluable.

A letter of resignation should be simple and direct, stating the fact that you are resigning, the effective date, giving the reasons (elaborate details are unnecessary), and closing on a positive note. A sample is shown in Figure 14-5.

DISMISSAL

Dismissal from a position is not always based on employer–employee incompatibility. There are economic and other reasons for cutting staff positions, and you have no control over them. If you "fall under the ax" of budget cuts or other administrative changes, such as consolidation of departments, you must accept them. Often, an employer who adjusts staff will have alternative jobs within the institution or, if not, will try to help employees find new positions. However, employers are under no obligation to do so.

On the other hand, a dismissal for cause, based on dishonesty, improper performance of duty, insubordination, illegal acts, excessive lateness or absences, or other substantiated causes is something every nurse can do something about

Your address and date of letter

Supervisor's name, title and address

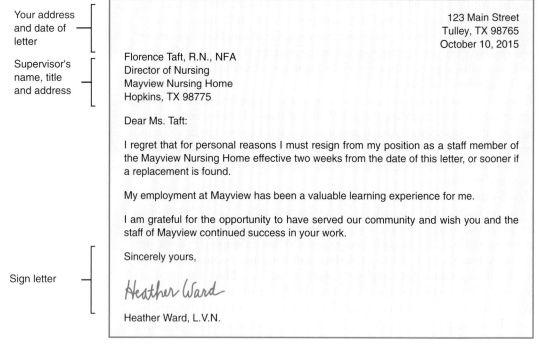

123 Main Street
Tulley, TX 98765
October 10, 2015

Florence Taft, R.N., NFA
Director of Nursing
Mayview Nursing Home
Hopkins, TX 98775

Dear Ms. Taft:

I regret that for personal reasons I must resign from my position as a staff member of the Mayview Nursing Home effective two weeks from the date of this letter, or sooner if a replacement is found.

My employment at Mayview has been a valuable learning experience for me.

I am grateful for the opportunity to have served our community and wish you and the staff of Mayview continued success in your work.

Sincerely yours,

Sign letter

Heather Ward

Heather Ward, L.V.N.

FIGURE 14-5. ● Sample resignation letter.

before it happens. Adherence to high standards is the best defense against charges of any kind.

If a dismissal is warranted, even though it might be disputed by the employee, the employer has certain options, depending on the nature of the cause for dismissal. Options will vary from employer to employer. A serious charge such as theft can result in an immediate dismissal with forfeiture of all benefits. A less serious matter, such as constantly arriving late for work, although grounds for dismissal if not corrected, is not likely to result in such drastic measures. In most cases, the dismissed employee may have the right to appeal.

YOUR BUDGET

Budgeting your income is largely a personal matter. You may already have a system for managing your money. If not, seek help for your specific needs from someone who understands the process. A budget does not have to be complex, but it should cover all areas of your income and expenses, the two major divisions of any budget.

If your position as an LP/VN is your first major employment, be sure to make the distinction between personal and professional (or business) expenses in your budget. Also, because you may be paying local, state, or federal taxes for the first time, get advice from an expert regarding what records you have to keep, how much you must pay, and how the taxes are to be paid. Private duty nurses are responsible for paying their own taxes and for getting licenses required for private duty practice.

✔ *It is never too early to begin planning for retirement.*

Other money matters for you to consider include savings or investment programs, planning for retirement, personal insurance (life, health, liability), and the establishment of a good credit rating. Guidance in these matters is recommended, even if you must consult a professional.

YOUR CAREER

As your nursing education program draws to an end, you should feel secure that your career as a nurse is well on its way. Now is a good time to think of what the future might hold. Goals are incentives to self-fulfillment and to a better, more comfortable life. Earning your license and position as an LP/VN may be one of the goals you have always wanted and you expect to be very satisfied to work in this position for a long time. Or you may have a little voice in the back of your mind telling you that you have just begun to show what you can do. Whether you choose to work as an LP/VN for a long time or are already planning to advance your education, you must maintain clinical competency in your current position.

There are many ways to maintain and improve your clinical skills. Keep up on new developments by reading printed and electronic nursing journals and other professional publications. Watch televised news documentaries about advances in the field of medicine.

Various organizations sponsor conventions and workshops. They may be offered locally or in another city. Attend them whenever possible, even if you must do so on your own time. If you show your determination to keep pace with nursing and a willingness to go out of your way to do so, you may get cooperation and time off from your employer. The least you will get will be your employer's respect for your enthusiasm and interest.

Refresher courses are also a means to maintain and improve skills and knowledge. They may be offered by your own program and by your employer. Treat them as opportunities to advance.

Some of the educational programs you attend might offer continuing education units (CEUs). The national standard is that one CEU equals 10 hours of qualified instruction in an approved program. Earned CEUs are an indication to your employer and others of your career commitment. CEUs are also required for license renewal in some states.

✔ *One CEU represents 10 hours of qualified instruction.*

If you have a specific clinical interest, you might want to enroll in an accredited course offered by a college or university. Accredited means that a course or program has been reviewed by an organization or accrediting body and has been found to meet the standards set by that body. Accreditation generally means that standards are above minimum standards as set, for example, by a state licensing authority. The course may be offered on a campus, at a satellite campus, or electronically through the Internet. Before registering for any course, know how much each credit will cost and if those credits can be transferred to another college or university.

✔ *Keep good records of all of the professional development, continuing education, and other educational programs you attend.*

Earning a clinical certification validates your clinical knowledge, as well as enhances your opportunity for advancement or promotion. Several agencies offer certification examinations for LP/VNs; for example, NAPNES sponsors certification exams in pharmacology, intravenous therapy, and long-term care. Chapter 13 offers a detailed discussion of clinical certifications for LP/VNs.

Finally, you may wish to make a major advance in your nursing career by becoming an RN. RN programs vary in length and complexity. A 4-year course of study at a college or university will lead to a bachelor of science in nursing (BSN) degree. An associate degree in nursing (ADN) is usually earned in 2 years at a college, university, junior college, or community college. Diploma programs are sponsored by hospitals, last about 26 to 30 months, and generally include up to 60 college credits. Graduates of all three of these types of nursing education programs are qualified to take the NCLEX-RN.

✔ *Before you enroll in any registered nursing program, be sure it is accredited by the Accreditation Commission for Education in Nursing or the Commission on Collegiate Nursing Education.*

You may already be enrolled in an articulated nursing program. An articulated nursing education program provides a sequence of courses that offers flexibility and choice. Some students choose to leave the program after completing the LP/VN portion of the curriculum; others choose to leave after completing the ADN portion of the curriculum; and others choose to leave after completing the BSN portion of the curriculum. These students may also have an option of returning to the next level of nursing education within a specific time period.

The LP/VN who was not enrolled in an articulated program and who wants to enroll in a professional nursing program should look for programs that offer advanced standing. Many professional nursing education programs provide a mechanism for LP/VN students to challenge—by examination, experience, and performance—certain professional nursing courses. Those who successfully meet the challenge criteria are exempt from taking the course and are granted advanced standing. Most nursing organizations are actively encouraging nursing educators to find innovative ways of providing a nursing career ladder. Some believe the ladder should begin with the certified nursing assistant and continue through doctoral studies. Because the number of innovative programs is rapidly increasing, people who want to continue their education in nursing should review all of their options by carefully studying college catalogs and talking with guidance counselors.

NURSING ORGANIZATIONS

Being active as a nurse and being active in nursing are not the same. Being active as a nurse means working as a nurse. Being active in nursing means participating in nursing organizations. Belonging to nursing organizations is important to your development as an LP/VN and also to the future of practical/vocational nursing as a career. The specific purpose of each organization is unique, but the intention of all such organizations is to benefit the membership through activities that advance the occupation.

Practical/Vocational Nursing Organizations

Two national organizations designed to meet the particular needs of practical/vocational nurses are the National Federation of Licensed Practical Nurses (NFLPN) and the National Association for Practical Nurse Education and Service (NAPNES).

The NFLPN was founded in 1949, and full membership is limited to LP/VNs and student practical/vocational nurses. In September, 1991, a category of affiliate membership was established to allow those who have an interest in the work of NFLPN but who are neither LP/VNs nor PN/VN students to join. Affiliate members receive all communications and may attend all NFLPN meetings but do not have the right to vote or hold office. This organization's primary purpose is to promote the practice of practical/vocational nursing. The NFLPN, through its organizational structure and membership, develops positions on educational requirements for the practice of practical/vocational nursing, makes recommendations related to continuing education, defines ethical conduct, and outlines standards and scope of practical/vocational nursing practice, all of which are based on a clearly defined philosophy of practical vocational nursing. In addition, the NFLPN attempts to influence legislation affecting the LP/VN through national and state lobbying programs.

✔ *Be actively involved in at least one professional organization.*

NAPNES was founded in 1941 to promote the special interests of practical/vocational nurses and to assist schools in developing educational programs. Membership is open to LP/VNs, practical/vocational nursing students, practical/vocational nursing school faculty and directors, and others interested in promoting the practice of practical/vocational nursing. The primary purpose of NAPNES is to promote an understanding of practical/vocational nursing and to develop continuing education opportunities for LP/VNs. NAPNES also develops positions on practical/vocational nurse education, defines ethical conduct, and publishes standards of nursing practice and education. The NAPNES official publication, the *Journal of Practical Nursing*, keeps members informed of organizational activities.

The future of practical/vocational nursing depends a great deal on the effectiveness of these two organizations. Because organizations are made up of people who share a common goal, it is important to your future as an LP/VN that you actively participate in one of these organizations.

National League for Nursing

The National League for Nursing (NLN) was founded in 1950, and membership is open to anyone interested in promoting health care through nursing service. This national organization is primarily concerned with education of nurses and improving the quality of health care. The official publication of the NLN is *Nursing Education Perspectives*.

✔ *Nursing organizations represent the interests of their members in society, politics, and the law as well as in nursing.*

The NLN is a large organization, and many of its activities are conducted through special divisions called Advisory Councils. One of the Advisory Councils of special interest is the Nursing Education Advisory Council.

American Nurses Association

The origins of the American Nurses Association (ANA), the professional association for RNs and students in professional nursing programs, can be traced to 1890. The ANA is deeply involved in issues important to professional nurses such as establishing a credentialing system for specialized practice, developing and administering specialty certification examinations, publishing a Code for Nurses, approving continuing education programs, and lobbying for nurses, nursing, and health care. Although LP/VNs cannot join the ANA, some of the activities of the ANA can have a direct influence on practical/vocational nursing. Reading the ANA official publication, the *American Journal of Nursing*, as well as NLN and practical/vocational nursing publications, will help you keep informed of the positions of all of these national organizations on issues that will affect you and how you practice nursing.

✔ *Visit nursing organization Web sites at least once a month to keep up on the latest developments and issues.*

Whichever organizations you choose to join, do so with the intention of being an active member. It can be an investment in your future, as well as a help to others in improving theirs. Remember, organizations depend on their members to provide direction and give strength.

POLITICAL PROCESS

President Obama's efforts related to making changes in how we pay for health care in this country provide a good example of how complex our political processes can be. As a member of the health care team and as a citizen of this country, you are now and will continue to be affected by political decisions. For example, political efforts to control rising health care costs may affect your salary; political efforts to revise the Medicare system may make it necessary for you to care for an aging or ill parent in your home; health care services may be reduced as a result of political actions; your job may be eliminated; or political action establishing new health care services may increase your personal income taxes.

✔ *One of the most effective ways to influence your future in nursing is to be involved in politics.*

As a nurse, you are in a unique position to see problems from a patient's viewpoint, the health care system's viewpoint, and a personal viewpoint. You must share your opinions and recommendations with your legislators.

You can affect the political process in several ways. The best-known way is to vote. Many elected officials keep in touch with their constitutions through Facebook, Twitter, Linkedin, Tumblr, and other social media. Social media along with television and newspaper reports help you learn a candidate's positions on various issues. Knowing a candidate's position will help you vote for those you think will best serve the interests of yourself and your patients.

THE *Web*

You can find the postal and e-mail addresses along with telephone numbers of elected federal officials at the House of Representatives and Senate Web sites. You can find addresses for state and local elected officials on your state and local government Web sites.

Another way to affect the political process is to e-mail, write, or telephone your legislator. Elected officials need and want to know your views and opinions. When writing, be sure to include your name and address. Senators and representatives usually respond only to their own constituents. If you present a matter that should be considered by someone other than your own senator or representative, he or she will forward it to the appropriate person. When you send an elected official an e-mail, be sure to address him or her properly. Begin your e-mail with a formal greeting such as "Dear Senator Jones." Guidelines on how to address written correspondence to various levels of state and national legislators are shown in Box 14-1.

BOX 14-1 Forms of Address in Written Correspondence

State Senators	Envelope: The Honorable (first and last name) Address City, State, Zip Code Salutation: Dear Senator (last name):
State Representatives or State Assembly Members	Envelope: The Honorable (first and last name) Address City, State, Zip Code Salutation: Dear Representative (last name):
US Senators	Envelope: The Honorable (first and last name) Address Washington, DC, 20510 Salutation: Dear Senator (last name):
US Representatives	Envelope: The Honorable (first and last name) Address Washington, DC, 20515 Salutation: Dear Representative (last name):

Other ways of affecting the political process include lobbying, negotiating, and demonstrating. Lobbying activities are conducted by organizations on behalf of their members. For example, NFLPN and NAPNES frequently lobby for or against legislation affecting LP/VNs.

Negotiating is the art of persuasion. In the political process, much time and energy is spent negotiating with and between legislators. Promises are made, positions are changed, and decisions are eventually reached.

Demonstrating is a technique that sometimes influences the political process. Demonstrations call attention to a particular problem or issue in a dramatic fashion. Demonstrations, whether peaceful or violent, usually attract public attention. They generally occur when the political process has been unresponsive to an issue of critical importance to a group of people.

Keeping informed of legislation that may affect you is not as difficult as it may seem. Your organizations, through their publications, keep members informed of current legislative events in both state and national governments. Your local newspaper and national news magazines are also sources of information on political issues.

✔ *Do you have the talent to be a politician who puts health issues high on his or her agenda?*

If you become politically active as a nurse and a concerned citizen, you should exercise care to avoid offending your employer. Your political convictions are personal, and you have no right to impose those convictions on your employer or your patients. For example, if you are actively working to pass pro-life legislation and your employer provides legal abortion services, it would be inappropriate for you to conduct political activities against your employer. Such conduct is unethical, and it puts both you and your employer in a difficult position.

The following fundamental tools are at your disposal to help you affect the processes that influence your life and career:

- Be informed. Stay abreast of what is happening in nursing by reading newspapers and nursing journals, listening to news broadcasts, and watching television programs that address current issues in health care.
- Participate. Join nursing organizations and activist groups and be active in their work.
- Vote. Express your opinions, and vote for those you want to represent you in elections in your organizations, your community, your state, and your country.
- Communicate. Let your representatives know your views through letters or meetings, and support their efforts to pass laws and make changes you favor.
- Influence others. Share your opinions with friends, colleagues, neighbors, and others.

To affect the political process, and thereby to affect decisions that have a direct bearing on your life, you must first realize that your opinion is important and that you have the right to express it. Even though an individual may seem insignificant in a large group, the group is made of nothing but individuals and you are one of them.

COLLECTIVE BARGAINING

Certain issues regarding your employment will be out of your direct control but within your indirect control. These include conditions affecting your job such as wage scales, work hours, working conditions, and other matters that are of daily concern. Nurses' and health care workers' unions are organizations

✔ *It is estimated that about 17% of nurses belong to a union.*

that, by representing nurses and bargaining with employers, reach agreements that ideally are in everyone's best interest. The process is called collective bargaining.

If you join a union, and if that union is acknowledged as the bargaining representative at your place of employment, your wishes will be conveyed to management (your employer) through the activities of the union. But you must first join the union and then be active in it for the process to be effective.

Unions work for the benefit of their members. Any issue can be advanced by a union, but in general, unions are involved in wage and hour matters, health and safety issues, discrimination issues of all kinds, and formulation of contracts between employers and union members that incorporate these items.

Joining a union is a personal choice. Whether you accept an offer to join is up to you. Before deciding either to join or not to join, look closely into what your decision would mean to you, your employment, and your career.

GRIEVANCES

No occupation or job is without its grievances (problems). It's not a good idea to look for them, especially at the beginning of your career when your attention should be on learning and performance, but you should be aware that they may appear from time to time. They may cover a range of serious matters, such as health and safety or discrimination on the basis of sex, race, religion, or other factors. There may be less serious issues of only passing concern. Some can be solved on the spot; others may require a lengthy process to settle.

✔ *Handle grievances through the correct channels and protocols.*

Most employers will have some form of grievance procedure (problem resolution process) for employees to rectify problems. In some institutions, the process may be a part of a contract worked out by the union representing workers there. At other establishments, it may be as simple as calling the problem to the attention of a supervisor.

Learn the process used at your institution or place of employment because without it, small, even petty, problems could grow out of proportion, and already large problems could become serious. Complaining about a problem accomplishes nothing if it's not done through the proper channels, whereas a legitimate complaint that reaches an authority that can do something about it gets action.

SUMMARY

Finishing your formal nursing education, getting your nursing license, and getting your first job as a licensed nurse is a time of excitement and anticipation. It is also a time of apprehension and concern. Questions race through your mind. What type of nursing do I want to do? Should I look for a job where I grew up or should I move away from home? Will I be able to do the job if I manage to get one? Will I get along with my coworkers? What organizations should I join? What can I do to improve health care?

As you begin answering these questions and making decisions about your career and your future, know that you are entering a career that offers you many options and opportunities. Take time to explore all of them so that the decisions you make are right for you.

1. In the opening story at the beginning of this chapter, the students heard a "lecture" about the importance of moving "into the future by listening, watching, and preparing for it." Find a nurse who has been working for more than 20 years. Ask that nurse to list equipment or procedures (or both) that are common today that he or she was not taught in school. How did this nurse learn about these new things? What does this nurse have to say about the importance of continuing education?

2. In addition to the places listed in this chapter, list other places where LP/VNs may work in your community.

3. What is the salary range for LP/VNs in various health care facilities in your community? (Web sites of local employers and health facility personnel offices can help you answer this question.)

4. Prepare your résumé for a prospective employer.

5. Ask a classmate to conduct a mock interview with you. Videotape the session, and then critique how well you presented yourself.

6. Think about how you will dress for an interview. If you are unsure of how you should dress, ask your instructor for advice.

7. Ask one or two experienced nurses about their transition from student to employee. What did they find most difficult? What would they recommend to make this transition less difficult?

8. List several things that you can do now to prepare for the transition from student to employee.

9. Select a problem related to health care that is currently being discussed in your state legislature. What are the issues? What are the positions of various special interest groups on the proposed legislation? Some topics that may be appropriate are catastrophic health insurance, regulating the cost of health insurance, repeal of the Affordable Care Act, genetic testing, or the future of Medicare.

10. After you investigate a political issue and reach a personal conclusion, e-mail or write a letter to your congressperson, giving your reasons for urging support or nonsupport of the proposed legislation.

11. Prepare a list of the pros and cons of union membership. Compare your list with those of your classmates.

12. Describe your nursing career goals. What position and responsibility do you want in 1 year, in 5 years, and in 10 years? What will you have to do to achieve these goals? Are these goals realistic? Do you have the ability to achieve them? What changes (personal, educational, and social) might you have to make to achieve your goals?

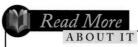

Read More
ABOUT IT

Benner P: From Novice to Expert: Excellence and Power in Clinical Nursing Practice, Commemorative ed. 2001. Upper Saddle River, NJ: Prentice-Hall, 2002.

Claywell L: LPN to RN Transitions, 3rd ed. St. Louis, MO: Mosby, 2014.

Harrington N, Terry CL: LPN to RN Transitions: Achieving Success in Your New Role, 4th ed. Philadelphia, PA: Lippincott Williams & Wilkins, 2012.

Kennedy JL: Job Interviews for Dummies, 4th ed. Hoboken, NJ: Wiley Publishing, 2012.

Mason DJ, Leavitt JK, Chaffee MW: Policy and Politics in Nursing and Health Care, Revised Reprint, 6th ed. St. Louis, MO: Saunders, 2013.

Nursing 2015: Philadelphia, PA: Lippincott Williams & Wilkins, 2015.

Yate MJ: Knock 'Em Dead Résumés: A Killer Resume Gets More Job Interviews, 11th ed. Avon, MA: Adams Media, 2014.

Yate M: Knock 'Em Dead Cover Letters: Cover Letters and Strategies to Get the Job You Want, 11th ed. Avon, MA: Adams Media, 2014.

Challenges in the Workplace

CHAPTER CONTENTS

LEARNING OBJECTIVES

When you complete this chapter, you will be able to:

1. Describe and give examples of several work-related challenges.

2. Describe and give examples of several occupational challenges.

3. Describe and give examples of several public health challenges.

4. Describe and give examples of several environmental challenges.

5. Given a challenging situation develop a step-by-step plan, including the rationale for each step, to resolve the situation.

It was a beautiful summer day, and all of the practical nursing students were sitting outside enjoying their lunch break and the warm weather. Classes would be finished soon; they would take the **NCLEX-PN** exam and then finally start working as nurses. It had been a long and difficult year, and they couldn't wait for it to be finished.

The subject of several classes the past few weeks had been about getting ready for that first job as a nurse. Where to apply, what type of nursing to look for, and when to start working were questions everyone was asking. This lunchtime conversation was no different.

"I have been working at a fast food restaurant after classes since school started and I can't wait to get out of that stressful place!" said Ethan. "I sure hope my first nursing job is not that stressful."

Isabella joined in and said, "I don't know about that. I've been working as a nurse aide for 5 years and let me tell you, there's a lot of stress in that job!" Antonio said, "I worked for 4 years as a computer technician and that job is no picnic! My boss was a real terror." Jena, by far the most upbeat and positive person in the class said, "I worked for 10 years in a couple of different jobs before I started school and I loved every minute of it. I worked with terrific people and had lots of fun AND we did a great job. If I didn't want to be a nurse so badly, I would have never left. I hope I get lucky enough to work with great people when I get my first nursing job!"

Jena's comment about enjoying her previous job set off a debate among the students about why some jobs are so stressful and others are so great.

As you prepare to join the health care team as a practical or vocational nurse, you will be faced with a number of workplace challenges. Some of these challenges are specific to nurses; others affect all workers regardless of their occupational choice. How you and your coworkers handle these challenges will determine whether your workplace is a healthy one or one that could make you sick.

As you read this chapter, try to clarify your thoughts and feelings about these different challenges and then think about what actions you might take if you found yourself in any of these situations. Learn about what resources are available to you and how you might use them if necessary. It is far healthier, both mentally and physically, to be actively involved in solving challenges than it is to be complaining and whining about them.

WORK-RELATED CHALLENGES

A healthy workplace is one in which the cultural and social environment is fair and supportive, workers feel safe from injury and harm, the physical environment is efficient and comfortable, and coworkers practice healthy behaviors. In an ideal world, all workplaces would be healthy workplaces.

Unfortunately, not all workplaces are healthy. Work-related challenges confront workers in all occupations—nursing included. Learn to recognize the challenges and be aware of what resources are available.

Abusive Work Environment

An abusive work environment is an environment in which a person feels threatened or intimidated by the boss or by coworkers. Yelling and screaming at others, throwing things, temper tantrums, and threats of firing are the more obvious abusive behaviors. Less obvious are looks, sighs, shrugs, and other body language that indicates disapproval of your work, your questions, or your conversations.

Regardless of the reasons why bosses or coworkers behave in this way, it creates an environment in which workers cannot do their best work. People dread going to work when they work in an abusive environment, and they are constantly wondering when the next outburst or threat will occur. They go home tired, drained, and frustrated.

✔ *Abusive behaviors by bosses or coworkers reduce the potential for high levels of productivity.*

Workers who want to report such behavior should first provide written complaints to their human resources managers or others who are in a position to stop the abuse. If the situation does not improve, the U.S. Equal Employment Opportunity Commission may be able to help. If the abusive work environment is occurring in a small independent office and the abusers have no bosses or no way of stopping the behaviors, it might be best to find a more comfortable and productive place of employment.

Abusive work environments take a toll on workers, their families, and their customers. Your actions and awareness can contribute to stopping the behaviors that make the workplace so uncomfortable.

THE *Web*

Equal Employment Opportunity Commission (EEOC) offices are located around the country. To find the office nearest you, go to the government's EEOC Web site.

Whistleblowing

Whistleblowing is the term used to describe a person who reports unethical or illegal workplace practices to the employer, a government agency, or the public. Workers, including nurses, sometimes observe behaviors and events that might jeopardize public health, the environment, or clients but are afraid to blow the whistle on these practices for fear of retaliation from the employer or coworkers.

✔ *Find out if your state has a whistleblower law.*

People who decide to blow the whistle must have sufficient documentation to substantiate their claim and should take their concerns to the employer prior to going public with the information. A whistleblower should also consider seeking legal advice prior to blowing the whistle. False allegations ruin reputations and careers and could result in a defamation of character suit against the whistleblower.

To protect those who report unethical or illegal practices, the federal government and at least 34 states have passed "whistleblower" legislation that protects nurses and others from retaliation by employers. Whether to blow the whistle is a difficult decision and one that must be carefully thought through. If you make a decision to report unethical or illegal practices, be prepared to do what is required of you throughout the investigations and trials—if it comes to that.

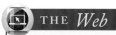

> THE *Web*
>
> The U.S. Department of Labor's division of Occupational Safety and Health Administration's (OSHA) Web site describes the Whistleblower Protection Program.

Bullying

A Workforce Bullying Institute survey revealed that approximately 56% of bullies are bosses and 33% of bullies are coworkers.

Bullying is described as aggressive behavior that is intended to gain power over or hurt another person (the target). Bullying behaviors include name calling, snubbing from social gatherings or conversations, belittling, coercing, gossiping, criticizing, shunning, spreading lies and rumors, withholding information, making insinuations, scapegoating, staring, giggling, or laughing at a person.

Workplace bullying affects approximately 65 million American workers. The victim can suffer from stress-related health conditions such as hypertension, depression, nervousness and anxiety, loss of sleep, and deteriorating family relationships. It can result in the victim quitting a job or a career.

You can and should do something when either you are the target of a bully or you know a target. If you are the target, seek help. Some behaviors that can help stop the bullying include giving a name to what is happening to you and telling someone you trust. Coworkers who are aware that you are being bullied can be a source of support. Sometimes, just telling the bully that you are not going to be his or her victim will stop the bully's behavior toward you. Refusing to be terrorized might also work.

If you know a target, be supportive and corroborate your observations of bullying. Let others know that you will not tolerate or participate in bullying of others. Volunteer to work on committees to address and correct situations that lead to bullying in the workplace. Work with your local legislators to determine how to legally stop bullying. Learn about how legislation related to bullying in schools has affected the learning environment for children and use that knowledge in developing workplace laws, policies, and procedures.

Learn about pending laws related to bullying in your state.

Workplace bullying, unlike workplace discrimination, is not covered by any existing federal or state laws. The Healthy Workplace Bill is a model bill that can be used by legislative groups to develop laws that provide legal recourse for those who are bullied at work. At least 28 states are considering antibullying legislation.

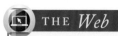

> THE *Web*
>
> An organization called Workplace Bullying offers suggestions on what you can do if you believe you are being bullied at work.

Violence

The National Institute for Occupational Safety and Health defines *workplace violence* as violent acts (including stalking, domestic violence, physical assaults, and threats of assaults) directed toward persons at work or on duty. While sensational stories of homicide in the workplace are media-intensive events, these stories do not inform us of the extent of the problem. The Department of Labor's Bureau of Labor Statistics reports that in 2013, there were 397 workplace homicides, the lowest annual rate ever reported. While the homicide rate is going down, the incidence of other forms of violence in the workplace is increasing.

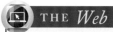
THE *Web*

> The National Institute for Occupational Safety and Health Web site provides suggestions on actions that can help prevent violence in the workplace.

Stalking and domestic violence are of grave concern. Women are usually the victims of these crimes and might have to leave their job to escape the situation. It is estimated that one in every four women will be the victim of domestic violence and that violence occasionally follows the woman to work. According to the U.S. Occupational Safety and Health Administration, there are about two million incidents of violence in the workplace each year, and about 20,000 of those cases are related to domestic disputes.

✔ *The National Domestic Violence Hotline (1-800-799-7233), operates 24/7, is available in 170 languages, and live chat is available every day from 7:00 to 2:00 am (CST).*

As the issue of violence in the workplace gains attention, measures to prevent it are being put in place. Security measures such as screening devices, security cameras, and security guards help prevent unauthorized entry into workplaces. Security lighting in parking lots, security escorts, and emergency action plans help deter violent acts. Conflict resolution programs and getting help for employees who appear to be troubled also aid in reducing violent acts in the workplace.

THE *Web*

> The National Network to End Domestic Violence and most individual states maintain Web sites that provide information, assistance, and links to organizations that can assist victims of domestic violence.

Diversity

The term *diversity* (in the workplace) refers to similarities and differences among workers in terms of age, cultural background, disabilities, spirituality and religion, race, gender, sexual orientation, and genetics. When workers allow these differences to control their interpersonal relationships with coworkers, they allow diversity to become a limiting factor in their personal growth and professional development.

✔ *Value and appreciate the uniqueness of each person and each patient.*

Age

During difficult economic times, many people who would not be working are working. Older workers who cannot afford to retire are working longer than they expected. This creates challenges for both younger and older workers because older workers' work ethics and loyalty, their skill in the use of technology, and communication styles may be quite different from those of younger workers. Older workers may have bosses and supervisors who are younger than themselves. Some older workers feel that text and e-mail messages and other forms of electronic communication are impersonal, while younger workers regularly use these forms of communication.

Intergenerational differences have the potential to create conflicts among workers. Avoid having disparaging thoughts, making critical comments, and attributing the behaviors and values of people to their age. Showing respect for the choices of others and properly addressing coworkers will go far in establishing mutually respectful relationships among people of widely varying ages.

Culture

People from different cultural backgrounds, as we discussed in Chapter 9, practice everyday activities in different ways. Every culture manages time, money, work, and personal space differently. Body language and social customs may also be different. While diversity can sometime lead to conflicts among workers, the benefits of working with people who are different are enormous. Coworkers from diverse cultural backgrounds add their different perspectives to the work environment. As you learn about their cultural practices, you become more able to live with, work with, and provide services to those who are different from you.

Disabilities

People with disabilities, whether physical, intellectual, or emotional, are found in many workplaces. These employees bring a wide range of talents to the workplace and, given the right accommodations, can be real assets. They provide a point of view to the work that others don't have. Their abilities far outweigh their disabilities.

Spirituality and Religion

There is a difference between religion and spirituality. Being religious means you are following a religion that has a set of organized beliefs and practices. It includes attending religious services, observing religious holidays, wearing religious garb, and having a place to pray. Because so many people work in occupations that operate on a 24/7 schedule, time to attend religious services or observe religious holidays may create conflicts in the workplace. Wearing religious garb may be a health or safety concern in some occupations. Providing a place to pray may not be possible in some work environments. Currently, employers are required to make reasonable accommodations for religious practices so long as those accommodations do not create an undue hardship on the employer. Congress is considering a bill to protect religious expression in the workplace, but the bill, which has been presented for more than 10 years, continues to draw opposition from businesses that say it will limit their ability to do their work.

Spirituality is a self-understanding of your own reality through your submission to whatever your higher power is. Spirituality is more of an individual quest than it is about practicing a set of organized beliefs. Self-understanding can come from meditation and thoughtful reflection, which is usually done in a quiet and private place. Practicing spirituality can go a long way in creating pleasant and productive relationships with coworkers.

Race

Working with people from diverse racial groups contributes to the development of a well-rounded work environment. The U.S. Census Bureau reports that in 2014, approximately 62.1% of the population of the United States was non-Hispanic White. The Census Bureau predicts that in 2043, that number will drop to 46%, meaning that non-Hispanic White will no longer be a racial majority. When racial diversity is valued and differing ideas are shared, the work environment becomes one of collaboration rather than one of conflict.

Gender

Gender differences occur in salary and benefits, being hired and fired, and advancement and training. While practices are slowly changing, men get promotions more quickly than do women, men continue to make more money than do women, and men get more job training than do women.

✔ *The Americans with Disabilities Act prohibits discrimination and ensures equal opportunity for persons with disabilities in employment, state and local government services, public accommodations, commercial facilities, and transportation.*

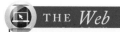

THE *Web*

The Lambda Legal Web site provides current information on civil rights issues of LGBT people and those with HIV.

Working with lesbian, gay, bisexual, or transgender (LGBT) people may be a challenge for some workers. LGBT workers are sometimes harassed, bullied, and discriminated against much like others we have discussed in the previous few paragraphs. The challenge is usually not with the quality or quantity of work but with the person's sexual orientation. Four states have laws that prohibit discrimination based on sexual orientation: 20 states and the District of Columbia have laws that prohibit discrimination based on sexual orientation and gender identity.

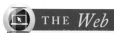

THE *Web*

The Equal Employment Opportunity Commission (EEOC) provides fact sheets and information on the laws that apply to diversity and discrimination practices in the workplace.

Discrimination

Discrimination is treating people based on a class or category rather than on their individual qualities and abilities. Workplace discrimination is such a serious problem that a number of federal laws have been passed to protect workers. While these laws are helpful, subtle forms of discrimination still exist in many workplaces.

Women executives may be excluded from male executive social functions. Promotions may be denied because of race. An older worker may be the brunt of office jokes. Many people make false assumptions about the abilities of physically handicapped workers. People who wear religious garb may be ostracized from the social aspects of the work environment.

One goal of the Human Genome Project is to make it possible to treat, cure, or prevent thousands of disease and illness that affect people. Based on findings from this project, biotechnology companies are rapidly developing tests that can be used to determine if a person has a gene that could cause a particular disease or illness. The public became very concerned that this information would be used to discriminate against people who were applying for health insurance and for jobs. Title II of the Genetic Information Nondiscrimination Act of 2008 was signed into law by President Bush on May 21, 2008. This law prohibits employment and health insurance discrimination based on genetic information about an applicant, an employee, or a former employee.

Welcoming the contributions of people of diverse and distinct physical, social, economic, political, racial, cultural, and religious backgrounds brings points of view to the workplace that would not otherwise be heard. This collaborative work environment improves relationships, expands one's understanding of the world, and improves customer service.

Sexual Harassment

As a historically predominately female profession with physicians and administrators being primarily male, nurses had first-hand knowledge of sexual harassment and discrimination well before this term became popular in the 1970s.

The U.S. Equal Employment Opportunity Commission describes sexual harassment as follows:

> *Unwelcome sexual advances, requests for sexual favors, and other verbal or physical conduct of a sexual nature constitutes sexual harassment when submission to or rejection of this conduct explicitly or implicitly affects an individual's employment, unreasonably interferes with an individual's work performance or creates an intimidating, hostile or offensive work environment.*

When the source of sexual harassment is a patient, there are several measures that might help the situation. First is to tell the patient that you do not accept comments of a sexual nature and he or she has to stop. If that doesn't work, you might consider taking another staff member with you when you need to go into the patient's room. You could request that you not be assigned to that patient, and if the situation gets too uncomfortable for all the team members, the patient could be transferred to another unit. Patients come and go, so these situations are generally resolved upon discharge.

✔ Title VII of the 1964 Civil Rights Act prohibits discrimination on the basis of race, color, religion, sex, or national origin.

The more difficult situations are those that occur between coworkers. Actions that might stop sexual harassment from a coworker include telling the harasser that his or her behavior constitutes sexual harassment, that sexual advances are unwanted, saying "Stop" in an aggressive voice, talking about the harassment to those you trust, documenting the harassment in writing, and, if all else fails, filing a formal complaint.

Sexual harassment in the workplace can have a number of detrimental effects on the victim. It can cause physical illnesses, it can put extreme stress on relationships with others, it can subject the victim to public humiliation, it can result in the loss of a job, and it can even force the victim to relocate to another city.

Do all you can to contribute to a friendly and supportive working team so that no one has to be afraid to go to work.

Job Stress

✔ Stress is a highly personalized experience and can vary widely even in identical situations for different people.

The Center for Disease Control defines *job stress* as the "harmful physical and emotional responses that occur when the requirements of the job do not match the capabilities, resources, or needs of the worker. Job stress can lead to poor health and even injury."

Causes of job stress include working conditions, conditions in the environment, and an individual's temperament and situation. What might cause job stress for one person might not cause it for another.

There has been much research about the causes and effects of job stress because of the negative effects on workers. Causes of job stress include bullying, violence, discrimination, unreasonable deadlines, inadequate staffing, job insecurity, long shifts, missed meals and breaks, low or inadequate pay, and inadequate training. Effects of job stress include elevated blood pressure, a depressed immune system, pain, weight problems, sleep disturbances, poor social relationships, physical injuries, quitting the job or the occupation, and psychological disturbances, to name a few.

All of the research seems to indicate that how you perceive a situation or what you think about a situation is the key to how you will respond to it. Two people in an identical situation could have very different feelings about it. One person may see the situation as very stressful and experience the effects of job stress. Another person in the same situation may see the situation as a challenge that he or she can overcome. Figure 15-1 shows that stress bounces off of some, while it penetrates others and has the potential to lead to injury and illness. The person

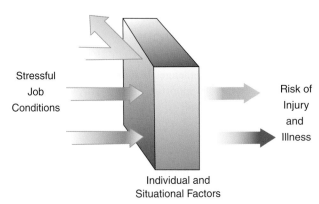

FIGURE 15-1. ● NIOSH model of job stress. (From DHHS Publication Number 99-101.)

who views a situation as a challenge is generally more positive and believes that he or she can improve conditions.

Many health care professionals blame stress for their addiction to prescription and illegal drugs, over-the-counter products, and alcohol. Nurses need to know that there is help not only for their stress but also for their addiction. State boards of nursing, support groups, peer assistance programs, private practitioners, and several organizations provide rehabilitation and recovery programs for nurses. Participation in these programs often leads to recovery and the opportunity to once again practice nursing.

Safety

OSHA is the federal agency that oversees the safety of about 130 million workers employed at more than 8 million worksites around the nation. Four thousand four hundred and five workers were killed on the job in 2013. In health care and social services, workers experienced more than 290,000 days away from work in 2013 and are second only to transportation and warehousing workers in musculoskeletal injuries.

It is important for everyone to take responsibility for safety in the workplace. From closing cabinet doors and drawers, promptly wiping up spills, reporting dangerous situations to supervisors, or even reporting employer negligence in providing a safe work environment to OSHA, safety is everyone's responsibility.

Information Technology

Information technology is a term that is used to describe technology that helps to produce, manipulate, store, communicate, and/or disseminate information. Smartphones, iPads, personal digital assistants (PDAs), wireless computers, and digital cameras all make it very easy to search for information on the Internet, to store our work, and to record our history.

As helpful as information technology is to our lives, there are concerns about how this technology is used in the workplace. Gaining unauthorized access to controlled areas, gaining access to computer-stored data by unauthorized users, breaching the confidentiality of financial and medical records, and the general failure of technology systems are all of great concern.

Many workers are concerned that they will be able to learn to use new systems and use systems properly, and fear that new technology could eliminate their

✔ *OSHA is a U.S. Department of Labor agency that has responsibility for administration and enforcement of laws enacted to protect the safety and health of workers in America.*

✔ *The rewards that come from helping patients and families during a difficult time in their life far outweigh the challenges that sometime occur in the workplace.*

jobs. They are concerned about the reliability of information gained through the Internet and about what would happen if the systems failed.

OCCUPATIONAL CHALLENGES

In addition to facing the general work-related challenges we just discussed, nurses are also confronted by challenges that are unique to nurses and nursing. Looking at these challenges as opportunities for discovery and growth rather than as obstacles and adversity will go a long way toward developing a healthy mental and physical connection between your work and your life.

Diversity

It is reasonable that the nursing team will increasingly reflect the diversity of the nation as a whole. Working with people who have different values, attitudes, religions, social systems, beliefs about health and illness, food preferences, sexual orientation, gender identity, languages, and role relationships offers many opportunities to explore our own values and beliefs and to learn to accept and appreciate the values and beliefs of others.

✔ *Value and appreciate the uniqueness each person and each patient brings to your life.*

Resolving conflicting cultural manifestations at work will be a continuing challenge for all of the nursing team members. For example, the cultural manifestations of time are different for different groups. For some cultural groups, time is flexible, and arriving at work around 7:00 am (between 6:30 and 7:30) is acceptable, whereas for other groups, time is not flexible, and arriving after 7:00 am is unacceptable. These cultural differences, unless discussed and understood by all workers, can create tension among the nursing team members.

A challenge for the future will be for nurses to develop an awareness of not only how culture affects a patient's response to health care but also how cultural diversity affects their own relationships with their coworkers.

 THE *Web*

> The following five national ethnic nurses' associations represent 350,000 nurses:
>
> Philippine Nurses Association of America, Inc. (PNAA)
> National Black Nurses Association, Inc. (NBNA)
> National Association of Hispanic Nurses, Inc. (NAHN)
> National Alaska Native American Indian Nurses Association, Inc. (NANAINA)
> Asian American/Pacific Islander Nurses Association, Inc. (AAPINA)

Work Fatigue

Nurses are very vulnerable to work fatigue because the work is not only physically challenging but also mentally challenging. Mental and physical fatigue put nurses at risk for personal injury and patients at risk for errors in care.

A number of different research studies have explored the causes of work fatigue in nurses. Nurses, usually because of family responsibilities, average only 6.7 hours of sleep on the days they work. They frequently work about 49 minutes longer than their scheduled shift. Errors are likely to occur when nurses work more than 12 consecutive hours. The National Institute of Medicine recommends that nurses should not work more than 12 hours in 24 hours and no more than 60 hours in a 7-day period.

Nurses need to be healthy and alert and functioning at the highest level not only for themselves but also for their patients. While it is tempting to volunteer for overtime shifts, work extra hours here and there, take a second job, and skip sleep to meet family expectations, over time this lifestyle will take a toll and could lead to stress, burnout, and compassion fatigue (CF).

Stress

Increased stress—up to a point—is good and improves performance. Some stress before an exam or before assisting in a critical procedure can actually improve functioning. For some, the stress of an exam is a challenge that they enjoy; for others, the stress of an exam can cause physical illness. What is stressful for one person may have little effect on another person.

Acute stress is the reaction to a real or perceived threat. Virtually all systems (e.g., the heart and blood vessels, the immune system, the lungs, the digestive system, the sensory organs, and brain) are modified to meet the perceived danger. The blood pressure goes up, the heart rate increases, and the digestive system slows down. This emergency response, first described by Walter Cannon in the 1920s, was referred to as "fight or flight." Body systems prepare to fight the perceived threat or to run away from the threat.

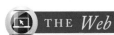 THE *Web*

> The American Holistic Nurses Association Web site provides excellent resources for learning about stress and what you can do to manage it. You might find the section titled "For Students" under the "Membership" tab especially helpful.

When people say they are "stressed," they are generally referring to the negative aspects of stress. They are feeling frustrated and angry or that they feel they have little control over their situation. We discussed stress in some detail in Chapter 2.

Nurses work in an occupation in which the potential for stress is high. Box 15-1 indicates some of the conditions that create stress for nurses. As a result of the many negative physical and psychological consequences of stress, some nurses may prematurely quit working in the profession. Surveys conducted over the past few years indicate that more than 50% of the nurses surveyed said they were considering leaving their current position and about 22% said they were considering leaving nursing altogether.

You are working hard to earn your nursing license, so you want to learn early on to manage stress rather than letting it manage you. Learn the symptoms of stress and get help to become skilled in applying effective coping strategies.

Burnout

The term *burnout* describes a condition characterized by a sense of hopelessness about one's job and is brought about by chronic stress. It decreases performance on the job and carries over into one's personal life. It can be the result of highly stressful working conditions or stressful relationships among staff.

Physical and psychological symptoms accompany burnout. Physical symptoms may include exhaustion, fatigue, headaches, susceptibility to colds, and the inability to sleep. Psychological symptoms may include quick loss of temper, decreased ability to make decisions, guilt, anger, and depression.

✔ *Burnout is often a result of working in a highly stressful work environment over an extended period of time.*

BOX 15-1   Causes of Stress for Nurses

- Understaffing
- Role conflict and ambiguity
- Inadequate resources
- Working in unfamiliar areas
- Excessive noise
- Lack of control and participation in planning and decision making
- Hostile work environment
- Technology
- Relationships with coworkers
- Lack of administrative rewards
- Underutilization of talents and abilities
- Rotating shift work
- Exposure to toxic substances
- Exposure to infectious patients
- Emotional needs of patients
- Poor leadership and management styles

At least part of the stress that produces burnout comes from the inability of those who suffer it to match what they expect of themselves to what time and conditions let them deliver. Candidates for burnout include nurses who want to provide ideal nursing care but are prevented from doing so because there isn't enough time for each patient or nurses who want to promote health but are faced every day with dying patients.

All too frequently, a nurse who has reached this point quits nursing to resolve the problem. This is a dramatic and sometimes unnecessary solution. As a new member of the health care team, you can do something now to avoid experiencing the kind of stress that could lead to burnout.

Discuss problems openly with coworkers and supervisors. Learn to share your feelings and listen to others in return. If the area of health care you are about to enter is one of known high stress, find out from the beginning what those who are already in it do to manage theirs. Don't shoulder a burden that is not yours to carry alone.

✔ *Having a friend who is a good listener can help you during periods of high stress.*

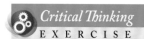
Critical Thinking
E X E R C I S E

You have been working full time for the past 3 years on the surgical unit of a general hospital. Because of staff shortages, you have worked an average of three extra 8-hour shifts each month for almost a year. You have also been taking a 3- or 4-credit college course each semester for the past 2 years. Six months ago, your father had a slight stroke, and you have been taking care of his house, shopping for him, and managing his finances. You have two children, ages 10 and 12, who have started to complain that you never spend any time with them. You feel exhausted all the time and have reached the point at which you feel as though you just can't keep up this pace even 1 more day. One morning as you are struggling to get out of bed, you decide that this is the day you are going to do something about how you feel. As you are getting dressed, you decide to start by making some changes related to the care of your father and to the number of extra shifts you have been working. Now that you have decided where you need to make some changes, what do you do next? In your thinking, consider the effects of your decision on others, the timeline for meeting the goals you establish, the financial and emotional costs, the effects on relationships, and other related issues. Use appropriate Characteristics of Critical Thinkers in Box 1-2 on pages 18–19 to develop your responses to these questions.

Compassion Fatigue

CF is not the same as "burnout." CF comes from caring too much for an individual patient. It can be described as physical, emotional, and spiritual exhaustion as a result of caring too much. Nurses who suffer from CF hear the stories of pain and suffering and trauma from a patient and then essentially feel that patient's pain. When this response is repeated patient after patient, the nurse begins to experience CF. Some describe CF as secondary posttraumatic stress.

Nurses who have CF make mistakes at work, their job performance goes down, morale drops, personal relationships are affected, and personality deteriorates. There is help for nurses who suffer from CF, and it is important to seek professional help as soon as you think you might be developing it. You should also exercise and eat properly, get enough sleep, develop a hobby or interest outside of nursing, connect with family and friends, take a job in a less traumatic clinical setting, or even take some time off from work. Left untreated, CF will render you incapable of being the kind and caring nurse you always wanted to be.

Violence

Violence in health care is of increasing concern. Nurses are particularly vulnerable because they are at times involved in caring for people who are involuntarily admitted or do not want treatment even though their problems may be life-threatening. Nurses have to set limits on visitors and visiting hours, on eating in patient rooms, and on the use of tobacco, alcohol, and illegal drugs. Nurses also care for patients who may be combative due to mental or physical illnesses.

✔ *Violence in health care occurs most often in waiting rooms, geriatric units, emergency rooms, and psychiatric units.*

Coworkers may also be a source of violence. People who are volatile for whatever reason may take out their frustrations and anger on coworkers. They may be verbally abusive or physically violent or may even use weapons that could injure others.

The Occupational and Safety Health Administration reported that 25 of every 10,000 nurses are the victims of violence while only 2 in 10,000 of all workers in all fields of work are the victims of violence. It is important to watch for signals of impending violence and to use behaviors that help diffuse anger. When a patient, visitor, or coworker appears agitated or displays a weapon, it is important to present a calm attitude, acknowledge the person's feelings, avoid aggressive behavior, and use your ingenuity to get help as soon as possible. If you feel you will not be able to lower the risks of injury, remove yourself and your patients from the situation as quickly and as safely as possible. Even if the situation ends without injury, it is very important that every incident of violence be reported to your immediate supervisor.

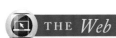 THE *Web*

These Web sites provide additional information on workplace violence:
Occupational Safety and Health Administration
Bureau of Labor Statistics
Centers for Disease Control

Safety

Nurses often express concerns for their personal safety. Some nurses say they do not have the training or protective equipment needed to be safe at work. Violence certainly compromises personal safety. Home care nurses are sometimes concerned about the safety of the neighborhoods and homes in which they treat their patients. Weapons and drugs inside health care facilities can pose a serious threat to the personal safety of nurses. Malfunctioning equipment can cause serious physical injuries. Fire in a health care facility that contains gases and other chemicals could lead to a devastating explosion and release of toxic gases. Radiation and radioisotope hazards, laser plumes, airborne toxins, aerosolized drugs, germicidal solutions, magnetic fields, medical waste, hazardous drugs, excessive overtime and sleep deprivation, failed ventilation systems, and infectious and contagious diseases constitute an incomplete list of potential safety hazards for nurses.

To be safe at work, nurses should learn all they can about the environment in which they work. Nurses should know everything from how to use a fire extinguisher to how to react to toxic fumes. Nurses should continually update their competence in self-protection procedures. Nurses should be able to implement disaster plans, security training, and personal safety practices. Nurses should contribute to making the workplace safer by serving on committees and workgroups organized to address these issues.

An accident due to disregarding safety procedures could result in physical injuries and the loss of your career in nursing. Focusing on the task at hand and taking the time to do it correctly will go a long way in keeping you safe at work.

Health Risks

Working in health care imposes a number of risks to nurses. A recent government study found that nurses rank 10th for musculoskeletal injuries among all occupations. Research has shown that 48% of nurses complain of chronic back pain and 12% say they had to quit nursing because of back pain.

Because musculoskeletal injuries are so prevalent in the nursing population and because lifting a patient can cause serious injuries to the nurse and the patient, 11 states have passed laws or resolutions supporting various aspects of safe patient handling. Ten states have pending legislation. The Nurse and Health Care Worker Protection Act of 2013 is a proposed federal law that would require employers to provide the equipment and personnel necessary to safely lift, move, and position patients. The law has been introduced several times but has yet to pass either the House or the Senate.

✔ *Find out if your state has legislation or regulations related to safe lifting and handling in place.*

Whether laws or regulations are in place or not, it is important that you learn all you can about how to safely lift and move a patient. You must also learn to use assistive devices, equipment, and new technologies. The more you know about these procedures, the less likely you are to develop a painful and enduring back injury.

THE *Web*

You can access a broad picture of the safe lifting issue at the Occupational Safety and Health Administration using the keywords "Safety and Health Topics Healthcare". This site provides links to current Web sites and publications related to this topic.

Accidental needle sticks are of extreme concern. The federal Needlestick Safety and Prevention Act (Pub.L.106–430) was signed into law on November 6, 2000. The number of occupational exposures to blood-borne pathogens from accidental sharps injuries in health care has declined over the years due to safer needle devices that are engineered to eliminate or at least minimize exposure. Even with legislation and safer devices, needlesticks continue to be a concern among health care workers.

Exposure to contagious diseases, radiation, latex allergies, contaminated air, chemicals, and antineoplastic drugs and other pharmaceuticals is also a concern to nurses. Regardless of where you work and your clinical specialty, you will be exposed to things in your work environment that may make you sick. You must use every possible precaution to protect yourself.

✔ *Take time to comply with all of the rules that are intended to protect you from disease or injury while at work.*

OSHA develops guidelines that employers must follow to ensure the health of health care workers, but not even OSHA can prevent nurses from contracting diseases or being exposed to environmental toxins that have not yet been identified. New products used in new ways have the potential to cause harm to those who handle them.

The efforts of OSHA, the Centers for Disease Control (CDC), state health agencies, and employers to deal with current problems are commendable and do increase health and safety in the workplace. However, not even these agencies can anticipate future risks.

It is important that you keep up with current events that have a direct impact on your own health in your workplace. It is also important that you follow all recommended protocols and precautions especially when your patient's illness has not yet been diagnosed.

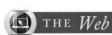

THE *Web*

> Visit the Occupational Safety and Health Administration Web site and use the search term "health care" to access federal documents related to safety and health in the workplace. Go to the Centers for Disease Control Web site then go to Workplace Safety and Health to learn more about federal guidelines related to workplace safety and health.

PUBLIC HEALTH CHALLENGES

Events that create public health concerns include acts of terrorism, bioterrorism, accidents or bombings that cause mass causalities, chemical emergencies whether intentional or accidental, natural disasters and severe weather conditions, and radiation emergencies (Fig. 15-2). While each of these events is distinct, the outcome is usually a large number of deaths and injuries that can create an enormous demand for health care services. We hear of bombings or plane or train crashes that kill and injure hundreds of people almost every day. Chemical disasters resulting from train and truck accidents make headlines on the evening news. It is estimated that one in four Americans lives within three miles of a

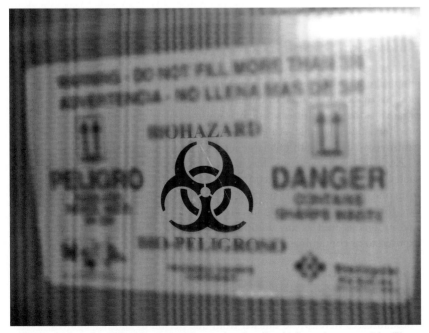

FIGURE 15-2. ● Carefully follow procedures when handling biohazardous materials. (Photo courtesy of Susan Roxandich, RN, BS, CNOR.)

hazardous waste site. We are all too aware of the devastating effects of natural disasters and severe weather conditions such as earthquakes, floods, hurricanes, and tornados. Radiation emergencies caused by a leak from a nuclear energy plant, fallout from a nuclear bomb, or from a "dirty" bomb that contains explosives and radioactive powder are rare but have long-term threats to public health.

✔ *The Environmental Protection Agency (EPA) provides detailed information to the public on many of the issues that threaten our environment and safety.*

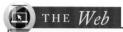 THE *Web*

The U.S. Environmental Protection Agency's "My Environment" Web site provides information about the environment in your community.

Terrorism

Since September 11, 2001, and the attacks on the New York World Trade Center, the Pentagon, and the crash of a plane in Pennsylvania that was intending to bomb the White House, the term *terrorism* has become an all-too-frequent word used in America. Because the purpose of terrorism is to use force or violence against a group of people or a society or government, terroristic acts using weapons of mass destruction, explosives, or poisons provide the potential for an enormous number of human injuries and deaths.

Nurses themselves may be the victims of acts of terrorism and, as such, will have all of the needs and concerns of other victims. They will be concerned about their physical injuries, they will wonder about the safety of their families and friends, they will be confused and scared, they may suffer from posttraumatic stress disorders, and they may wonder why they survived.

Nurses who are not physically injured will most likely be involved in caring for people who have been injured by these acts. Being prepared for a huge influx of people into a health care facility who need immediate emergency care requires preparation and planning. It is important for all nurses to participate in emergency preparedness training programs offered by employers and community groups.

Bioterrorism

OSHA defines bioterrorism as "the intentional use of micro-organisms to bring about ill effects or death to humans, livestock, or crops." Some of the microorganisms that could be used by bioterrorists include ricin along with those microorganisms that cause diseases such as anthrax, plague, viral hemorrhagic fevers, smallpox, and tularemia. An extremely small amount of any of these microorganisms can cause death to a large number of people in a short period of time.

✔ *Use all available precautions when caring for someone who may be the victim of bioterrorism.*

Each of these "weapons" has a different way of being transmitted. Some, such as anthrax, are transmitted through air. Others are transmitted by droplets from one person to another or through food or water. Because nurses commonly care for patients before a diagnosis is made, it is important to follow Standard Precautions as well as any additional appropriate precautions to avoid being exposed to or contaminated by one of these agents.

Contagious Diseases

Prior to vaccines, diseases such as measles, mumps, rubella, whooping cough, polio, chickenpox, diphtheria, and tetanus caused serious public health concerns. These diseases were spread quickly from one person to another, epidemics were not uncommon, and the mortality rate of those who contracted one of these

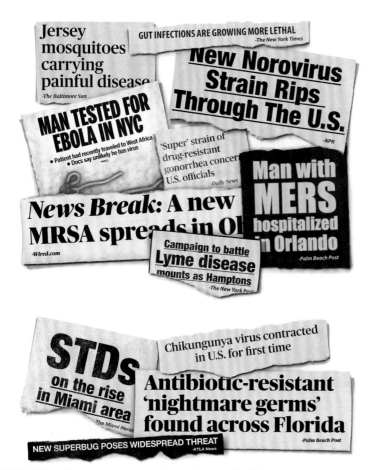

FIGURE 15-3. ● Contagious diseases often make news headlines.

diseases was high. While these diseases in the United States have been largely eradicated because of vaccinations, others have emerged.

With the increase in global travel, contagious illnesses spread farther and faster than ever before. The World Health Organization reported that new diseases are emerging at the rate of one per year. Public health threats in recent years include severe acute respiratory syndrome (SARS), *Escherichia coli*, methicillin-resistant *Staphylococcus aureus* (MRSA), Ebola, influenzas, Middle East respiratory syndrome (MERS), and Marburg hemorrhagic fever, to name a few (Fig. 15-3). The US government has 20 Quarantine Stations located throughout the country, which are staffed with medical and public health officers. It is hoped that quarantining those entering the country who are ill or who may be traveling from areas where the incidence of contagious diseases is high will reduce the health threat to citizens of the United States.

The CDC's National Center for Emerging and Zoonotic Infectious Diseases Web site provides current information on the location of current contagious outbreaks, health information for travelers including recommended vaccines and medicines for worldwide destinations, as well as health care–associated infections. Nurses and other health care workers who come in close contact with people can obtain the most up-to-date knowledge about contagious diseases that could affect their own health at this Web site.

Emergency Preparedness

Emergency preparedness is a term that is used to describe the processes involved in planning for a public health emergency. Federal, state, and local agencies develop procedures that would be used during different types of public health emergencies. Health care facilities are also involved in planning for emergencies since that is where the causalities are taken for treatment.

Many health care employers conduct annual mock disaster drills that are designed to provide workers with practice and experience in coping with the sudden increase in the need for health care services that natural and man-made disasters would demand. If you are asked to participate in a mock disaster drill, it is important that you provide your observations of the strengths and weaknesses you noticed during the evaluation phase of the drill. If you are not a direct participant, you can ask yourself those "What would I do if...?" questions as you go about your regular assignments. You are also responsible for knowing what you will be expected to do should a disaster occur.

While practice and experience prepares health care workers to handle a variety of emergency situations, there are always those situations that no one imagined. The best response to the unknown is to use what you know, use common sense, remain calm, use critical thinking skills, and follow the instructions given by those in charge of the situation.

✔ *A Family Emergency Plan is important because your family may not be together when disaster strikes.*

THE *Web*

The Federal Emergency Management Agency Web site provides ideas on their *Ready* page about how you can prepare and protect yourself and your family during an emergency.

Nurse's Role

Nursing services are critical to recovery from any public health emergency. Many organizations welcome nurses who speak the language of the people affected, who have previous disaster relief experience, who have disaster training, who are ex-military, or who have certain specialties such as OR, ER, pediatrics, or trauma. The American Red Cross is only one of hundreds of organizations that trains and assigns volunteers to help survivors in a variety of disasters.

It is important that you continue to learn about public health emergencies and how they could affect you, your family, and your work. If volunteering to help those who have suffered from a disaster is something you might want to do, now is the time to prepare. To be accepted as a volunteer, training is necessary and being able to speak another language is a key asset.

✔ *Use Standard Precautions to protect yourself and others from inadvertent exposure to life-threatening microorganisms.*

THE *Web*

For more information on terrorism, bioterrorism, mass causalities, chemical emergencies, natural disasters, severe weather, and radiation emergencies, go to the Emergency Preparedness page of the Centers for Disease Control Web site.

ENVIRONMENTAL CHALLENGES

It is well known that we must tackle the global environmental issues that threaten all of us. Climate change, soil conservation and a dwindling food supply, population increases, pollution, changing ecosystems, nuclear testing, and the destruction of forests are just some of the issues that will, unless changes are made, adversely affect our future as well as the future of our children and our grandchildren.

In addition to global concerns, nurses have very real and immediate environmental concerns at work. Nurses are subject to health risks that come from unsafe equipment and procedures, from long-term noise and light pollution, and from working night shifts. Nurses are also subject to illnesses caused by toxic substances and escaping radiation that is present in their work environment.

Toxic Substances

Exposure to toxic substances comes from handling drugs including antineoplastic drugs and antibiotics, from gases that escape during anesthesia, from gases used to cold sterilize equipment, and from mercury gases that could escape from certain medical equipment. Other toxic substances include cleaning products used to disinfect work areas, plastics, latex, biological materials, and air pollution.

✔ *Look at some of the MSDS sheets during your next clinical assignment.*

While toxic substances may be essential to treating and curing diseases, the inappropriate or improper use and disposal of these substances can cause substantial injury or illness. For this reason, the U.S. Department of Labor's division of OSHA requires that all employers make the Material Safety Data Sheets (MSDS) available to all employees (Fig. 15-4). The law requires that there be an MSDS sheet on file for every chemical used in the facility. Among the information you can learn from an MSDS is what first aid measures are appropriate for that toxic substance, what to do in the event of an accidental release, what

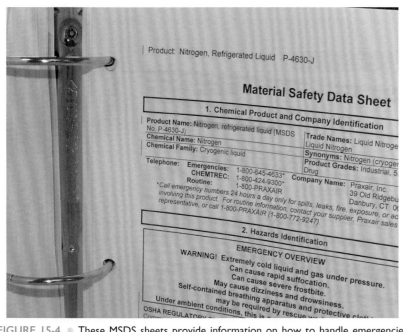

FIGURE 15-4. ● These MSDS sheets provide information on how to handle emergencies involving specific dangerous materials. (Photo Courtesy of Susan Roxandich, RN, BS, CNOR.)

measures to take to protect yourself when handling this substance, and how to dispose of the substance.

Radiation

Radiation is used in health care facilities to diagnose and treat disease. X-ray machines, radioactive materials, and radioactive drugs are the usual sources of radiation. Many radioactive materials are potential sources of contamination and are kept in a locked and secured area of the treatment facility. Uncontrolled exposure to any radiation must be immediately reported and treated. A pamphlet published by the American Association for Physics in Medicine provides helpful information for health care workers.

Pollution

Pollution generated by health care facilities is a serious employee and public health concern. The EPA found that medical waste incinerators are a leading source of dioxin, a toxic substance that is linked to cancer, reproductive disorders, and immune system dysfunction.

Allergies to latex gloves and powder, mercury gases, air pollution from medical gases, asbestos, radon, and biohazardous materials are just a few examples of other pollutants that abound in health care facilities. In addition to pollutants, an organization named *Practice Greenhealth* estimates that hospitals generate more that 5.9 million tons of waste each year.

✔ *"Pollution prevention means not polluting in the first place." EPA*

Practice Greenhealth was created to educate health care professionals about pollution prevention opportunities. Many hospitals and other health care facilities are working to recycle as much nonhazardous waste as possible. As a worker in the health care industry, you have a responsibility to comply with your employer's procedures for recycling and reducing waste.

Learn all you can about your working environment so that your own health and the health of your patients are not put in jeopardy. Work with your employer and community agencies to create a healthy and pollution-free environment.

 THE *Web*

The federal government has passed a number of laws and regulations related to medical hazards. A description of potential hazards and possible solutions can be reviewed on the Occupational Safety and Health Administration Web site under the heading *Hazards*.

SUMMARY

The issues that were discussed in this chapter confront workers every day. Knowing what the challenges are and knowing that there are things we can do to diminish their impact on us as individuals and on our workplace goes a long way toward creating a pleasant and productive working environment.

Use good communication skills to overcome differences and defuse stress. Be actively involved in making your workplace and your community safer and cleaner. Prepare yourself and your family for the unexpected and hope that it never happens. Practice self-care activities that will help you balance your work and your life. Get help from others if you feel as though you need it.

APPLY
Critical Thinking Skills

1. Go to the Employees and Applicants section of the Equal Employment Opportunity Commission's Web site, and review some of the Discrimination by Type listings that are relevant to work-related challenges.

2. Search the Internet for current cases involving nurses who blew the whistle on illegal or incompetent health care.

3. Keep a stress journal. For 1 week, note which events and situations cause a negative physical, mental, or emotional response. Record the day and time. Give a brief description of the situation. Where were you? Who was involved? What seemed to cause the stress? Also, describe your reaction. What were your physical symptoms? How did you feel? What did you say or do? Finally, on a scale of 1 (not very intense) to 5 (very intense), rate the intensity of your stress. Is it time to take the next step and develop a plan to reduce or eliminate some of the stressors in your life?

4. What stress management techniques would help you avoid "burnout?"

5. Make a conscious effort to learn one thing every day about a culture different from yours. For example, you might learn about what foods Muslim people do not eat or how Latinos view time and punctuality. Record your findings in a journal.

6. Volunteer to participate in a mock disaster drill in your clinical facility or your community.

7. Make a list of things you can do if you think your working environment is hazardous to your health.

8. Find out what happens to biohazardous medical waste in your clinical facility.

9. Choose a chemical cleaning product used in your home (e.g., Simple Green) and a product used in health care (e.g., Cidex). Locate these products on the Internet, and read the MSDS sheet related to that product. Is it hazardous? How is it disposed of? What happens if it is ingested? What first aid measures are recommended? Is personal protection required when using the product?

Read More
ABOUT IT

Byrd MY, Scott CL: Diversity in the Workforce: Current Issues and Emerging Trends. New York, NY: Routledge, 2014.

Chapman GD, White PE, Harold M: Rising Above a Toxic Workplace: Taking Care of Yourself in an Unhealthy Environment. Chicago, IL: Northfield Publishing, 2014.

Humphries J, Campbell JC: Family Violence and Nursing Practice, 2nd ed. New York, NY: Springer, 2010.

Hunt S: The Practical Preppers Complete Guide to Disaster Preparedness. New York, NY: St. Martin's Griffin, 2014.

Thomas SP: Transforming Nurses' Stress and Anger: Steps toward Healing, 3rd ed. New York, NY: Springer, 2008.

Todaro-Franceschi V: Compassion Fatigue and Burnout in Nursing: Enhancing Professional Life. New York, NY: Springer, 2012.

Tweedy JT: Healthcare Safety for Nursing Personnel: An Organizational Guide to Achieving Results. Boca Raton, FL: CRC Press, 2015.

Weinstein S: B is for Balance: A Nurse's Guide for Enjoying Life at Work and at Home. Indianapolis, IN: Sigma Theta Tau, 2014.

Current Issues and Future Concerns

LEARNING OBJECTIVES

When you complete this chapter, you will be able to:

1. List techniques that will help you adapt to future changes in the workplace.

2. Identify sources of information related to occupational risks.

3. Discuss several methods through which you can maintain your competence to practice nursing.

4. Critically analyze an announcement for a continuing education program.

5. Identify the advantages and disadvantages of mandatory continuing education for nurse license renewal.

LEARNING OBJECTIVES *continued*

6. Analyze how changes in the health care system and new categories of health care workers affect patient care.

7. Identify how some of the major issues and future concerns of nurses and nursing will affect your career.

8. Defend your positions on current issues in nursing.

9. Use available resources and knowledge to provide individualized and high-quality nursing care to people with diverse needs and treatment options.

Aleshia is a practical nurse working in a research laboratory at a large medical center. On her way in to her house after work one day, her neighbor Carmen approached her, asking if she could spare a few minutes to talk. Aleshia could see that Carmen was upset about something and told Carmen that, of course, she could talk with her.

The two went in to Aleshia's house, and while Aleshia was making coffee, Carmen began describing a situation that was of great concern to her. Carmen described how she and her husband had been trying to conceive a child for the past 5 years and finally, she became pregnant. During her first prenatal visit, the doctor told Carmen that she was about 6 weeks pregnant. "Aleshia, I just don't know what to do. The doctor suggested that we have a genetic assessment of the baby. When I asked her why she would suggest this, she said that if there are any problems, we could decide whether we wanted to continue the pregnancy or not. To tell the truth, we really want this baby and I don't know if we should do the testing or not. Aleshia, please tell me what you think we should do." Aleshia fussed with her coffee for what seemed like a long time and finally said, "You know I won't tell you what to do, but I will make a suggestion. It might be very helpful for you and your husband to meet with a genetic counselor. These folks can help you sort out your feelings about genetic testing and explain why you should or should not have it and what you can do with the results. It is a difficult decision, and getting help in making the decision will help both of you to understand your choices." As their conversation moved to talking about how exciting it was to be finally expecting a child and how Carmen planned to decorate the baby's room, the issue of genetic testing was put in the back of Aleshia's mind for at least a little while.

It was not all that long ago that organ transplants, immunizations against serious illnesses, arthroscopic surgery, gene therapy, and implants to control diabetes were unheard of. What the future holds for us is unknown, but what we know from history is that it will be very different from what we know today.

Many of the issues and concerns that are presented in this chapter have been examined in more detail in other chapters in this book. The purpose of this chapter is to talk about current issues and concerns that will most likely confront you when you begin your first job as a licensed practical or vocational nurse (LP/VN). What you know today will get you started, but you will have to continually strive to adapt to social, cultural, scientific, and technological changes. You must actively participate in resolving issues and concerns that will affect your career as an LP/VN now and in the future.

CHANGE

It is not whether there will be changes during your career and life, but how you manage them that will make a difference. People who see change as an opportunity to do things better and more efficiently will make better personal adjustments at home and at work. Those who do not like change and either actively or passively resist it will experience a tremendous amount of stress.

It will help you in your career as a nurse to learn to expect changes in how you work and to do all that you can to be involved in helping to decide what those changes may be. You can do so by participating in political activities, voting in political elections, serving on policy and procedure committees, continuing your education both formally and informally, joining professional organizations, and maintaining a positive and optimistic attitude that proposed changes will improve how things are done.

✔ *Change provides opportunities for personal and professional growth.*

People who have difficulty accepting change often make statements such as "We've never done it that way before," "We don't have enough staff to do that," "Sounds good, but…," and "I've always done it this way and it works just fine." Just imagine where we would be today if everyone thought this way.

New technology, the invention of new equipment, new categories of health care workers, and new diseases are just a few changes that nurses will experience in the next few years. People who ask questions such as "How can we do this better?" "What are the alternatives to how things are now?" "How many different methods can we think of to achieve our goal?" are creative thinkers who are open-minded and able to accept change in stride. Creative thinking will go a long way toward smoothing your transition to the future. Use the self-assessment exercise "How Do You View Creativity?" on pages 342–347 to explore your creativity.

Now is the time to pay attention to how you respond to change. If you find that your first reaction to change is to resist it, begin analyzing your responses and try replacing negative reactions with thinking that is more open-minded, creative, and positive. Consider change as an opportunity to grow as a person and to learn as a nurse.

GREEN HEALTH CARE

Green health care—the incorporation of environmentally friendly practices into health care delivery—is essential to preventing air, water, and land pollution. According to Practice Greenhealth, hospitals generate more than 5.9 million tons of waste each year.

Latex gloves, mercury, polyvinyl chloride, medical gases, pharmaceuticals, medical waste, and hazardous materials are just a few examples of pollutants that abound in health care facilities. Environmental Protection Agency research found that medical waste incinerators were the leading source of dioxin, a toxic substance that is linked to cancer, reproductive disorders, and immune system dysfunction.

✔ *Take an active role in protecting the environment from pollution.*

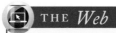

THE *Web*

A few of the many organizations working to promote healthy environ-
ments in health care include Practice Greenhealth, the U.S. Environmental
Protection Agency, state government environmental agencies, Health Care
Without Harm, the American Hospital Association, and the World Health
Organization.

Contaminated air, water, and land is a serious threat to you and your family. Learn all you can about your working environment, and work with your
employer and other agencies to create a nontoxic environment for yourself and
your patients.

ASSESS YOURSELF   How Do You View Creativity?

Creative/innovative thinking results in better problem-solving abilities that enhance your productivity, decrease
stress, and help you avoid future shocks. What is your understanding of creative/innovative attitudes?

A. SELF-ASSESSMENT

1. Do you consider yourself creative?
   a. Very
   b. Moderately
   c. Not at all

2. How many creative accomplishments have you achieved in the past?
   a. Many
   b. Some
   c. None

3. Do you want to be more creative?
   a. Yes
   b. No

4. Do you think it's your destiny to develop something creatively?
   a. Yes
   b. No

5. When you were growing up, did the following apply?
   a. Moved frequently.
   b. Given freedom and independence to think for yourself.
   c. Given clear standards of right and wrong.
   d. Parents were independent and effective in their work.
   e. Parents respected you and your abilities.
   f. Intense closeness was avoided.
   g. Consistent and effective discipline.
   h. Many positive models to identify with.
   i. Lack of pressure to find professional identity.
   j. Parents had more artistic, cultural, and intellectual interests than did neighbors

6. Do you
   a. Allow free time during the day to do nothing?
   b. Feel guilty when not working?
   c. Alternate between work and play?

7. Do you love the work that you want to be creative?
   a. Yes
   b. No

8. Do you ask questions that might be thought stupid by others?
   a. Yes
   b. No

9. Do you
   a. "Strike while the iron is hot?"
   b. "Make the iron hot by striking?"
   c. "Strike out?"

10. Which do you believe?
    a. "If it ain't broke, don't fix it."
    b. "It's always broke."

11. Do you
    a. Need a logical explanation for everything?
    b. Delight in uncertainty and mystery?

12. Do you
    a. Prefer to work alone?
    b. Prefer to work in groups?

13. Do you
    a. Need to put everything in its proper place?
    b. Tolerate ambiguous situations well?

14. In problem solving, do you
    a. Need to have a clear plan before moving ahead?
    b. Try anything to find a direction to move?

15. When someone suggests a new idea, do you
    a. Immediately evaluate it, looking for weaknesses?
    b. Defend it, trying to find its strengths?
    c. Play with the possibilities suggested by the idea?

16. In solving problems, do you
    a. Logically figure the situation out?
    b. Look for as many possibilities as you can think of?
    c. Rely on hunches that you check out later?

17. Do you believe that intuition is
    a. A reality worth relying on?
    b. The inability to be logical?

18. Do you
    a. Like excitement and change?
    b. Prefer peace and a reliable routine?

19. How willing are you to take a chance?
    a. Comfortable with risking
    b. Depends on the situation

continued on page 344

20. If you were given a new toy or game to play, would you
   a. Always go by the instructions?
   b. Play around, improvising with the materials?
   c. Devise variations after learning the correct way?

21. Do you agree (A) or disagree (D) with the following?
   a. What others think about you is important.
   b. Rules are made to be broken.
   c. Dreams are useless.
   d. It's bad to change your mind frequently.
   e. Wishing makes it happen.
   f. Curiosity killed the cat.

22. Do you most go by
   a. A situation's potential
   b. The practical consequences
   c. How others might react
   d. The beauty of the solution

B. YOUR UNDERSTANDING OF CREATIVITY

23. Which of the following are characteristics of creativity?
   a. Spontaneity
   b. Deliberateness
   c. Newness
   d. Value
   e. Skills
   f. Play
   g. Work
   h. Convergence
   i. Divergence

24. Does an idea have to be carried out to be considered "creative"?
   a. Yes
   b. No

25. Do you believe creative production
   a. Is best rewarded?
   b. Is hindered by rewards?

26. Do you believe creative behavior
   a. Is a sign of compensation for unmet emotional needs?
   b. Is an expression of the healthy personality?

27. Creativity
   a. Is an all-or-none phenomenon—you're creative or you're not?
   b. Exists on a continuum?

28. Which is more important to originality?
   a. Asking the right question
   b. Finding the right answer

C. SOME CHALLENGES

29. Count the squares.

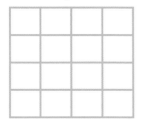

30. Connect the dots with four straight lines.

31. What different uses can you find for a plastic milk bottle?

32. Take a word beginning with "C." Then consider the problem of war. Force-fit as many metaphoric solutions using your "C" word. For example, how is war "cow-like"? "Car-like"? "Candle-like"? What new perspectives can you come up with for solving the problem of war?

DISCUSSION OF EACH QUESTION BY NUMBER

1. If you think you're creative, chances are you're right.
2. Your history of creative accomplishments, even more than "creativity test" scores, tends to indicate how creative you will be in the future.
3. If you want to be more creative, you must know your field and understand creative problem-solving approaches; then, with the right motivation, you will meet your goals. Desire is as important as ability. Those who don't care or dare to be creative won't.
4. Those who are gifted in creativity have a sense of destiny about what they are trying to do. It helps them persist when others might give up.
5. All these characteristics have been found in the early lives of creative people.
6. Paying attention to ideas that pop up during free time leads to imaginative breakthroughs. Alternation between work and play is important to creative fitness. Innovation often results from purposeful play.
7. If you don't love what you are doing, it is unlikely you will ever be inspired.
8. Only those who don't ask questions are stupid.
9. You need to do both (a) and (b)/or you'll strike out creatively.
10. Those who believe (a) will always fall into the adequacy trap.
11. The drive to find a logical explanation often motivates creative individuals, but frequently they do not get original solutions through a logical route. The nonlogical, sometimes random, but purposeful play of the creative individual is fueled by curiosity and delight in uncertainty and mystery.
12. Although many creative ideas come in brainstorming groups, highly creative individuals often are introverts who value working alone with a problem more than gaining approval and acceptance from others.
13. A rigidly ordered life is governed too closely by outmoded rules from the past. Because creative people have one foot in current reality and another in the future, they have to tolerate ambiguity well. They seek ambiguous situations to impose their particular order on the world.

continued on page 346

ASSESS YOURSELF   How Do You View Creativity? *continued*

14. Innovators question the way even when it seems right. They continually seek a better way. Consequently, they stir things up just to see what might happen. Plans are primarily useful to get you going; then you readjust as you see the results.

15. Immediate evaluation—any kind of judgment—will kill off the next creative idea. Be curious rather than critical. Creative people play with others' ideas and build on them if they can. Then everyone gains.

16. Logic can be useful if the logical system is up-to-date. But if you want to get ahead of the crowd, you need to find new possibilities and new paradigms. Hunches are OK, if you check them out later.

17. Intuition is a sudden wholistic insight, not processed serially like logical thinking. One who is creative uses both logical and nonlogical methods. Anything is OK in creative thinking if it is the means to a better end.

18. Creative people must seek change where they hope to be creative, but change in every area of life can be chaotic. The more internal stability individuals have, the more freedom they have to change externally. Rigidity, however, is anathema to creativity.

19. Those who dare to take a chance will be creative. Luck comes to those who work hard and to those who see what others are afraid to see. Creativity is often persistence with a twist.

20. When everything fails, reread the instructions. But innovative solutions do not come with instructions for their discovery. So practice the improvising lifestyle, trying things out, just to see what might happen. Then you will be ready to deal with unexpected events.

21. Creative people cannot be too dependent on another's judgments, which are often based on past criteria, for the future has its own requirements that others might not yet understand. To the innovator, rules are made to be broken. Imaginative solutions often come to those who pay attention to the metaphors of their dreams. Be willing to change your mind—it shows you are learning something new. Your wishes drive imaginative solutions to the surface. Although curiosity killed the cat, information brought it back to investigate further.

22. Innovators look to the situation's potential and the beauty of a solution. Yet, the practical consequences and how others react often decide if an idea ever gets a hearing.

23. All these are characteristics of creativity.

24. If you do not try to carry out a new idea, how will you know how good it is? Besides, you may never get valuable feedback to make improvements.

25. Rewards tend to alter the focus from the creative process to externals. Intrinsic motivation from the joy of the work stirs most creativity.

26. Some people create to compensate for unmet needs, but they sustain little joy in the work. Healthy people express creative attitudes in all they do. As they fulfill the creative potential in the work they do, they fulfill themselves.

27. Creativity exists on a continuum. Although some people have more creative talent than do others, all can become more creative.

28. The most original thinkers spend more time analyzing the problem than trying to find a quick answer to an inadequate question.

29. Sometimes, the right answer is not always the best solution. Too often, it causes us to stop investigating further. If you answered 16 (counting all the small squares), you were right. If you answered 25 (adding also the nine four-box squares), you were right. If you said 29 (adding also the four nine-box squares), you were right. If you said 30 (adding the large sixteen-box square), you may have the best answer possible… till someone comes along with a better one.

30. Sometimes, you have to go outside your internal boundaries, challenging the assumptions and the unconscious gestalt of the square. Can you find ways to connect the dots with three lines or even one line?

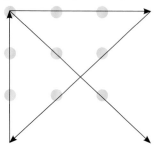

31. To put milk in, water in, anything in. To use as a buoy, a plant holder, a club, a bat. Cut it up and use it as a bailer, a funnel. The more you list, the more likely you will come up with original answers. Usually, these are toward the end when you run out of remembered solutions.

32. Any word can be used as a metaphor to serve as a bridge to a better solution. Shifting perspective through the right metaphor may help us find some paths to ending war. We all need to be more creative, or we are not going to live on this planet much longer. I hope you came up with some good new ideas.

Printed with permission from Young JG: Creativity Self-Assessment. Adventures in Creativity. Available on-line at jgyoungmd.net then the search term "Creativity Self Assessment."

OCCUPATIONAL RISKS

Working in health care imposes a number of risks to nurses. Accidental needle-sticks are of extreme concern. Musculoskeletal injuries, overexposure to radiation, latex allergies, exposure to the human immunodeficiency virus, hepatitis, tuberculosis, rare viruses, drug-resistant superbugs, and as yet unknown diseases are concerns that confront nurses now and will continue to do so in the future.

The issue of safe lifting and handling and concerns about needlestick injuries to health care workers continue to receive the attention of nursing organizations, health care administrators, and politicians. A number of state and federal legislative actions are being or have recently been introduced. Know what policies, procedures, and legislation are being proposed on these issues and actively work to implement new safety guidelines.

✔ *Be involved in protecting your own safety and the safety of your coworkers.*

OSHA develops guidelines that employers must follow to ensure the safety of health care workers, but not even OSHA can prevent nurses from contracting diseases or being exposed to environmental toxins that have not yet been identified. New products used in new ways have the potential to cause harm to those who handle them.

The efforts of OSHA, the Centers for Disease Control, state health agencies, politicians, and employers to deal with current problems are commendable and do increase safety in the workplace. Prudent nurses will do everything possible to know as much as they can about their working environment. Careful attention to handling medications and understanding the implications of a medical diagnosis will go a long way toward helping you maintain your own health. Educate yourself on the latest self-protective procedures and assertively demand that the necessary training and equipment be available in your workplace.

CHEMICALLY IMPAIRED NURSES

It is estimated that 10% to 15% of nurses have or are currently using illegal drugs and abusing alcohol and incorrectly using prescription and nonprescription drugs. Some of the excuses so many nurses give for resorting to using drugs, alcohol, or both include job-related stress, inability to cope with changes in the workplace, overwhelming personal responsibilities, a feeling of frustration and helplessness in their personal and professional lives, and easy access to drugs.

✔ *Drug and alcohol abuse destroys careers and families.*

In an effort to help those who are impaired, each state board of nursing has developed a disciplinary program. These disciplinary programs are intended to give the impaired nurse an opportunity to rehabilitate himself or herself and avoid losing their nursing license. Those who fail to complete the prescribed treatment program are subject to further action against the license. Final disciplinary actions taken by boards of nursing are reported to the National Practitioner Data Bank and are public information.

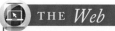

THE *Web*

Go to the Web site for your state board of nursing, and read about voluntary recovery programs, reporting procedures, and resources available to impaired nurses. You can also find the names, license numbers, and reasons why nurses have had their license suspended or revoked.

It is your responsibility to yourself, your family, and your patients to avoid the use of addictive substances. If you or someone you know does become addicted to drugs or alcohol, the only option is to seek immediate assistance. Referring yourself or someone else to your state board of nursing for the voluntary treatment and rehabilitation program may not only save a career—it may save a life.

MAINTAINING COMPETENCE

Many of the techniques and skills you learned this year will, in the next few years, be replaced by new techniques and skills. Your nursing program has prepared you with the minimum competencies needed to enter the practice of practical/vocational nursing, but maintaining and expanding your competencies will require attention throughout your entire career.

Maintaining competence through informal educational experiences is one of the most frequently used methods for keeping up with changes in nursing. Reading journals, attending staff development programs offered by your employer, learning new procedures or techniques from those skilled in their performance, reading patient health records, listening to physicians as they discuss treatment options, and learning to use new and different equipment will help you remain competent in your nursing skills (Fig. 16-1).

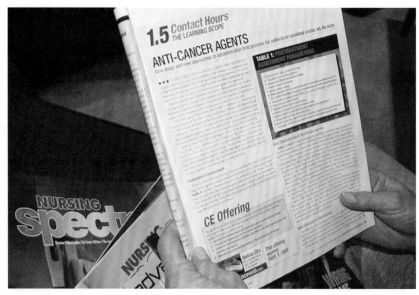

FIGURE 16-1. ● Journals provide current information that can help you keep up with changes in the field of nursing.

Another method for maintaining competence is through formal continuing education. Formal continuing education includes lectures, workshops, seminars, college courses, and independent study programs. Sponsors of continuing education programs include hospitals, nursing homes, colleges and universities, and nursing and health care associations. Sponsors can apply to nursing organizations, such as the American Nurses Association, the National Federation of Licensed Practical Nurses, the National Association for Practical Nurse Education and Service, the National League for Nursing, and individual state boards of nursing for program approval. Approved programs may offer continuing education units (CEUs). One CEU is the equivalent of 10 contact hours of participation in an approved continuing education program.

When selecting a continuing education program, you should consider those that apply directly to your learning needs. You will want to determine the program's purpose, objectives, content, teaching–learning methods, and faculty qualifications. You will also want to know whether the program is approved to offer CEUs and which organization gave that approval. The cost of the program, including registration fees, meals, and materials, as well as the refund policy should be clearly written on the brochure. The cancellation policy should indicate that registration fees are refunded if the company cancels the program.

✔ *Keeping good records of your participation in continuing education is essential.*

It is as important to keep good records of your participation in continuing education programs as it is to participate. Your records can be presented to prospective employers as evidence of your commitment to your career. These records can also be presented to your state board of nursing to document that you have met the continuing education requirement for license renewal (if your state has such a law).

If you decide not to work for a period of time, your state board of nursing has a procedure for inactivating your nursing license. When you decide to return to your career in nursing, your board has requirements for reactivation. Most boards require evidence that you have completed a refresher course that is approved by the board and that meets their specific requirements before your license can be reactivated. The thinking is that a refresher course will update the competence you had prior to inactivating your license. Be sure you know the renewal requirements before you decide to place your license on inactive status.

CONTINUING EDUCATION FOR LICENSE RENEWAL

A current issue that will no doubt become more important in the future is the controversy over whether continuing education for license renewal should be voluntary or mandated by law. People who believe that continuing education should be voluntary assert that continuing education is a responsibility of all nurses and that laws should not dictate how this responsibility is met. Those who favor laws that define the minimum hours of continuing education required for license renewal believe that this is the only way to ensure that nurses will keep their knowledge current.

✔ *What are the continuing education requirements for license renewal in your state?*

The nurse practice acts of 34 states require a specific number of contact hours in continuing education for license renewal as a practical/vocational nurse. Of these, some states additionally require a minimum number of hours of practice as a nurse for license renewal. If you practice nursing in a state that does not yet have a mandatory continuing education requirement for license renewal, this is one of the current issues in which you should become involved. Learn the reasons for both mandatory and voluntary continuing education and the implications of each. When this issue is presented in your state or place of employment, you will be prepared to help influence decisions that will benefit you, your colleagues, and your future.

INFORMATION TECHNOLOGY IN HEALTH CARE

The computer is the most visible example of technology in health care. Computers provide the technology for voice-activated charting, customized nursing care plans, assessment of acuity levels, and reminders to staff of treatment and medication schedules. Computer technology aids in ordering supplies, equipment, diagnostic tests, and medications. Computers assist in developing clinical pathways and care maps. Computer programs provide quick access to drug incompatibilities and food interactions, treatment modalities, and suggested interventions related to specific nursing diagnoses.

Even more outstanding advances are expected in the future. Knowledge discovery through analyzing data from different perspectives and summarizing it into useful information will lead to early detection of disease outbreaks and drug reactions. Computer assistive devices will allow the disabled and elderly to remain independent and in their homes longer. Computer programs will develop treatment plans based on an individual's DNA rather than on a general treatment plan prescribed for thousands of people. Telemedicine will treat people in remote and rural areas that do not have ready access to health care providers. Robots controlled by computers will be used more routinely in surgery and will be developed to provide mobility to those who have sustained a spinal cord injury. The ways in which computers can and will be used in health care continue to be mind boggling with the most amazing applications yet to come.

The widespread use of computer technology in health care poses many future concerns. Questions about maintaining the confidentiality of individually identifiable health information and how to protect the integrity of the system from hackers and cybercriminals are already big concerns. What effect the temporary failure of a computer system on which the staff is totally dependent will have on the ability of the nursing staff to carry out scheduled medication and treatment plans remains to be seen. What effect would a natural disaster that destroys Internet and phone cables have on health care in a heavily populated region? Will excessive reliance on computers lead to a loss of skill in treating patients the "old-fashioned way"? Will critical thinking and communication skills be diminished? There are many "what ifs," yet better diagnostic tools and treatment regimens continue to improve our health and well-being.

Being proficient in using current computer technology in health care settings today does not guarantee success in the future. New programs, new systems, and new applications will require continued education and training.

✔ Computers quickly provide access to information to manage and improve health care.

ELECTRONIC HEALTH RECORDS

An electronic health record (EHR) records medical history, medications, illnesses, results of physical exams, radiology images, notes by doctors and nurses, as well as results of diagnostic and laboratory tests in a digital format. The EHR can be shared among health care providers in a variety of settings. Some of the advantages of the EHR were discussed in Chapter 7.

The Affordable Care Act instituted regulations beginning October 1, 2012, that requires health plans to begin adopting and implementing rules for the secure and confidential electronic exchange of health information. These rules are being implemented over a period of years and provide monetary reimbursement to health care providers who had to purchase equipment and train staff to implement electronic records.

While EHRs improve communication between health care providers, there are several issues and concerns surrounding this type of health record. The greatest concern is confidentiality of patient information. It is estimated that 150 people have access to at least a part of a patient's medical record during a hospitalization. Another concern is cost. Implementing an EHR system is very expensive due to the need to purchase equipment and provide training programs for staff. There are some concerns that patients whose records are lost or incorrectly transferred to an EHR may sue for damages as a result of this type of error.

Nurses express concern about software design and programming issues that have caused medication and treatment errors. Some say systems are complicated and difficult to use. There is concern about how to correct a human error when incorrect information is entered or correct information is entered on an incorrect record. Nurses are concerned about delays in the availability of the EHR for new and emergency admissions and how those delays could affect treatment. Over time, the sheer volume of information in an EHR may make it difficult to find pertinent information that was entered in the distant past.

While EHRs are good, they still present many challenges to those who use them and to the patient. It will be important for you to express any concerns you might have about EHRs to your supervisor so that implementation of this system does not compromise quality of patient care or confidentiality of health records.

EMPLOYMENT

The nursing shortage that occurred in the early 2000s brought a lot of national attention to the importance of nurses in our society and in having a sufficient number of nurses to work in health care facilities. The various task forces that were created to solve this problem made a number of recommendations and as a result, the number of people who graduated from nursing school between 2000 and 2010 more than doubled. The increase in the number of graduates along with an economic recession in 2007 has led to a more-than-adequate supply of nurses. But the plentiful supply of nurses is expected to gradually disappear before 2020, and some predict that the shortage will be larger than ever. The median age of LP/VNs is 43.6 years with nearly half over the age of 50. Those nurses will most likely be retiring in a few years. More than 32 million Americans will gain medical insurance under the provisions of the Affordable Care Act, and baby boomers (those born between 1946 and 1964) began turning 65 in 2011. By 2030, 20% of the population will be over 65 years of age. And when the economy is good, nurses (primarily female) tend to not work, and when the economy recovers, many nurses exit the workforce to stay home and care for children causing the shortage to return.

THE *Web*

Go to the Occupational Outlook Handbook Web site, and use the search term *Licensed Practical/Vocational Nurse* to learn more about the projected job openings for LP/VNs.

The Bureau of Labor Statistics projects a 25% growth rate for LP/VNs between 2012 and 2022, so now is the time, when you are defining your clinical interests and exploring your employment options, to think about what you want to be doing 5 and 10 years from now.

✔ *Accept a job that will help you achieve your long-term career goals.*

Opportunities for employment in all areas of health care are becoming more plentiful. If you have limited knowledge and experience in an area in which you want to work, you will need to prepare yourself with the special skills needed in that setting. You can do this by volunteering your services a few hours a week, by attending continuing education activities, by finding a mentor (a tutor or coach) in the setting in which you want to work, and by accepting a position on a trial basis at perhaps a lower rate of pay.

Your nursing education probably included experiences in a variety of clinical settings. It is well known that most new graduates get their first job through contacts made during a clinical rotation. It is in your best interest to demonstrate to the staff and supervisors in these clinical rotations that you have the characteristics and qualities of an effective team member. When the time comes for you to seek employment, you will be remembered.

✔ *Remember to keep your portfolio up-to-date.*

Some health care facilities are reducing the total number of employees as a way of controlling costs. When job openings do occur, employers have many applicants from which to choose. Having an excellent academic background, strong clinical skills, and an ability to present yourself well during an interview will make you a convincing candidate. Being flexible in the hours and shifts you can work and demonstrating a strong desire to learn will go a long way toward securing employment.

EDUCATION

The curriculum of nursing education programs changed from the few models that were widely used from the 1950s through the 1990s. The current curriculum is preparing nurses to work not only in acute care but also in long-term care, special acute care units, and community health care settings. This curriculum is more accommodating to older students, minority students, and students who cannot attend class during traditional hours and days. It includes seamless, integrated courses of study that acknowledge prior knowledge, skills, and related work experience. This curriculum is also using nontraditional teaching methods such as simulations, distance learning, and interactive Web-based instruction to incorporate different learning styles in instruction.

✔ *It is absolutely essential that you expand your knowledge and skills throughout your nursing career.*

The use of computer technology in nursing education is providing many opportunities for learners to be actively involved in acquiring knowledge and skills. Traditional lectures in which the teacher talks and the learner listens will become a rare rather than a usual method of teaching. Nursing students, as well as graduate nurses, are beginning to enroll in distance learning classes, join content-related list serves, participate in sophisticated clinical simulation laboratories, attend teleconferences, and use the Internet for research.

The nurse who subscribes to a philosophy of lifelong learning can expect to have a long and rewarding career. The skills of today will be inadequate for the future. Patient care will be based on new knowledge, and it will be skill intensive. Those whose skills and knowledge remain at the level they are today will be quickly left behind.

LONG-TERM CARE FACILITIES

The number of long-term care facilities, as well as the number of residents living in these facilities, is expected to increase rapidly between now and 2030, as baby boomers enter their elderly years.

In 2002, approximately 14% of Americans were age 65 or older, and that number is expected to increase to over 20% in just 15 years. The number of those aged

85 and older is expected to almost triple from 6.3 million now to 17.9 million in 2050. Studies show that more than 50% of people older than 85 need assistance with some activities of daily living and that about 15% live in nursing homes. While age alone does not predict a need for assistance, the older a person gets the more likely it is that he or she will need some assistance with activities of daily living. It is fairly easy to conclude that there will be a tremendous increase in the need for a wide variety of long-term care services for the elderly.

Younger people with injuries or debilitating diseases whose families cannot care for them at home will create an additional need for services in long-term care facilities. These younger people may be paralyzed, or they may have Parkinson's disease, Down syndrome, acquired immunodeficiency syndrome, or chronic and crippling diseases.

The addition of subacute units to long-term care facilities is changing the perception of facilities or nursing homes. Traditionally, resident units were classified as skilled care, intermediate care, or custodial care. People living in custodial care units usually need some assistance with a few activities of daily living; those living in intermediate care units need assistance with several activities of daily living plus medications and minor treatments; and those living in skilled care units need treatments, procedures, and frequent assessments that must be performed by licensed nurses.

✔ *Opportunities to provide care for older people will be available in many different kinds of settings, including long-term care facilities.*

These subacute units in long-term care facilities care for people who, in the past, were often admitted to acute care hospitals. Patients who are dependent on a ventilator, who need monitoring during medication adjustments, and who have unstable diabetes are just a few examples of those who might be admitted to a subacute unit.

These changes in the types of health care services provided in long-term care facilities will provide many employment opportunities for LP/VNs in the future.

CULTURAL DIVERSITY AND THE NURSING TEAM

While much attention has been devoted to learning to meet the needs of diverse patient populations, less has been discussed about relationships among diverse team members. Just over half of the LP/VNs were White in 2013, while 23.6% were Black/African American, 7.5% were Hispanic/Latino, 3.6% were Asian, 0.6% were American Indian/Alaska Native, and 1.4% were multiple or other races. About 7.6% of LP/VNs are men and about 15% of registered nurses are foreign-born. Given these numbers plus other differences discussed elsewhere in this book, it is quite likely that, regardless of the setting in which you choose to work, your coworkers will be quite different from you and also quite different from one another in many ways.

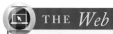
THE *Web*

> The U.S. Department of Agriculture offers a program titled *Handling Diversity in the Workplace*. This short course offers valuable suggestions on how to communicate and work across cultural differences.

Creating a positive work environment that is made up of people from different cultures requires that individual nurses take personal responsibility for learning about the culture of others. Knowing that different cultures relate differently to peers, supervisors, and patients will explain why some team members will not challenge an apparently incorrect directive from a supervisor while others do not hesitate to "speak up." Some are not bothered by conflict and others will do everything they can to avoid it. How different cultures define a "good employee" varies from culture to culture as does touching others and the boundaries of personal space. Some people use formal communication styles while people from some cultures routinely use slang.

Open communication, sensitivity, respect, and an interest in understanding others will go a long way toward creating an environment that will help culturally diverse staff learn appropriate ways to behave and interact.

DISCRIMINATION

Discrimination is defined as showing partiality or prejudice in actions or policies. Direct discrimination is based on age, race, color, sex, national origin, religion, marital status, pregnancy, sexual orientation, membership in organizations, or qualified handicaps. Subtle, indirect discrimination consists of the unequal or preferential treatment or favoritism of some individuals over others. A common subtle discriminatory practice is to always assign the nurse who doesn't complain to care for those patients who are the most difficult or require the most care. A few other examples include paying male nurses more than female nurses for the same job; promoting unqualified nurses over more highly qualified nurses; always granting a certain nurse's request for a religious holiday; asking only male nurses to assist in lifting and moving patients; offering all continuing education opportunities to a single individual; or denying a promotion because of a physical issue such as obesity or HIV-positive status.

✔ *Work to eliminate direct as well as subtle forms of discrimination.*

Complying with discrimination laws will not prevent subtle discriminatory behavior in the workplace. Knowing that subtle discrimination occurs is the first step toward stopping it. Pay attention to the body language of those with whom you work. If you notice that someone looks uncomfortable, ask them why. Suggest actions that will result in equal treatment.

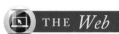

THE *Web*

Questions and answers about federal laws prohibiting job discrimination can be reviewed at the Equal Employment Opportunity Commission Web site.

NURSE LICENSURE COMPACT

Nurse Licensure Compact is the term used to describe interstate licensing of nurses. Having a nursing license that is valid in your state of residence as well as in other states will give you increased flexibility when moving from state to state. For you to have your nursing license recognized in other states, your state of residence must sign an interstate compact. An interstate compact is an agreement between two or more states in which each agrees to recognize the validity of the nursing license issued by the other state. As of January 2015, 24 states had enacted legislation that provides for interstate licensure of nurses; seven states have pending legislation.

✔ *Twenty-four states currently belong to the Nurse Licensure Compact.*

While many believe that interstate licensure is positive, others are concerned that inconsistencies between licensing requirements in individual states will undermine the state's ability to ensure that residents receive safe nursing care. Interstate licensure is an issue that will affect you as you enter into the practice of nursing. Use your favorite Internet search engine and the search term "Nurse licensure compact" to learn more about both sides of this issue.

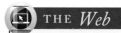

THE *Web*

Visit the National Council of State Boards of Nursing Web site, and click on Licensure Compacts to get the latest information on this issue.

If your state is a participating state, learn about how the interstate compact might affect you in your employment. If your state does not participate, learn about activities related to this issue. Determine your position, and work with other nurses and your legislators to pass or defeat proposed legislation.

DELEGATION AND CROSS-TRAINING

Legal issues related to the delegation of nursing tasks to unlicensed assistive personnel (UAP), the use of multipurpose workers, and cross-training of nurses will continue to concern licensed nurses well into the future.

Go to the National Council of State Boards of Nursing or to your state board of nursing Web site, and use the search word "Delegation," "Decision Making Model," "Nurse Practice Act," or similar term, to read the latest regulations and guidelines related to delegating or assigning tasks to UAP. When a nurse delegates his or her tasks to a UAP, he or she must be absolutely certain that the person to whom the task is delegated is competent to perform it. (See Chapter 13, "Planning and Delegating Patient Care," to review the process involved in delegating nursing duties to others.) Delegating or assigning tasks to an unlicensed person does not remove liability from the licensed nurse. Licensed nurses must use great caution and follow state and agency guidelines when delegating tasks.

The legal issues associated with delegating tasks that by law belong to licensed nurses to UAPs and multipurpose workers will expose the patient to a multitude of caregivers, each with their own tasks to perform. Employers who expect to save money by replacing licensed nurses with other, less knowledgeable workers may in the long run lose money because of patient dissatisfaction with the quality of their care, the large number of people who provide that care, and because of claims of malpractice as a result of negligent care.

The cross-training of nurses and other health care workers is an issue that has stimulated a lot of discussion. The LP/VN who is working in a hospital and can provide respiratory therapy treatments, do electrocardiograms (ECGs), draw blood, and start intravenous (IV) therapy fluids may be considered cross-trained. The LP/VN in this scenario is performing jobs normally performed by the respiratory care practitioner, the ECG technician, and the IV team. Cross-training is also used to describe the nurse who is trained to work in several different clinical specialties, such as the postpartum unit, the normal and intensive care nursery, and the delivery room.

There are advantages and disadvantages to being cross-trained. One advantage is that the person who is cross-trained is a valuable employee. If the time comes to decrease the size of the staff, the cross-trained person may be retained, whereas those with limited skills would be let go. A second advantage is for the employer. Because the cross-trained person can work in several different areas of the facility or do the jobs of several other people, an employer can save the money that would be paid to others.

✔ *Keep current on new laws, regulations, and employer policies that affect delegating your nursing tasks to others and accepting new tasks for yourself.*

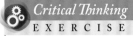

Critical Thinking
E X E R C I S E

Suppose your state passes a law that says the nurse-to-patient ratio on an acute care medical surgical unit must be 1:4. At the time the law was passed, 1:4 was a good ratio and provided adequate staff and sufficient time for nurses to provide safe care. Over the past few years, the patients admitted to this patient unit became progressively sicker and required more care. The 1:4 ratio is no longer adequate, but because the law only requires one nurse for every four patients, cost-conscious owners and managers refuse to hire more staff. They are complying with the law and see no reason to add the expense of additional staff nurses. Short of changing the law (which usually takes several years), propose some possible solutions or courses of action that you believe could deal with this issue. Use Appropriate Characteristics of Critical Thinkers in Box 1-2 on pages 18–19 to develop your response to this situation.

A major disadvantage to cross-training is based on the quality of the training the person receives for these additional duties. Almost anyone can quickly learn the manipulative skills needed to perform treatments and procedures. Acquiring the knowledge essential to understanding the implications and side effects of procedures and how to cope with potential complications takes much longer. The respiratory care practitioner, for example, spends up to 4 years learning to provide respiratory therapy services.

Another disadvantage to cross-training is related to safety. The nurse who is cross-trained to work in the four different divisions of the maternity department may have difficulty maintaining competency in all four areas. It would be even more difficult to maintain competency if the licensed nurse who usually worked on a medical unit was cross-trained to work in the maternity postpartum unit but was only assigned to work in that unit once or twice a month. The LP/VN who can, in addition to providing patient care, provide respiratory therapy treatments, do ECGs, draw blood, and start IV therapy fluids may find that this added workload is more than he or she can safely handle.

It is likely that you will be personally confronted with the issues of delegation of duties and cross-training as you continue your career in nursing. Remember to base your actions on state nursing practice laws as well as your competence to perform additional duties.

SAFE STAFFING

Insurance companies and owners of health care facilities have taken drastic measures, including reducing the number of licensed nurses, to lower their costs. One of the results of cutting costs by reducing nursing staff has been increasing complaints from nurses and consumers that nurse staffing is inadequate for providing safe care. Although many states recognize that nurses and patients are concerned, California was the first state to pass a law that related to the nurse staffing issues.

On October 10, 1999, the governor of California signed into law the first bill that set the stage for mandating nurse-to-patient or safe staffing ratios. The California Department of Health Services then worked with the California Nurses Association for almost 4 years to develop regulations that establish minimum, specific, and numerical registered nurse-to-patient ratios for all hospital units. These regulations took effect in January 2004 and were revised in January 2008. Examples of nurse-to-patient ratios include 1 nurse to 2 patients in intensive care units, 1:1 in the operating room, 1:4 in the emergency room, and 1:5 in medical–surgical units.

THE *Web*

The American Nurses Association maintains current information on staffing issues on their Web site. Use the search term *Nurse Staffing Plans & Ratios* to learn more about what individual states are doing in regard to staffing issues.

Currently, 13 states have enacted legislation or adopted some form of regulation regarding nurse staffing. Nurses and others opposed to legally mandated ratios believe that the government should not determine ratios and that laws do not allow the flexibility needed to deal with real practice issues. Those who support safe staffing ratios believe that patient safety will be improved, job and patient satisfaction will improve, and care errors will decrease.

Higher numbers of patients per nurse puts nurses in a stressful situation. Many nurses who are suffering from heavy workloads leave nursing, which makes the situation even worse. Find out what if any activities related to RN and LP/VNs and safe staffing are occurring in your state, and get involved in helping to address this issue.

NURSE SHORTAGE

While the shortage of nurses that began in the late 1990s has eased, experts are warning that this is a temporary condition and that the shortage could become even more serious over the next 15 years.

When the economy improves, nurses who returned to work to supplement family income during the recession will stop working and the number of working nurses will decline. As discussed earlier in this chapter, employed nurses are getting older with the average age of registered nurses now at 47 years and LP/VNs at 43.6 years. Baby boomers are getting older and will be using more health care services. Practical nursing schools report that in 2013, they could not accept 41% of qualified applicants because of lack of faculty and clinical sites. Nurses who are suffering from burnout, compassion fatigue, and job dissatisfaction and who quit their jobs also contribute to the shortage. Expanded career options for women reduce the number of women interested in entering a career in nursing. The Bureau of Labor Statistics predicts that more than 200,000 new and replacement LP/VNs will be needed by 2022.

A shortage of working nurses would have a significant impact on health care as well as on you individually. How will you handle a heavy workload? What will you do to relieve the stress you might experience from short staffing? Will you be asked to perform duties beyond your scope of practice? Do you know how to refuse an assignment that you know you are not competent to perform? Will you be able to provide the quality of care you believe is essential for patient safety? What will you do to recruit young people to a career in nursing?

There are a number of initiatives designed to prevent the pending shortage of nurses. Private corporations such as the Robert Wood Johnson Foundation, the Institute of Medicine, and the American Association of Retired Persons committed millions of dollars to ongoing research into the conditions that create the supply and demand for nurses and have developed projections and recommendations for the future of nursing. Most individual states have task forces that monitor the status of the nursing workforce in their state. The federal government, civic and health care organizations, private organizations, unions, and minority organizations offer various forms of financial grants and loans to pay for a nursing education. Improving working conditions and salaries are helping to keep nurses working in nursing. Government-sponsored financial incentives that encourage nurses to earn advanced degrees and become faculty members are beginning to pay off. The availability of qualified faculty means nursing schools can enroll more students. Simulations are becoming more sophisticated and capable of providing clinical experiences. The future is unknown, but research shows that adequate staffing improves the quality of care for patients and the job satisfaction of nurses.

✔ *The Bureau of Labor Statistics predicts a 25% growth in jobs for licensed practical/vocational nurses between now and 2022.*

✔ *Discover Nursing and Nurses for a Healthier Tomorrow are two Web sites that provide career materials appropriate for recruiting activities.*

COMPLEMENTARY AND ALTERNATIVE THERAPIES

Most physicians in the United States practice traditional Western medicine. This approach, often referred to as the *medical model* of treatment, is focused on diagnosing and treating the physical aspects of a dysfunction with surgery, medications, or general medical protocols.

Complementary and alternative therapies are terms used to describe a variety of health care approaches that are outside the medical model. Complementary therapy generally refers to using a nonmedical approach *together with* traditional medicine. Alternative therapy generally refers to using a nonmedical approach *in place of* traditional medicine. Aromatherapy, basic neuromuscular integration, foot reflexology, hypnotherapy, massage, therapeutic touch, meditation, dietary supplements, and Reiki are just a few of the many complementary and alternate therapies being offered today (Fig. 16-2). Many more therapies are described in Appendix D.

The National Institutes of Health (NIH), recognizing the potential for both the use and misuse of alternatives, established the Office of Alternative Medicine in 1992. The focus of this agency is on the scientific investigation of the value of using alternative and complementary interventions to improve health and health care.

The name of the office has changed several times, and in December 2014, it became known as the National Center for Complementary and Integrative Health. Integrative health is the term used to describe treatment that is based on the medical model with the addition of complementary and alternative therapies. For example, patients who are receiving radiation treatments often suffer severe nausea. Traditional medicine prescribes an antinausea medication. Those who practice integrative medicine might add cannabis, acupuncture, or Reiki therapy to the antinausea medication.

As a health care consumer, you may or may not at some time in the future consider complementary or alternative therapies for yourself and your family

✔ *Consumers spent more than $34 billion on vitamins, minerals, and dietary supplements in 2013.*

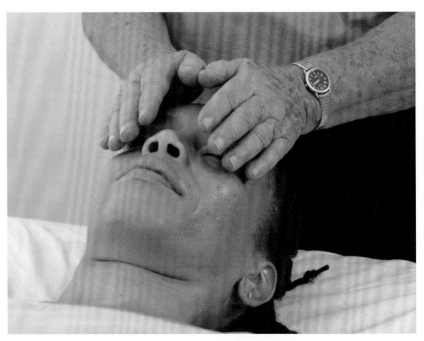

FIGURE 16-2. ● Reiki practitioner with a patient. (© Bob Stockfield.)

or you may expect appropriate nonmedical therapies be integrated into your medical plan of care. As a nurse, you will have more and more patients who find that combining different treatments and therapies is best for them. People are beginning to expect their physicians to integrate complementary and alternative methods of treatment into their therapy, so it is important that you learn all you can and use that knowledge to support patient decisions regarding their own plan of care.

 THE *Web*

> The National Center for Complementary and Integrative Health's Web site provides information on the effectiveness of complementary, alternative, and integrative health treatments as well as on breaking news and current research in this field of medicine.

CRITICAL THINKING

A current issue and an even greater future concern is the ability of nurses to apply critical thinking skills in their nursing practice. Knowledge in nursing and medicine is growing by leaps and bounds, and health care situations are becoming more complex every day so that being able to identify problems, propose solutions, and make good decisions will be an essential characteristic of tomorrow's nurse.

Great critical thinking skills do not just happen. The longer you work as a nurse, the more experience you will gain. But experience can only improve your critical thinking skills if you take the time to reflect on the results of your nursing behaviors. What assessments did you make, what additional data should you have had, and are there additional interventions that you did not think of? Determine why certain outcomes happened and what actions might lead to a better outcome. Look for opportunities to discuss the reasoning behind an expert nurse's clinical decisions. Ask the "What if" question to figure out potential events. Ask your instructors to critique your critical thinking skills while you are still a student.

The characteristics of critical thinkers described in Box 1-2 on pages 18–19 are worth reviewing on occasion. A good foundation in effective critical thinking and problem-solving skills plus experience, a willingness to learn, applying evidence-based practices in your nursing practice, and a questioning approach to your work will help you become a skilled critical thinker.

BIOETHICS

Advances in biology and medicine are creating new bioethical issues every day. The use of genetic information and genomics for a variety of purposes is an area of medicine that is already beginning to affect our lives. The use of genetic patterns to anticipate disease conditions and the use of genetic engineering to alter cell structure are just the beginning.

✔ *The Human Genome Project provides the foundation for developing new treatments for many diseases.*

President Obama asked Congress for $215 million in the 2016 federal budget to support research in what he calls the "precision medicine initiative" or individualized medicine. Currently, treatment is designed for average persons but very few people are average. Precision medicine would use an individual's genetic code to develop more effective individualized therapeutic and preventive strategies.

Pharmacogenomics, an extension of this approach, prescribes drugs based on the genetic makeup of an individual. Individualize medicine and pharmacogenomics are the future; however, that future may be years away because of needed research and the cost of this approach to treating diseases.

What effects will tinkering with genetic structures, making custom DNA on a computer, a national DNA data bank, ectogenesis (growing an embryo or fetus outside the human womb), and growing human organs in animals for later transplant have on us as individuals and on our society?

How will future breakthrough advances in biology and medicine be viewed by individuals and cultures and religions? Some are excited to see how far scientists can go, while others believe that we should not disturb the complex makeup of the human body. You have a responsibility as a nurse and as a person to keep yourself informed about the ramifications of proposed therapies. Use critical thinking skills to evaluate different points of view. Join organizations that support your beliefs and vote for those who support your position. Be an informed and involved citizen and nurse.

ETHICAL ISSUES

Our complex society creates many opportunities to question whether certain behaviors are ethical or not. Sex selective abortion, designer babies, minor children forced into medical treatment by the courts, mandated surgery to correct diseases that are costly to society and insurance companies, and the use of genetic information to treat potential diseases are just a few ethical issues that are going to become more prevalent in the future.

Maternal–fetal issues have been around for many years but are increasing in complexity. Sperm banks create questions about paternal rights. Questions about the rights of surrogate mothers, the ethics of genetic counseling and genetic engineering, termination of pregnancy, rights of the father, and rights of the fetus will continue to be asked now and in the future.

Organ transplants are not new, but new sources of donor organs and new ways of obtaining donor organs will present an ethical concern for many people. Killing animals for their organs and buying and selling organs are real issues that will face us more frequently in the future.

The National Institutes of Health announced on April 14, 2003, that the Human Genome Project had been completed. Having information about genetic disorders will raise many ethical questions. Will people be denied jobs or life insurance or health insurance because of a genetic disorder? Will people use sperm banks, donor eggs, or both when genetic testing predicts that two people's genetic makeup will produce a child that is undesirable to them? Will people have elective surgery based on a genetic possibility of acquiring a particular disease, and should health insurance companies pay for that surgery?

These are just a few examples of ethical questions that are important to us now or will be in the future. Learn as much as you can about ethical issues, and develop the nursing skills that will enable you to support the legal decisions of your patients regardless of your personal beliefs.

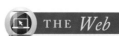
THE *Web*

The National Human Genome Research Institute Web site contains a section titled "My Family Health Portrait" in which you can enter you family health history. This history can help you and your health care provider discover your genetic heritage and guide you in making healthy environment and lifestyle choices.

END-OF-LIFE ISSUES

Reaching the end of life (EOL) because of a serious illness is difficult for patients as well as for their families and significant others. People have talked openly about quality of life for years yet have been very reluctant to discuss what might be termed the "quality of death." And nurses were no different.

But that has changed dramatically over the past 15 years so that virtually all nursing schools now include a course or courses in end-of-life care. The September 2014 National League for Nursing end-of-program competencies for a graduate of a practical nursing program include the ability to:

> *function in a collaborative role to provide care in multiple settings with an emphasis on community-based chronic care management and palliative/end-of-life care (team/ collaboration).*

Palliative care is the term used to describe care that is intended to provide comfort during this time. Palliative care does not offer a cure or treat a disease. The goal of palliative care is to prevent and relieve suffering and to improve the quality of life for people who are terminally ill (Fig. 16-3).

The World Health Organization defines palliative care as follows:

> *Palliative care is an approach that improves the quality of life of patients and their families facing the problem associated with life-threatening illness, through the prevention and relief of suffering by means of early identification and impeccable assessment and treatment of pain and other problems, physical, psychosocial, and spiritual. Palliative care*

- *Provides relief from pain and other distressing symptoms*
- *Affirms life and regards dying as a normal process*
- *Intends neither to hasten nor postpone death*
- *Integrates the psychological and spiritual aspects of patient care*
- *Offers a support system to help patients live as actively as possible until death*
- *Offers a support system to help the family cope during the patient's illness and in their own bereavement*

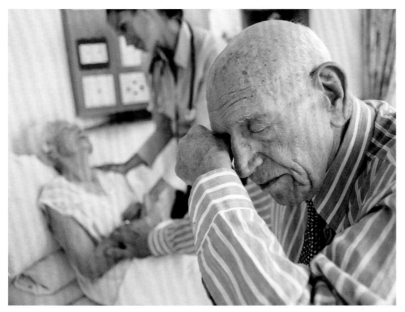

FIGURE 16-3. ● Hospice care encourages family members to be with terminally ill patients.

- *Uses a team approach to address the needs of patients and their families, including bereavement counseling, if indicated*
- *Will enhance quality of life and may also positively influence the course of illness*
- *Is applicable early in the course of illness, in conjunction with other therapies that are intended to prolong life, such as chemotherapy or radiation therapy, and includes those investigations needed to better understand and manage distressing clinical complications*

✔ *You must uncover and understand your own feelings about the EOL before you can help others.*

Nurses can access hundreds of workshops and online end-of-life continuing education courses, and a number of organizations including the National Board for Certification of Hospice and Palliative Nurses offer LP/VNs a certification examination in end-of-life care.

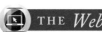

THE *Web*

> Medline Plus is a service of the National Institutes of Health and the National Library of Medicine. This site includes more than 2,000 links to information about the many aspects of EOL issues. The Practical Bioethics organization publishes a pamphlet titled *Caring Conversations* on their Web site.

✔ *It takes effort and thought and a good understanding of yourself to encourage others to make decisions that are best for them and their families.*

Because so many patients have had to suffer severe pain during a terminal illness, families are demanding that their loved ones be made as comfortable as possible as they approach the end of their life. All 50 states have laws that allow people to write an advanced directive or a living will that specifies their health care preferences if they are incapacitated. People can also designate a health care proxy to make decisions for them.

Information about advanced directives and living wills in your state can be obtained from the Web site of your state bar association, state medical association, state nursing association, and from most hospitals or medical centers.

Learn as much as you can about these and other issues. Look at each issue from your personal viewpoint and from society's viewpoint. When you can accept the rights of people and society to have opinions different from yours, you will be able to provide nursing care to all your patients, regardless of their personal decisions.

The future is either alarming or reassuring—depending on your personal point of view. Some people with terminal illnesses have already decided when and where and how they will die. Will physician-assisted suicide become a common medical practice? Will financial disparity in health care make lifesaving treatments unavailable to the poor? Will cryonic suspension (frozen) become more common? How long should a person be permitted to remain on life support? These are just a few of what are sure to be more issues in the future.

HEALTH CARE REFORM

One of Barack Obama's top presidential campaign issues was health care. As soon as he took office in January 2009, he began working with legislators to pass legislation that would reform health care in the United States. After much debate, health care reform passed the House and Senate with the Democrats voting for these bills and Republicans voting against these bills. Comprehensive health care reform legislation was signed into law by President Obama in March 2010. The Patient Protection and Affordable Care Act was signed into law on March 23, 2010, and was amended by the Health Care and Education Reconciliation Act on March 30, 2010. The name "Affordable Care Act" (ACA) is used to refer to the final amended version of the law.

Following are a few of the main provisions of the ACA:

- 48 million uninsured Americans will have access to affordable health insurance options.
- 5.6 million people with preexisting conditions will no longer be denied health insurance.
- 500,000 families will be saved from bankruptcy caused by medical bills.
- People who cannot get health insurance through their work will get a tax credit toward purchasing their own insurance.
- Lifetime limits on insurance coverage will be eliminated.
- The gap in Medicare prescription drug coverage will be reduced.
- Payments to medical professionals who work in underserved communities will be increased.

Not everyone in the country is in agreement with this legislation. A number of people, politicians, insurance companies, and organizations are working to repeal all or parts of the Act. Whether the ACA is repealed or replaced remains to be seen.

Future issues related to health care reform include the following:

- Who should be covered?
- What medical test, treatments, and services should be paid for, and who should make those decisions?
- Should services be denied?
- Should dental and vision exams be included?
- Should preventative care be covered?
- Should people be able to move to another state or change jobs without having to change coverage?
- Is health care a right or a privilege?

You will need to use your best critical thinking skills as you attempt to understand all of the concerns and issues related to the ACA and health care reform. With a good knowledge of all of the issues, you will be able to decide what laws and regulations are best for you and your family and to express those decisions when you elect public officials.

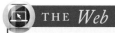

THE *Web*

Use government Web sites to learn about the contents of the Affordable Care Act and the issues surrounding this legislation.

There is no doubt that during your career as a nurse, you will see many changes in how health care is delivered. What role will the federal and state governments have in controlling and delivering health care? What will the future health care system look like? Will there be national health insurance? What the future holds is unknown, but we can be sure that the health care system will change and that it will never again be what it is today.

VIOLENCE AND BULLYING IN THE WORKPLACE

Violence and bullying among nursing team members are not uncommon. Bullying is not often reported, but estimates speculate that between 27% and 85% of staff nurse have been bullied at work. As many as 90% of new nurses report some form of treatment that could be classified as bullying. As many as 67% of nurses in one survey said they witnessed one or more episodes of violence between coworkers, and in another survey, nearly 28% of nurses witnessed bullying. Violence and bullying in the workplace are detrimental to the effective care of patients and must be openly discussed by nurses.

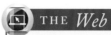 THE *Web*

> The Occupational Safety and Health Administration provides possible solutions to different types of violence in health care in the Workplace Violence section of their Web site.

The first step toward ending these behaviors is to acknowledge they exist. Following this, team members need to develop a good understanding of why people become bullies, how to avoid being a target, and how to build a strong sense of community on the nursing unit. Nurses should look out for each other and take action when they observe a situation in which a fellow team member is being bullied. Because the observers usually outnumber the bullies, bullies soon have no one to intimidate.

✔ *An organization called the Workplace Bullying Institute provides suggestions on what to do if you are the target of a bully.*

It is important that experienced nurses mentor new and inexperienced nurses, that nurses develop positive relationships with one another, that nurses have mutual respect for one another, and that each team member does his or her share of the work. It is also important that managers set a positive example for their team. Creating a work environment free of bullying and violence will go a long way toward reducing nursing staff turnover and shortages.

WORKPLACE CONFLICTS

An issue that will become more prevalent in the future will be conflicts in the workplace. As we have seen in previous chapters and also in previous topics in this chapter, the workforce is becoming more diverse in many aspects. As the workforce becomes more diverse, so does the opportunity for misunderstandings among coworkers.

Real and imagined differences in how coworkers are treated can lead to conflicts. If a conflict is not recognized and quickly dealt with, the work environment can become very toxic. The most logical person to address coworker conflict is the nurse manager of the team or unit. If that person is perceived to be the cause of the conflict, then a supervisor might be the most appropriate person.

The first step in the resolution of conflict is to be sure it is a mutual problem and not just your problem. If it is just your problem, then discuss your concerns with those in your chain of command. If it is a group problem, suggest meeting as a group to identify the issues that seem to be creating the conflict.

Those who want to resolve a conflict must abide by certain "rules." They must listen to the opinions of other people in the group. They must be courteous in allowing others to talk without interruption. They must practice active listening, pay attention to other points of view, list facts, and examine the work issues—not personalities. They must keep an open mind and try to see issues from different points of view.

Sometimes a conflict is resolved just by following the above rules. The path to a resolution becomes clear, and all of the coworkers believe there should no longer be a conflict over that issue.

Other times, it takes an extra step or two to resolve the conflict. Brainstorming is a good way to encourage everyone in the group to suggest solutions. List all possible solutions, and then eliminate those that everyone agrees can be eliminated. Then, from the statements that are left, develop a mutually acceptable compromise statement or two that describes what actions will resolve the conflict. At this point, everyone in the group should clearly understand what to expect going forward.

The most effective tools in reducing conflict among coworkers are to practice fairness, good listening and communication skills, and respect for others. Following these simple guidelines will go a long way toward creating a positive and constructive work environment.

PERSONAL WELL-BEING

Most nurses are quite willing to give all of their time and energy to meet the needs of their patients, their families, and their friends. They volunteer to help with all the school and church events, they willingly work extra shifts, and they give up much needed sleep so they have time to do things for others. They are always trying to meet the needs of others and rarely if ever of themselves. This lifestyle of constant stress will eventually lead to resenting the people who take all of your time and energy. You will begin to feel used and abused by those around you. You will not enjoy going to work, and you will feel frustrated and drained most of the time. You will think about quitting nursing.

Be a healthy nurse by taking care of yourself. Create a balance between physical, emotional, personal, social, spiritual, and professional activities. Eat well, sleep well, play well, and maintain a healthy weight. Create a network of friends, nurses and nonnurses, who support each other and you in all kinds of ways. Learn to let others help you when you need it. Know that everything is not a priority. Learn to say "No" to requests that would take the little bit of time you have for yourself. Plan your day—don't let the day plan you.

If you are not taking care of yourself, start by taking 5 minutes a day to do something for yourself. Read suggestions and tips from nurses about how to improve your own well-being. You are working hard to become a nurse. Don't let mismanagement of your own self force you to leave a career you are working so hard to obtain.

THE FUTURE

How illness is diagnosed and treated will be very different in the future. New tools to maintain and monitor health and prevent illness will be readily available. It will be a challenge to keep up-to-date on how to use these technologies and the data that are generated in your personal life as well as in your nursing practice.

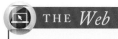

THE *Web*

There are many Web sites that describe how technological advances are changing the future of health care.

✔ *Get involved in helping to resolve issues that affect you, your working conditions, and the health and well-being of your patients.*

The future of the health care system (facility owners, administrators, employees, and the public) will be affected in unpredictable ways by federal legislation and guidelines. Will setting aside pretax dollars in a Health Spending Account actually help individuals pay for the cost of health care? Will consumers use health care transparency (making information on the cost of procedures and services and the quality of individual providers available to the public) to make informed choices for health care? Will legislation related to nursing education and practice be passed, and if so, is the federal government the agency that should control nursing practice?

What is in the future of medical care? Smartphones have attachments that can diagnose and monitor physical and mental health, little lab attachments perform routine lab tests, apps let you consult with a doctor any time of the day or night, and smartphones expand the use of selfies to aid in diagnosing a variety of physical illnesses. Handheld ultrasound, MRI, and x-ray devices are already available. A variety of commercial wristband sensors monitor a number of physical parameters. 3D printers can use living cells to create transplantable organs. DNA sequencing will make personalized medical care routine. Ultrasound surgery will eliminate surgical cuts. This may sound like science fiction, but it is not.

What will be the job of the nurse in the future? Smartphone technology will certainly change how nurses assess their patient's vital signs and blood values. Preparation for diagnostic procedures will be different, how medications are administered will be changed, and the postoperative care of ultrasound surgery patients will be different from those who had a surgical cut. Most people will receive medical care at home or in an outpatient office. Many countries, including the Unites States, are working to improve the skills of robotic nurses that have already been built.

Nursing students will learn differently in the future. They will use extremely realistic human patient simulators for clinical practice. They will learn to use new methods and devices to administer medications. Learning will be enhanced by true-to-life color images of wounds and skin conditions. Students will use handheld digital technology to access protocols for patient care. Much of the learning will be Web based, and many courses will be completed online. Nursing students will be more independent and self-directed in their learning.

There is no doubt that advances in technology and science are going to continue to improve our health and make our lives better. But there are issues surrounding all of these advances. Will only the wealthy be able to afford to purchase the technology? Will people have the physical and/or mental ability to use and maintain the equipment and understand the data that are generated? Can breaches in the security of Web-based protected health information be absolutely prevented? Will relying on digital technology reduce the nurse's ability to use critical thinking, logic, and common sense? Will artificial intelligences make critical thinking obsolete? Will the future bring isolation from coworkers, or will it become more important than ever to work in teams? How, when, and where will workers learn how to use the new technology for the benefit of the patient? Will the nurse still be there to comfort the grieving mother, rock a crying baby, or hold the hand of the person who is dying?

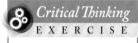

Critical Thinking
E X E R C I S E

Make your own predictions about what two or three issues will be hot topics in the next 5 and 10 years. How will you be affected by these issues, what is your position on each issue, and how do you plan to be involved in influencing the outcome of each issue? Use appropriate Characteristics of Critical Thinkers in Box 1-2 on pages 18–19 to develop your response to these questions.

SUMMARY

This chapter has touched on just a few current issues and future concerns. What the future holds is unknown. There will no doubt be new issues and new concerns. Technology will continue to have an impact on how we live our lives and where. Some ethical dilemmas will be resolved, and new ones will develop. The health care system will be different from what it is today. How you practice your profession and where you practice it will continue to change over time.

Your best plan for enjoying a long and rewarding career in nursing is to take advantage of every educational opportunity you can and to be deeply involved in anything and everything that affects you as a nurse and your patient as a person.

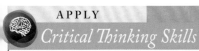

APPLY
Critical Thinking Skills

1. In the opening story at the beginning of this chapter, Aleshia suggested that Carmen learn more about genetic testing. In the search section of your favorite search engine, type the words "genetic testing." What are the current and future concerns related to gene testing? Would you ask for genetic testing of a fetus for yourself or a member of your family? Explain your answer.

2. Assess how well you think you adapt to change. What makes you uncomfortable when a change is about to occur? What can you do to make better adjustments to change?

3. Make a list of things you can do if you think your working environment is hazardous to your health.

4. Review several brochures announcing continuing education programs. How much do these programs cost, where are they held, are they accredited by a recognized accrediting agency, are continuing education credits offered, and what audience are they designed to attract? Would attending any of these programs improve your nursing practice?

5. Does your state require continuing education for renewal of the LP/VN license? How many hours are required? Are the requirements specific or general?

6. Plan a debate on specific points of the Affordable Care Act with your classmates.

7. In addition to the issues discussed in this chapter, what other issues and future concerns can you identify and describe?

8. Take a position on any current issue in nursing and defend it. Include facts and figures to support your position.

9. Do an Internet search using the search team "future of medicine." What findings surprised you the most? What was the most unbelievable thing you read?

10. What is your greatest concern for your future as a nurse? What can you do to influence the outcome?

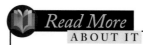

ABOUT IT

Berlinger N, Jennings B, Wolf SM: The Hastings Center Guidelines for Decision on Life-Sustaining Treatment and Care Near the End of Life: Revised and Expanded Second Edition, 2nd ed. New York, NY: Oxford University Press, 2013.

Dayer-Berenson L: Cultural Competencies for Nurses: Impact on Health and Illness, 2nd ed. Sudbury, MA: Jones and Bartlett Learning, 2013.

Fontaine KL: Complementary and Alternative Therapies for Nursing Practice, 4th ed. Upper Saddle River, NJ: Prentice-Hall, 2014.

Jacobs JR, Skocpol T: Health Care Reform and American Politics: What Everyone Needs to Know, Rev Upd ed. New York, NY: Oxford University Press, 2012.

Matzo M, Sherman DW: Palliative Care Nursing: Quality Care to the End of Life, 4th ed. New York, NY: Springer Publishing, 2015.

Niles NJ: Basics of the U.S. Health Care System, 2nd ed. Burlington, MA: Jones and Bartlett Learning, 2014.

Phyde IT: The Dark Side of Nursing. Bloomington, IN: Balbou Press, 2014.

Rubenfeld MG, Scheffer B: Critical Thinking TACTICS for Nurses: Achieving the IOM Competencies, 3rd ed. Burlington, MA: Jones and Bartlett Learning, 2015.

Wilson A: Wellbeing for Nurses Magazine. Available in the App Store.

Zerwekh J, Claborn JC: Nursing Today: Transition and Trends, 8th ed. St. Louis, MO: Saunders, 2014.

A few of the many journals of particular interest to LP/VNs include the following:
    Journal of Aging Health
    Complementary Therapies in Clinical Practice
    Journal of Transcultural Nursing
    Holistic Nursing Practice
    Home Healthcare Now
    Journal of Practical Nursing-Online
    Men in Nursing
    Nursing Ethics
    Nursing Made Incredibly Easy
    And many, many more

Essential Online Resources for Practical and Vocational Nursing Students

Because of the dynamic nature of the Internet, any Web addresses or links contained in this listing may have changed since publication or may no longer be valid. If an address is not valid, try locating the site by using a major search engine and key words. Many Web sites listed in this directory will require the entry of a key word or phrase to get to the content. Be aware that some Web sites may transmit viruses to your computer. Be sure your antivirus software is up to date, and heed any warnings that might appear on your screen.

Within these major headings, you will find Web sites that provide additional information on these topics:

CAREER LINKS
COMMUNICATION SKILLS
DICTIONARIES
EDUCATION AND ACCREDITATION
ETHICAL AND BIOETHICAL CASE STUDIES
GOVERNMENT RESOURCES
HUMOR
LEADERSHIP AND MANAGEMENT
LEARNING TOOLS
LEGAL CASE STUDIES
ORGANIZATIONS
PERSONAL INTEREST
TESTING

CAREER LINKS

Worker's skills	http://wdr.doleportfolita.gov/SCANS/whatwork/
Templates for creating a resume	www.office.microsoft.com/en-us/templates
The National Practitioner Data Bank	www.npdb.hrsa.gov
Job searching tools	www.jobsearch.about.com
Career Planning	www.quintcareers.com/career_planning_tips.html
Personal Finance (Money Essentials)	http://money.cnn.com
Online resume development	http://resume.monster.com
Workplace Bullying	www.workplacebullying.org
National Network for Domestic Violence	www.nnedv.org
Safe Patient Handling Professionals	www.asphp.org
Safe Patient Handling	www.osha.gov
Needlesticks	http://www.cdc.gov/niosh/topics/bbp/sharps.html
Tool Kit of articles related to work activities	www.mindtools.com

COMMUNICATION SKILLS

Communicating with blind/vision impaired	www.nfb.org
Communicating with GLBT Parents, Family, Friends	www.community.pflag.org
Communicating with people with disabilities	www.dol.gov/odep/pubs/fact/comucate.htm
Communicating with hearing impaired	www.hearingloss.org
Communication and team building through games	www.gamesforgroups.com/index.html
Communication style	www.communicationworks.com
Communication through body language	https://www.psychologytoday.com/blog/subliminal
National Caregivers Resources for speech	www.caregiverslibrary.org

DICTIONARIES

Pronouncing general dictionary	www.merriam-webster.com
Pronouncing medical dictionary	www.nlm.nih.gov/medlineplus/mplusdictionary.html
Taber's for mobile devices	www.tabers.com

EDUCATION AND ACCREDITATION

Accreditation Commission for Education in Nursing	www.acenursing.org
American Nurses Association	http://nursingworld.org
Commission on Collegiate Nursing Education	www.aacn.nche.edu
Institute for Credentialing Excellence	www.credentialingexcellence.org
National Association for Practical Nurse Education and Service	www.napnes.org
National Federation of Licensed Practical Nurses	www.nflpn.org

ETHICAL AND BIOETHICAL CASE STUDIES

Big Religion Comparison Chart	www.religionfacts.com
Center for Bioethics and Human Dignity	https://cbhd.org/resources/case-studies
Center for Practical Bioethics	www.practicalbioethics.org/resources/case-studies
Islamic Medicine	www.islamicmedicine.org
Jewish Virtual Library	www.jewishvirtuallibrary.org
National Library of Medicine	www.nlm.nih.gov
The Hastings Center	www.thehastingscenter.org

GOVERNMENT RESOURCES

2015 Dietary Guidelines for Americans	www.usda.gov
Affordable Care Act	www.healthcare.gov
Americans with Disabilities	www.ada.gov
Bureau of Labor Statistics	www.bls.gov
Canadian Mental Health Association	www.cmha.ca
Centers for Disease Control	www.cdc.gov
Centers for Medicare and Medicaid	www.cms.gov
Department of Health and Human Services	www.hhs.gov

Drug Abuse	www.drugabuse.gov
Environmental Protection Agency	www.epa.gov
Equal Employment Opportunity Commission	www.eeoc.gov
Disaster Planning	www.ready.gov.make-a-plan
Federal Dietary Guidelines	www.health.gov/dietaryguidelines
Federal Emergency Management Agency	www.fema.gov
Food and Drug Administration	www.fda.gov
Health Resources and Services Administration	www.hrsa.gov
Healthy People 2020	https://www.healthypeople.gov
HIPAA Guidelines	www.hhs.gov/ocr/privacy/
Human Genome Project	www.genome.gov
Indian Health Services	www.ihs.gov
Mailing address for Senators and Representatives	www.usa.gov
National Institutes of Health	www.nih.gov
Occupational Safety and Health Administration	www.osha.gov
Physical Activity Guidelines	www.health.gov/paguidelines
U. S. Department of Veterans Affairs	www.va.gov

HISTORY

A brief outline of major events in medicine since 2600 BC	www.datesandevents.org/events-timelines/10-history-of-medicine-timeline.htm
American Association for the History of Nursing	www.aahn.org
American Nurses Association	www.nursingworld.org/halloffame
History and Timelines	www.historyworld.net
International Council of Nurses	www.icn.ch

HUMOR

Great Clean Jokes	www.greatcleanjokes.com
Laughter is the best medicine	www.webmd.com
Laughter Prescription	http://www.ncbi.nlm.nih.gov/pmc/articles/PMC2762283/
Links to nursing humor	www.allnurses.com/nursing-humor-share/
Nursing Humor	www.nursinghumor.com

LEADERSHIP AND MANAGEMENT

Conflict Resolution	www.helpguide.org
Leadership and Management Skills	www.mindtools.com
Leadership and Management Skills, Techniques, and Tools	www.mindtools.com
Leadership Self-Assessment	http://nwlink.com/~donclark/leader/self.html
Leadership Style Quiz	http://psychology.about.com/library/quiz/bl-leadershipquiz.htm

LEARNING TOOLS

Critical Thinking	www.alfaroteachsmart.com
Graphic Organizers	www.eduplace.com
Learning Styles Assessments	http://marciaconner.com
Thinking Styles (Free Assessment)	www.thinkwatson.com
SQ3R Method of Reading	www.mindtools.com
Test Anxiety	www.mayoclinic.org
Thinkport Graphic Organizers	www.thinkport.org

LEGAL CASE STUDIES

Healthcare Providers Service Organization	www.hpso.com/case-studies
Legal case studies	www.nso.com
Legal case studies	www.nursingcasestudy.com
Legal Eagle Eye Newsletter for the Nursing Profession	www.nursinglaw.com

ORGANIZATIONS

Accreditation Commission for Education in Nursing	www.acenursing.org
American Association for Long Term Care Nursing	www.ltcnursing.org
American Association for the History of Nursing	www.aahn.org
American Association of Colleges of Nursing	www.aacn.org
American Holistic Nurses Association	www.ahna.org
American Hospital Association	www.naha.org
American Nurses Association	www.nursingworld.org
American Osteopathic Association	www.osteopathic.org
American Society for Healthcare Risk Management	www.ashrm.org
Asian American/Pacific Islander Nurses Association, Inc.	www.aapina.org
Community Health Accreditation Program	www.chapinc.org
End-of-life advice	www.compassionandchoices.org
Health Occupations Students of America	www.hosa.org
Joint Commission (Healthcare accreditation)	www.jointcommission.org
National Alaska Native American Indian Nurses Association	www.nanainanurses.org
National Association for Homecare and Hospice	www.nahc.org
National Association for Practical Nurse Education and Service	www.napnes.org
National Association of Hispanic Nurses	www.nahnnet.otg
National Black Nurses Association	www.nbna.org
National Council of State Boards of Nursing	http://www.ncsbn.org
National Federation of Licensed Practical Nurses	www.nflpn.org
National Hospice and Palliative Care Organization	www.nhpco.org
National League for Nursing	www.nln.org

Philippine Nurses Association of America, Inc.	www.mypnaa.org
Practice Greenhealth	www.practicegreenhealth.org
Tobacco Free Nurses	www.tobaccofreenurses.org
World Health Organization	www.who.org

PERSONAL INTEREST

2015 Dietary Guidelines for Americans	www.health.gov/dietaryguidelines
Charity Navigator	www.charitynavigator.org
End of Life	www.caregiverslibrary.org
Federal Student Financial Aid Application	www.fafsa-application.com
Healthy Living	www.webmd.com
Mental and Emotional Health	www.helpguide.org
Multi-state Nursing License	https://www.ncsbn.org/nurse-licensure-compact.htm
National Whistleblowers Center	www.whistleblowers.org
Physical Activity Guidelines	www.health.gov/PAGuidelines
Substance Abuse and Mental Health Administration	www.samhsa.gov
Tobacco Free Nurses	www.tobaccofreenurses.org
Whistleblowers Case Studies	www.whistleblowerlaws.com

TESTING

Administers NCLEX exams	www.pearsonvue.com
NCLEX-PN Exam	www.ncsbn.org
Test anxiety self-assessment	www.fredonia.edu/counseling

My favorite Web sites

_____

_____

_____

NFLPN Nursing Practice Standards for the Licensed Practical/Vocational Nurse[1]

PREFACE

The Standards were developed and adopted by the NFLPN to provide a basic model, whereby the quality of health service and nursing service and nursing care given by licensed practical/vocational nurses (LP/VNs) may be measured and evaluated.

These nursing practice standards are applicable in any practice setting. The degree to which individual standards are applied will vary according to the individual needs of the patient, the type of health care agency or services, and the community resources.

The scope of licensed practical nursing has extended into specialized nursing services. Therefore, specialized fields of nursing are included in this document.

THE CODE FOR LICENSED PRACTICAL/VOCATIONAL NURSES

The Code, adopted by NFLPN in 1961 and revised in 1979, provides a motivation for establishing, maintaining, and elevating professional standards. Each LP/VN, upon entering the profession, inherits the responsibility to adhere to the standards of ethical practice and conduct as set forth in this code.

1. Know the scope of maximum utilization of the LP/VN as specified by the nursing practice act and function within this scope.
2. Safeguard the confidential information acquired from any source about the patient.
3. Provide health care to all patients regardless of race, creed, cultural background, disease, or lifestyle.
4. Uphold the highest standards in personal appearance, language, dress, and demeanor.
5. Stay informed about issues affecting the practice of nursing and delivery of health care and, where appropriate, participate in government and policy decisions.
6. Accept the responsibility for safe nursing by keeping oneself mentally and physically fit and educationally prepared to practice.
7. Accept responsibility for membership in NFLPN and participate in its efforts to maintain the established standards of nursing practice and employment policies that lead to quality patient care.

INTRODUCTORY STATEMENT

Definition

Practical/Vocational nursing means the performance for compensation of authorized acts of nursing, which utilize specialized knowledge and skills and which

---

[1]Reprinted with permission of the National Federation of Licensed Practical Nurses, Inc. Copyright 2004.

meet the health needs of people in a variety of settings under the direction of qualified health professionals.

Scope

Licensed Practical/Vocational nurses represent the established entry into the nursing profession and include specialized fields of nursing practice.

Opportunities exist for practicing in a milieu where different professions unite their particular skills in a team effort: to preserve or improve an individual patient's functioning and to protect health and safety of patients.

Opportunities also exist for career advancement within the profession through academic education and for lateral expansion of knowledge and expertise through both academic/continuing education and certification.

STANDARDS

Education

The Licensed Practical/Vocational Nurse
1. Shall complete a formal education program in practical nursing approved by the appropriate nursing authority in a state
2. Shall successfully pass the National Council Licensure Examination for Practical Nurses
3. Shall participate in initial orientation within the employing institution

Legal/Ethical Status

The Licensed Practical/Vocational Nurse
1. Shall hold a current license to practice nursing as an LP/VN in accordance with the law of the state wherein employed
2. Shall know the scope of nursing practice authorized by the Nursing Practice Act in the state wherein employed
3. Shall have a personal commitment to fulfill the legal responsibilities inherent in good nursing practice
4. Shall take responsible actions in situations wherein there is unprofessional conduct by a peer or other health care provider
5. Shall recognize and have a commitment to meet the ethical and moral obligations of the practice of nursing
6. Shall not accept or perform professional responsibilities that the individual knows he or she is not competent to perform

Practice

The Licensed Practical/Vocational Nurse
1. Shall accept assigned responsibilities as an accountable member of the health care team
2. Shall function within the limits of educational preparation and experience as related to the assigned duties
3. Shall function with other members of the health care team in promoting and maintaining health, preventing disease and disability, caring for and rehabilitating individuals who are experiencing an altered health state, and contributing to the ultimate quality of life until death
4. Shall know and utilize the nursing process in planning, implementing, and evaluating health services and nursing care for the individual patient or group

   a. Planning: The planning of nursing includes:
      1) Assessment/data collection of health status of the individual patient, the family, and community groups
      2) Reporting information gained from assessment/data collection
      3) The identification of health goals
   b. Implementation: The plan for nursing care is put into practice to achieve the stated goals and includes:
      1) Observing, recording, and reporting significant changes, which require intervention or different goals
      2) Applying nursing knowledge and skills to promote and maintain health, to prevent disease and disability, and to optimize functional capabilities of an individual patient
      3) Assisting the patient and family with activities of daily living and encouraging self-care as appropriate
      4) Carrying out therapeutic regimens and protocols prescribed by personnel pursuant to authorized state law.
   c. Evaluations: The plan for nursing care and its implementations are evaluated to measure the progress toward the stated goals and will include appropriate persons and/or groups to determine:
      1) The relevancy of current goals in relation to the progress of the individual patient
      2) The involvement of the recipients of care in the evaluation process
      3) The quality of the nursing action in the implementation of the plan
      4) A reordering of priorities or new goal setting in the care plan
5. Shall participate in peer review and other evaluation processes
6. Shall participate in the development of policies concerning the health and nursing needs of society and in the roles and functions of the LP/VN

Continuing Education

The Licensed Practical/Vocational Nurse
1. Shall be responsible for maintaining the highest possible level of professional competence at all times
2. Shall periodically reassess career goals and select continuing education activities, which will help to achieve these goals
3. Shall take advantage of continuing education opportunities, which will lead to personal growth and professional development
4. Shall seek and participate in continuing education activities, which are approved for credit by appropriate organizations, such as the NFLPN

Specialized Nursing Practice

The Licensed Practical/Vocational Nurse
1. Shall have had at least one year experience in nursing at the staff level
2. Shall present personal qualifications that are indicative of potential abilities for practice in the chosen specialized nursing area
3. Shall present evidence of completion of a program or course that is approved by an appropriate agency to provide the knowledge and skills necessary for effective nursing services in the specialized field
4. Shall meet all of the standards of practice as set forth in this document

GLOSSARY

Authorized (acts of nursing) Those nursing activities made legal through State Nurse Practice Acts or other laws.

Lateral Expansion of Knowledge An extension of the basic core of information learned in the school of practical nursing.

Peer Review A formal evaluation of performance on the job by other LP/VNs.

Specialized Nursing Practice A restricted field of nursing in which a person is particularly skilled and has specific knowledge.

Therapeutic Regimens Regulated plans designed to bring about effective treatment of disease.

Career Advancement A change of career goal.

LP/VN A combined abbreviation for licensed practical and licensed vocational nurse. The LVN title is used in California and Texas for the nurses who are called LPNs in other states.

Milieu One's environment and surroundings.

Protocols Courses of treatment, which include specific steps to be performed in a stated order.

National Association for Practical Nurse Education and Service Standards of Practice and Educational Competencies of Graduates of Practical/Vocational Nursing Programs[1]

INTRODUCTION

These standards and competencies are intended to better define the range of capabilities, responsibilities, rights, and relationship to other health care providers for scope and content of practical/vocational nursing education programs. The guidelines will assist:

- Educators in development, implementation, and evaluation of practical, vocational nursing curricula.
- Students in understanding expectations of their competencies upon completion of the educational program.
- Prospective employers in appropriate utilization of the practical/vocational nurse.
- Consumers in understanding the scope of practice and level of responsibility of the practical/vocational nurse.

Professional Behaviors

Professional behaviors, within the scope of nursing practice for a practical/vocational nurse, are characterized by adherence to standards of care, accountability for one's own actions and behaviors, and use of legal and ethical principles in nursing practice. Professionalism includes a commitment to nursing and a concern for others demonstrated by an attitude of caring. Professionalism also involves participation in lifelong self-development activities to enhance and maintain current knowledge and skills for continuing competency in the practice of nursing for the licensed practical/vocational nurse (LP/VN), as well as individual, group, community, and societal endeavors to improve health care.

Upon completion of the practical/vocational nursing program, the graduate will display the following program outcome:

Demonstrate professional behaviors of accountability and professionalism according to the legal and ethical standards for a competent licensed practical/vocational nurse.

The following competencies demonstrate that this outcome has been attained:

1. Comply with the ethical, legal, and regulatory frameworks of nursing and the scope of practice as outlined in the LP/VN practice act of the specific state in which licensed.
2. Utilize educational opportunities for lifelong learning and maintenance of competence.
3. Identify personal capabilities and consider career mobility options.

---

[1]As approved and adopted by the NAPNES Board of Directors, May 6, 2007.

Reprinted with permission from the National Association for Practical Nurse Education and Service, Inc. Copyright 2007, http://www.napnes.org

4. Identify own LP/VN strengths and limitations for the purpose of improving nursing performance.
5. Demonstrate accountability for nursing care provided by self and/or directed to others.
6. Function as an advocate for the health care consumer, maintaining confidentiality as required.
7. Identify the impact of economic, political, social, cultural, spiritual, and demographic forces on the role of the LP/VN in the delivery of health care.
8. Serve as a positive role model within health care settings and the community.
9. Participate as a member of a practical/vocational nursing organization.

Communication

Communication is defined as the process by which information is exchanged between individuals verbally, nonverbally, and/or in writing or through information technology. Communication abilities are integral and essential to the nursing process. Those who are included in the nursing process are the LP/VN and other members of the nursing and health care team, client, and significant support person(s). Effective communication demonstrates caring, compassion, and cultural awareness and is directed toward promoting positive outcomes and establishing a trusting relationship.

Upon completion of the practical/vocational nursing program, the graduate will display the following program outcome:

Effectively communicate with patients, significant support person(s), and members of the interdisciplinary health care team incorporating interpersonal and therapeutic communication skills.

The following competencies demonstrate that this outcome has been attained:
1. Utilize effective communication skills when interacting with clients, significant others, and members of the interdisciplinary health care team.
2. Communicate relevant, accurate, and complete information.
3. Report to appropriate health care personnel and document assessments, interventions, and progress or impediments toward achieving client outcomes.
4. Maintain organizational and client confidentiality.
5. Utilize information technology to support and communicate the planning and provision of client care.
6. Utilize appropriate channels of communication.

Assessment

Assessment is the collection and processing of relevant data for the purposes of appraising the client's health status. Assessment provides a holistic view of the client, which includes physical, developmental, emotional, psychosocial, cultural, spiritual, and functional status. Assessment involves the collection of information from multiple sources to provide the foundation for nursing care. Initial assessment provides the baseline for future comparisons in order to individualize client care. Ongoing assessment is required to meet the client's changing needs.

Upon completion of the practical/vocational nursing program, the graduate will display the following program outcome:

Collect holistic assessment data from multiple sources, communicate the data to appropriate health care providers, and evaluate client responses to interventions.

The following competencies demonstrate that this outcome has been attained:

1. Assess data related to basic physical, developmental, spiritual, cultural, functional, and psychosocial needs of the client.
2. Collect data within established protocols and guidelines from various sources, including client interviews, observations, measurements, health care team members, family, significant other(s), and review of health records.
3. Assess data related to the client's health status, identify impediments to client progress, and evaluate response to interventions.
4. Document data collection and assessment, and communicate findings to appropriate members of the health care team.

Planning

Planning encompasses the collection of health status information, the use of multiple methods to access information, and the analysis and integration of knowledge and information to formulate nursing care plans and care actions. The nursing care plan provides direction for individualized care and assures the delivery of accurate, safe care through a definitive pathway that promotes the client and support person's progress toward positive outcomes.

Upon completion of the practical/vocational nursing program, the graduate will display the following program outcome:

Collaborate with the registered nurse or other members of the health care team to organize and incorporate assessment data to plan/revise patient care and actions based on established nursing diagnoses, nursing protocols, and assessment and evaluation data.

The following competencies demonstrate that this outcome has been attained:

1. Utilize knowledge of normal values to identify deviation in health status to plan care.
2. Contribute to formulation of a nursing care plan for clients with non-complex conditions and in a stable state, in consultation with the registered nurse and as appropriate in collaboration with the client or support person(s) as well as members of the interdisciplinary health care team using established nursing diagnoses and nursing protocols.
3. Prioritize nursing care needs of clients.
4. Assist in the review and revision of nursing care plans with the registered nurse to meet the changing needs of clients.
5. Modify client care as indicated by the evaluation of stated outcomes.
6. Provide information to client about aspects of the care plan within the LP/VN scope of practice.
7. Refer client as appropriate to other members of the health care team about care outside the scope of practice of the LP/VN.

Caring Interventions

Caring interventions are those nursing behaviors and actions that assist clients and significant others in meeting their needs and the identified outcomes of the plan of care. These interventions are based on knowledge of the natural sciences, behavioral sciences, and past nursing experiences. Caring is the "being with" and "doing for" that assists clients to achieve the desired outcomes. Caring behaviors are nurturing, protective, compassionate, and person centered. Caring creates an environment of hope and trust where client choices related to cultural, religious, and spiritual values, beliefs, and lifestyles are respected.

Upon completion of the practical/vocational nursing program, the graduate will display the following program outcome:

Demonstrate a caring and empathic approach to the safe, therapeutic, and individualized care of each client.

The following competencies demonstrate that this outcome has been attained:

1. Provide and promote the client's dignity.
2. Identify and honor the emotional, cultural, religious, and spiritual influences on the client's health.
3. Demonstrate caring behaviors toward the client and significant support person(s).
4. Provide competent, safe, therapeutic, and individualized nursing care in a variety of settings.
5. Provide a safe physical and psychosocial environment for the client and significant other(s).
6. Implement the prescribed care regimen within the legal, ethical, and regulatory framework of licensed practical/vocational nursing practice.
7. Assist the client and significant support person(s) to cope with and adapt to stressful events and changes in health status.
8. Assist the client and significant other(s) to achieve optimum comfort and functioning.
9. Instruct the client regarding individualized health needs in keeping with the licensed practical/ vocational nurse's knowledge, competence, and scope of practice.
10. Recognize the client's right to access information and refer requests to appropriate person(s).
11. Act in an advocacy role to protect client rights.

Managing

Managing care is the effective use of human, physical, financial, and technological resources to achieve the client-identified outcomes while supporting organizational outcomes. The LP/VN manages care through the processes of planning, organizing, and directing.

Upon completion of the practical/vocational nursing program, the graduate will display the following program outcome:

Implement patient care, at the direction of a registered nurse, licensed physician, or dentist through performance of nursing interventions or directing aspects of care, as appropriate, to unlicensed assistive personnel (UAP).

The following competencies demonstrate that this outcome has been attained:

1. Assist in the coordination and implementation of an individualized plan of care for clients and significant support person(s).
2. Direct aspects of client care to qualified UAPs commensurate with abilities and level of preparation and consistent with the state's legal and regulatory framework for the scope of practice for the LP/VN.
3. Supervise and evaluate the activities of UAPs and other personnel as appropriate within the state's legal and regulatory framework for the scope of practice for the LP/VN as well as for the facility policy.

4. Maintain accountability for outcomes of care directed to qualified UAPs.
5. Organize nursing activities in a meaningful and cost-effective manner when providing nursing care for individuals or groups.
6. Assist the client and significant support person(s) to access available resources and services.
7. Demonstrate competence with current technologies.
8. Function within the defined scope of practice for the LP/VN in the health care delivery system at the direction of a registered nurse, licensed physician, or dentist.

APPENDIX D

Complementary Health Approaches:
A Dictionary of Terms

Acupuncture involves placing pressure needles in specific channels throughout the body to relieve many symptoms and illnesses.

Alternative Medicine is used in place of conventional medicine. An example of an alternative therapy is using a special diet to treat cancer instead of undergoing surgery, radiation, or chemotherapy that has been recommended by a conventional doctor.

Aromatherapy ("ah-roam-uh-THER-ah-py") involves the use of essential oils (extracts or essences) from flowers, herbs, and trees to promote health and well-being.

Art Therapy helps people express inner feelings through drawing, painting, and craftwork.

Ayurveda ("ah-yur-VAY-dah") is an alternative medical system that has been practiced primarily in the Indian subcontinent for 5,000 years. Ayurveda deals with a complete approach to life and includes diet and herbal remedies and emphasizes the use of body, mind, and spirit in disease prevention and treatment.

Biofeedback is a way of learning to change the body's responses in a way that improves health using electronic instruments that measure and indicate various things that are happening in the body.

Chinese Medicine is an alternative medical system (for Westerners) that uses yin and yang, zang and fu organs, the eight principles, and other beliefs to help the body use its own potential to cure diseases.

Complementary Medicine is used together with conventional Western medicine. An example of a complementary therapy is using aromatherapy along with medications to help lessen a patient's discomfort following surgery.

Chiropractic ("ki-roh-PRAC-tic") is an alternative medical system. It focuses on the relationship between the bodily structure (primarily that of the spine) and the function, and how that relationship affects the preservation and restoration of health. Chiropractors use manipulative therapy as an integral treatment tool.

Dietary Supplements Congress defined the term *dietary supplement* in the Dietary Supplement Health and Education Act (DSHEA) of 1994 as a product (other than tobacco) taken by mouth that contains a "dietary ingredient" intended to supplement the diet. Dietary ingredients may include vitamins, minerals, herbs or other botanicals, amino acids, and substances such as enzymes, organ tissues, and metabolites. Dietary supplements come in many forms, including extracts, concentrates, tablets, capsules, gel caps, liquids, and powders. They have special requirements for labeling. Under DSHEA, dietary supplements are considered foods, not drugs.

Diets and Nutrition provide alternatives to traditional treatments or can be used along with (complementary to) traditional medical treatments. There are thousands of diets and nutritional programs ranging from macrobiotics to vegetarian to low carbohydrates to phytochemicals to the latest fad diet.

Electromagnetic Fields (EMFs, also called electric and magnetic fields) are invisible lines of force that surround all electrical devices. The earth also produces EMFs; electric fields are produced when there is thunderstorm activity, and magnetic fields are believed to be produced by electric currents flowing at the earth's core.

Environmental Medicine is an alternative medical system in which therapy is based on how factors in our environment—food, chemicals, water, and air quality—affect us. Treatment ranges from environmental control to immunotherapy.

Feldenkrais Method is an educational process that retrains the mind to move the body by knowing how the body works and to increase flexibility.

Guided Imagery in healing is probably best known for its direct effects on physiology. Through imagery, you can stimulate changes in many body functions usually considered inaccessible to conscious influence.

Holistic Medicine is an alternative medical system that emphasizes the mental, physical, emotional, and spiritual as well as personal responsibility and participation in one's own health care.

Homeopathic Medicine ("home-ee-oh-PATH-ic") is an alternative medical system. In homeopathic medicine, there is a belief that "like cures like" meaning that small, highly diluted quantities of medicinal substances are given to cure symptoms, when the same substances given at higher or more concentrated doses would actually cause those symptoms.

Humor Therapy is based on extensive research that provides evidence that humor and laughter positively affect healing and well-being.

Hypnosis includes hypersuggestibility, which means that under certain conditions, a person might be able to perform activities that he or she could not normally perform.

Magnet Therapy is sometimes used by patients on their own or is administered by health care providers. Magnet therapy may be applied to the whole body or only to areas affected by illness. Devices may be implanted or used externally. Some traditional Chinese medicine (TCM) practitioners suggest that magnets may affect patterns of flow of the body's life force, known as chi (qi).

Massage ("muh-SAHJ") therapists manipulate muscle and connective tissue to enhance function of those tissues and promote relaxation and well-being.

Music Therapy as a healing influence is as old as the writings of Aristotle and Plato. The positive physical and emotional responses to music work together to improve health.

Naturopathic ("nay-chur-o-PATH-ic") Medicine is an alternative medical system in which practitioners work with natural healing forces within the body, with a goal of helping the body heal from disease and attain better health. Practices may include dietary modifications, massage, exercise, acupuncture, minor surgery, and various other interventions.

Osteopathic ("ahs-tee-oh-PATH-ic") Medicine is a form of conventional medicine that, in part, emphasizes diseases arising in the musculoskeletal system. There is an underlying belief that all of the body's systems work together, and disturbances in one system may affect function elsewhere in the body. Some osteopathic physicians practice osteopathic manipulation, a full-body system of hands-on techniques to alleviate pain, restore function, and promote health and well-being.

Pet Therapy also known as animal-assisted therapy, is a guided interaction between an individual and a trained animal. This interaction can help people cope with depression, posttraumatic stress disorder, physical limitations, and unpleasant side effects of a variety of medical treatments.

Progressive Relaxation encourages the person to learn how to focus on each muscle, then tensing and relaxing to ultimately achieve total relaxation.

Qigong ("chee-GUNG") is a component of traditional Chinese medicine that combines movement, meditation, and regulation of breathing to enhance the flow of chi (qi) (an ancient term given to what is believed to be vital energy) in the body, improve blood circulation, and enhance immune function.

Reflexology is based on the theory that the body has "reflex areas" on the hands and feet that correspond to gland and organs.

Reiki ("RAY-kee") is a Japanese word representing universal life energy. Reiki is based on the belief that when spiritual energy is channeled through a Reiki practitioner, the patient's spirit is healed, which in turn heals the physical body.

Rolfing is a form of massage that promotes well-being through deep manipulation. This manipulation aims to balance the body and improve range of motion as well as energy level and mood.

Tai Chi aims to address the body and mind as an interconnected system and to improve mental and physical health while benefiting posture, balance, flexibility, and strength. Tai chi includes sequences of slow movements coordinated with deep breathing and mental focus.

Therapeutic Touch is derived from an ancient technique called laying-on of hands. It is based on the premise that it is the healing force of the therapist that affects the patient's recovery; healing is promoted when the body's energies are in balance; and by passing their hands over the patient, healers can identify energy imbalances.

Trager Method requires that the therapist employ gentle rocking, stretching, and swinging movements to achieve deep relaxation and a sense of well-being.

Yoga developed in India more than 5,000 years ago; calms the mind and emotions and tones the body through unification with the universal spirit. Participants perform a series of stretching, breathing, and meditation techniques to achieve internal harmony.

Zen Meditation is the study of self and combines posture, positioning, breathing, and meditation and has existed for at least 2,500 years.

These are just a few of the hundreds of terms related to complementary health practices. The Web site http://www.nccam.nih.gov is a comprehensive resource for reliable information on complementary and integrative health.

Index

Note: Page numbers followed by 'b' indicate boxes, 'f' indicate figures; those followed by 't' indicate tables.

CCS0618